Cardiac CT Imaging

Editors

SUHNY ABBARA
PRABHAKAR RAJIAH

RADIOLOGIC CLINICS
OF NORTH AMERICA

www.radiologic.theclinics.com

Consulting Editor
FRANK H. MILLER

January 2019 • Volume 57 • Number 1

ELSEVIER

1600 John F. Kennedy Boulevard • Suite 1800 • Philadelphia, Pennsylvania, 19103-2899

http://www.theclinics.com

RADIOLOGIC CLINICS OF NORTH AMERICA Volume 57, Number 1
January 2019 ISSN 0033-8389, ISBN 13: 978-0-323-65503-3

Editor: John Vassallo (j.vassallo@elsevier.com)
Developmental Editor: Donald Mumford

Radiologic Clinics of North America (ISSN 0033-8389) is published bimonthly by Elsevier Inc., 360 Park Avenue South, New York, NY 10010-1710. Months of issue are January, March, May, July, September, and November. Periodicals postage paid at New York, NY and additional mailing offices. Subscription prices are USD 508 per year for US individuals, USD 933 per year for US institutions, USD 100 per year for US students and residents, USD 594 per year for Canadian individuals, USD 1193 per year for Canadian institutions, USD 683 per year for international individuals, USD 1193 per year for international institutions, and USD 315 per year for Canadian and international students/residents. To receive student and resident rate, orders must be accompanied by name of affiliated institution, date of term and the signature of program/residency coordinator on institution letterhead. Orders will be billed at individual rate until proof of status is received. Foreign air speed delivery is included in all *Clinics* subscription prices. All prices are subject to change without notice. **POSTMASTER:** Send address changes to *Radiologic Clinics of North America*, Elsevier Health Sciences Division, Subscription Customer Service, 3251 Riverport Lane, Maryland Heights, MO63043. **Customer Service: Telephone: 1-800-654-2452** (U.S. and Canada); **1-314-447-8871** (outside U.S. and Canada). **Fax: 1-314-447-8029. E-mail: journalscustomerservice-usa@ elsevier.com (for print support); journalsonlinesupport-usa@elsevier.com (for online support)**.

Reprints. For copies of 100 or more of articles in this publication, please contact the Commercial Reprints Department, Elsevier Inc., 360 Park Avenue South, New York, New York 10010-1710. Tel.: +1-212-633-3874; Fax: +1-212-633-3820; E-mail: reprints@elsevier.com.

Radiologic Clinics of North America also published in Greek Paschalidis Medical Publications, Athens, Greece.

Radiologic Clinics of North America is covered in *MEDLINE/PubMed (Index Medicus)*, *EMBASE/Excerpta Medica, Current Contents/Life Sciences, Current Contents/Clinical Medicine, RSNA Index to Imaging Literature, BIOSIS, Science Citation Index,* and *ISI/BIOMED*.

Printed in the United States of America.

Contributors

CONSULTING EDITOR

FRANK H. MILLER, MD, FACR
Lee F. Rogers MD Professor of Medical
Education, Chief, Body Imaging Section and
Fellowship Program, Medical Director, MRI,
Department of Radiology, Northwestern
Memorial Hospital, Northwestern University
Feinberg School of Medicine, Chicago, Illinois,
USA

EDITORS

SUHNY ABBARA, MD, FACR, FSCCT
Professor and Chief, Cardiothoracic
Imaging, Department of Radiology, UT
Southwestern Medical Center, Dallas,
Texas, USA

**PRABHAKAR RAJIAH, MBBS, MD, FRCR,
FSCMR**
Associate Professor, Department of Radiology,
Cardiothoracic Imaging, Associate Director of
Cardiac CT and MRI, UT Southwestern
Medical Center, Dallas, Texas, USA

AUTHORS

SUHNY ABBARA, MD, FACR, FSCCT
Professor and Chief, Cardiothoracic
Imaging, Department of Radiology, UT
Southwestern Medical Center, Dallas,
Texas, USA

PRACHI P. AGARWAL, MD, MS
Professor, Department of Radiology, University
of Michigan, Ann Arbor, Michigan, USA

PHILIP A. ARAOZ, MD
Professor, Department of Radiology, Mayo
Clinic, Rochester, Minnesota, USA

SANJEEV BHALLA, MD
Mallinckrodt Institute of Radiology, St Louis,
Missouri, USA

PHILIPP BLANKE, MD
Department of Radiology, St Paul's Hospital,
University of British Columbia, Centre for Heart
Lung Innovation, St Paul's Hospital, University
of British Columbia, Vancouver, British
Columbia, Canada

JOHN JEFFREY CARR, MD, MSc
Cornelius Vanderbilt Professor of Radiology,
Departments of Biomedical Informatics and
Cardiovascular Medicine, Vanderbilt University
Medical Center, Nashville, Tennessee, USA

JONATHAN H. CHUNG, MD
Department of Radiology, The University of
Chicago, Chicago, Illinois, USA

ERIC R. FLAGG, MD
Clinical Fellow, Department of Radiology and
Biomedical Imaging, University of California,
San Francisco, San Francisco, California, USA

THOMAS A. FOLEY, MD
Assistant Professor, Department of Radiology,
Mayo Clinic, Rochester, Minnesota, USA

SHERIEF GARRANA, MD
Resident Physician, Department of Radiology,
University of Missouri in Kansas City (UKMC),
St Luke's Hospital of Kansas City, Kansas City,
Missouri, USA

BRIAN B. GHOSHHAJRA, MD, MBA
Cardiac MR PET CT Program, Department of
Radiology (Cardiovascular Imaging), Division of
Cardiology, Massachusetts General Hospital,
Harvard Medical School, Boston,
Massachusetts, USA

HAROLD GOERNE, MD
Cardiovascular Radiologist, Department of
Radiology, Cardiovascular Imaging Service, IMSS
Western National Medical Center, Cardiovascular
Imaging Service, Imaging and Diagnosis
Center (CID), Guadalajara, Jalisco, Mexico

AVANTI GULHANE, MD, DNB
Research Fellow, Cardiovascular Imaging,
Department of Radiology, Perelman School of
Medicine, University of Pennsylvania,
Philadelphia, Pennsylvania, USA

SANDEEP HEDGIRE, MD
Cardiac MR PET CT Program, Department of
Radiology (Cardiovascular Imaging), Division of
Cardiology, Massachusetts General Hospital,
Harvard Medical School, Boston,
Massachusetts, USA

KIMBERLY G. KALLIANOS, MD
Assistant Professor, Department of Radiology
and Biomedical Imaging, University of
California, San Francisco, San Francisco,
California, USA

JACOBO KIRSCH, MD, MBA, FAHA, FNASCI
Center Director, Hospital Specialties,
Vice-Chair, Department of Imaging, Section
Head, Cardiothoracic Imaging, Cleveland
Clinic Florida, Weston, Florida, USA

SETH KLIGERMAN, MD
Associate Professor, Diagnostic Radiology,
Division Chief of Cardiothoracic Radiology,
University of California San Diego, San Diego,
California, USA

LUIS A. LANDERAS, MD
Department of Radiology, The University of
Chicago, Chicago, Illinois, USA

JONATHON A. LEIPSIC, MD, FRCPC
Department of Radiology, St Paul's Hospital,
University of British Columbia, Centre for Heart
Lung Innovation, St Paul's Hospital, University
of British Columbia, Vancouver, British
Columbia, Canada

DIANA E. LITMANOVICH, MD
Director of Cardiac CT, Director of
Cardiothoracic Fellowship, Associate
Professor of Radiology, Harvard Medical
School, FNASCI, Diagnostic Radiology, Beth
Israel Deaconess Medical Center, Boston,
Massachusetts, USA

HAROLD LITT, MD, PhD
Chief, Cardiothoracic Imaging Division,
Department of Radiology, Perelman School of
Medicine, University of Pennsylvania,
Philadelphia, Pennsylvania, USA

XHORLINA MARKO, MD
Interventional Fellow, Miami Cardiac and
Vascular Institute, Baptist Health South Florida,
Miami, Florida, USA

SANTIAGO MARTÍNEZ-JIMÉNEZ, MD
Radiologist, Professor, Department of
Radiology, St Luke's Hospital of Kansas City,
Kansas City, Missouri, USA

CHARIS McNABNEY, MB BCh
Department of Radiology, St Paul's Hospital,
University of British Columbia, Vancouver,
British Columbia, Canada

ALASTAIR MOORE, MD
Assistant Instructor, Department of
Radiology, Cardiothoracic Imaging, UT
Southwestern Medical Center, Dallas,
Texas, USA

KAREN G. ORDOVAS, MD, MS
Professor, Department of Radiology and
Biomedical Imaging, University of California,
San Francisco, San Francisco, California,
USA

CONSTANTINO S. PEÑA, MD
Interventional Radiologist, Medical Director of
Vascular Imaging, Miami Cardiac and Vascular
Institute, Baptist Health South Florida, Miami,
Florida, USA

**PRABHAKAR RAJIAH, MBBS, MD, FRCR,
FSCMR**
Associate Professor, Department of
Radiology, Cardiothoracic Imaging, Associate
Director of Cardiac CT and MRI, UT
Southwestern Medical Center, Dallas, Texas,
USA

PRAVEEN RANGANATH, MD
Department of Radiology, Cardiothoracic Imaging, UT Southwestern Medical Center, Dallas, Texas, USA

CONSTANTINE A. RAPTIS, MD
Mallinckrodt Institute of Radiology, St Louis, Missouri, USA

DEMETRIOS A. RAPTIS, MD
Mallinckrodt Institute of Radiology, St Louis, Missouri, USA

SACHIN SABOO, MD
Department of Radiology, Cardiothoracic Imaging, UT Southwestern Medical Center, Dallas, Texas, USA

ANA PAULA SANTOS LIMA, MD
Associate Specialist, Department of Radiology and Biomedical Imaging, University of California, San Francisco, San Francisco, California, USA

JAN-ERIK SCHOLTZ, MD
Cardiac MR PET CT Program, Department of Radiology (Cardiovascular Imaging), Division of Cardiology, Massachusetts General Hospital, Harvard Medical School, Boston, Massachusetts, USA; Department for Diagnostic and Interventional Radiology, University Hospital Frankfurt, Frankfurt, Germany

STEPHANIE SELLERS, PhD
Department of Radiology, St Paul's Hospital, University of British Columbia, Centre for Heart Lung Innovation, St Paul's Hospital, University of British Columbia, Vancouver, British Columbia, Canada

SATINDER SINGH, MD, FCCP, FNASCI
Department of Radiology, University of Alabama at Birmingham, Birmingham, Alabama, USA

YUKI TANABE, MD
Department of Radiology, Cardiothoracic Imaging, UT Southwestern Medical Center, Dallas, Texas, USA

JONATHAN R. WEIR-MCCALL, MBChB, PhD
Department of Radiology, St Paul's Hospital, University of British Columbia, Vancouver, British Columbia, Canada

ERIC E. WILLIAMSON, MD
Professor, Department of Radiology, Mayo Clinic, Rochester, Minnesota, USA

RYAN WILSON, MB BCh
Department of Radiology, Vancouver General Hospital, University of British Columbia, Vancouver, British Columbia, Canada

PHILLIP M. YOUNG, MD
Associate Professor, Department of Radiology, Mayo Clinic, Rochester, Minnesota, USA

Contents

Cardiovascular disease is the leading cause of death in the United States and world-wide. Despite major advances in the treatment of acute myocardial infarction, enhanced prevention of ischemic heart disease remains critical to improving the health of individuals and communities. The computed tomographic coronary artery calcium score is an established imaging biomarker that identifies the presence and amount of coronary atherosclerosis in an individual and their future risk for clinical cardiovascular disease and premature cardiovascular death. This article describes the process of performing a computed tomography scan for coronary artery calcium, quantifying the score and interpreting the results.

Coronary computed tomography angiography (CTA) has become an important part of current cardiovascular care and is the first-choice imaging modality for noninvasive visualization of coronary artery plaque and stenosis. It has high sensitivity for the detection of coronary stenosis and excellent negative predictive value to rule out stenosis with consistently high image quality at low radiation doses. In this article, we point out the technical aspects of modern coronary CT imaging, give a comprehensive overview of coronary CTA interpretation, including standardized reporting, and point out body of evidence for current clinical use.

Multidetector-row computed tomography (MDCT) can provide crucial information and rapid triage of emergency department patients with suspected acute coronary syndrome (ACS) or acute aortic syndrome (AAS). Coronary computed tomography angiography has high negative predictive value to rule out ACS, and MDCT is diagnostic for AAS and its variants. Optimization of acquisition technique and up-to-date knowledge of the pathophysiology of these conditions can improve study and interpretation quality for diagnosis of ACS or AAS.

This article reviews the imaging manifestations of acute myocardial infarction (MI) on computed tomography (CT) accompanied by case examples and illustrations. This is preceded by a review of the pathophysiology of MI (acute and chronic), a summary of its clinical presentation, and a brief synopsis of the technical aspects of cardiac CT. Several examples of the appearance of acute MI and its complications are shown on routine and cardiac tailored CT, and a sample of the latest advances in imaging technique, including dual-energy CT, are introduced.

This article reviews the imaging manifestations of chronic myocardial infarction (MI) on computed tomography (CT) and the common mimickers of MI, clinically and on imaging. Several examples of the appearance of chronic MI, its complications, and mimickers of MI are shown on both routine and cardiac CT.

Computed tomography of the heart can characterize and differentiate various forms of nonischemic cardiomyopathy, which are covered individually in this article. With its excellent spatial and ever-improving temporal resolution, computed tomography scanning can delineate cardiac function, anatomy, and myocardial tissue characterization. Various cardiac computed tomography techniques can be tailored to the relevant clinical question, as discussed in the article. Although cardiac computed tomography scanning is not often the primary modality for myocardial evaluation, decreasing radiation doses and emerging applications make this fast and widely available examination a useful tool in the evaluation of the patient with cardiomyopathy.

Although not considered a first-line modality for assessing cardiac masses, computed tomography (CT) can provide clinically useful information and is underused for this purpose. In addition to characterizing masses with insights about presence of fat or calcification and the perfusion characteristics of a mass, CT produces high-resolution four-dimensional images depicting the mass and its relationship to chambers, valves, and coronaries. This is combined with imaging of the chest, abdomen, or coronaries. Advances in CT technology, such as dual-energy CT, dynamic perfusion imaging, and three-dimensional printing for preoperative planning, will increase the role of CT in assessment of cardiac masses.

The prevalence of adult congenital heart disease (ACHD) is increasing due to advances in surgical techniques, anesthesia, and perioperative care. Imaging plays an important role, not only in the surveillance of ACHD, but also in the initial evaluation of cases that have escaped detection early in life and present with symptoms later in adulthood. In this article, we review the role of computed tomography in the comprehensive evaluation of ACHD.

Congenital abnormalities of the thoracic aorta encompass a variety of disorders with variable clinical manifestations ranging from asymptomatic to life threatening. A variety of imaging modalities are available for the evaluation of these anomalies with computed tomography (CT) commonly preferred due to its excellent spatial resolution and rapid acquisitions, avoiding the need of general anesthesia or even sedation. We review the embryology, imaging findings, and associations of multiple congenital thoracic aorta malformations with emphasis in the role of CT angiography in the evaluation of these pathologies.

Computed tomography angiography (CTA) has the ability to evaluate the aortic wall and the lumen easily, quickly, and reproducibly without the need for invasive techniques. The images are isotropic, allowing several reconstructions. When imaging the aorta, CTA has replaced catheter angiography in the diagnosis of acquired disease such as aortoiliac disease, aneurysm, and infectious and inflammatory disease of the aorta.

Valvular heart disease is a common clinical problem. Although echocardiography is the standard technique for the noninvasive evaluation of the valves, cardiac CT has evolved to become a useful tool in the evaluation of the cardiac structures as well. Importantly, CT allows for improved quantification of valvular calcification due to its superior spatial resolution. It may improve the detection of small valvular or perivalvular pathology or the characterization of valvular masses and vegetations. This review describes the assessment of normal and diseased heart valves by cardiac CT and discusses its strengths and weaknesses.

Amid rapid growth in transcatheter valvular interventions computed tomography (CT) has emerged as a pivotal noninvasive imaging resource that can be used throughout many stages of the transcatheter heart valve process, enhancing procedural success and efficacy. It affords a three-dimensional assessment of the aortic and challenging saddle-shaped mitral annulus, facilitating appropriate device selection, sizing, and preprocedural prediction angles for prosthetic deployment. Postprocedural imaging allows documentation of procedural success, evaluation of prosthesis positioning, and identifying asymptomatic complications. This article provides an overview of the role of CT in both trancatheter aortic valve repair (TAVR) and transcatheter mitral valve replacement (TMVR).

Although the pericardium is simply a 2-layered membrane enveloping the heart and great vessels, there are numerous anatomic variations, congenital anomalies, and pathologic conditions that can occur. Although echocardiography is most often the first imaging modality used to assess the pericardium, computed tomography and MR imaging are frequently being used to aid in diagnosis and assess response to therapy. Therefore, detailed knowledge of the pericardium in both its normal and diseased states is important to best direct patient care and potentially improve patient outcomes.

Cardiac injury can occur in the setting of blunt and penetrating trauma resulting in significantly adverse clinical outcomes. Although the clinical presentation is variable and computed tomographic imaging is rarely performed to specifically evaluate for cardiac injury, the ability to recognize the findings of cardiac injury on computed tomographic examinations performed for thoracic trauma is essential to avoid misdiagnosis and direct potentially lifesaving interventions. This article reviews the direct and indirect computed tomographic findings of cardiac injury.

Various disease processes may affect the ascending thoracic aorta, aortic arch, and/or descending thoracic aorta, including aneurysms, dissections, intramural hematomas, penetrating atherosclerotic ulcers, and aortic transection/rupture. Many of those conditions require surgical intervention for repair. Multiple open and endovascular techniques are used for treatment of thoracic aortic pathology. It is imperative that the cardiothoracic radiologist have a thorough knowledge of the surgical techniques available, the expected postoperative imaging findings, and the complications that may occur to accurately diagnose life-threatening pathology when present, and avoid common pitfalls of misinterpreting normal postoperative findings as pathologic conditions.

PROGRAM OBJECTIVE

The objective of the *Radiologic Clinics of North America* is to keep practicing radiologists and radiology residents up to date with current clinical practice in radiology by providing timely articles reviewing the state of the art in patient care.

TARGET AUDIENCE

Practicing radiologists, radiology residents, and other healthcare professionals who provide patient care utilizing radiologic findings.

LEARNING OBJECTIVES

Upon completion of this activity, participants will be able to:

1. Review the pathophysiology of both acute and chronic myocardial infarction and imaging manifestations on computed tomography
2. Discuss the direct and indirect computed tomographic findings of cardiac injury
3. Recognize the role of computed tomography in the comprehensive evaluation of adult congenital heart disease

ACCREDITATION

The Elsevier Office of Continuing Medical Education (EOCME) is accredited by the Accreditation Council for Continuing Medical Education (ACCME) to provide continuing medical education for physicians.

The EOCME designates this enduring material for a maximum of 15 *AMA PRA Category 1 Credit*(s)™. Physicians should claim only the credit commensurate with the extent of their participation in the activity.

All other healthcare professionals requesting continuing education credit for this enduring material will be issued a certificate of participation.

DISCLOSURE OF CONFLICTS OF INTEREST

The EOCME assesses conflict of interest with its instructors, faculty, planners, and other individuals who are in a position to control the content of CME activities. All relevant conflicts of interest that are identified are thoroughly vetted by EOCME for fair balance, scientific objectivity, and patient care recommendations. EOCME is committed to providing its learners with CME activities that promote improvements or quality in healthcare and not a specific proprietary business or a commercial interest.

The planning committee, staff, authors and editors listed below have identified no financial relationships or relationships to products or devices they or their spouse/life partner have with commercial interest related to the content of this CME activity:

Suhny Abbara, MD, FACR, FSCCT; Prachi P. Agarwal, MD, MS; Philip A. Araoz, MD; Sanjeev Bhalla, MD; Philipp Blanke, MD; John Jeffrey Carr, MD, MSc; Jonathan H. Chung, MD; Eric R. Flagg, MD; Thomas A. Foley, MD; Sherief Garrana, MD; Harold Goerne, MD; Avanti Gulhane, MD, DNB; Sandeep Hedgire, MD; Kimberly G. Kallianos, MD; Alison Kemp; Jacobo Kirsch, MD, MBA, FAHA, FNASCI; Seth Kligerman, MD; Pradeep Kuttysankaran; Luis A. Landeras, MD; Diana E. Litmanovich, MD; Xhorlina Marko, MD; Charis McNabney, MB BCh; Frank H. Miller, MD, FACR; Alastair Moore, MD; Karen G. Ordovas, MD, FRCP; Prabhakar Rajiah, MBBS, MD, FRCR, FSCMR; Praveen Ranganath, MD; Constantine A. Raptis, MD; Demetrios A. Raptis, MD; Sachin Saboo, MD; Ana Paula Santos Lima, MD; Jan-Erik Scholtz, MD; Stephanie Sellers, PhD; Satinder Singh, MD, FCCP, FNASCI; Yuki Tanabe, MD; John Vassallo; Jonathan R. Weir-McCall, MBChB, PhD; Eric E. Williamson, MD; Ryan Wilson, MB BCh; Phillip M. Young, MD.

The planning committee, staff, authors and editors listed below have identified financial relationships or relationships to products or devices they or their spouse/life partner have with commercial interest related to the content of this CME activity:

Brian B. Ghoshhajra, MD, MBA: is a consultant/advisor and receives research support from Siemens Medical Solutions USA, Inc.

Jonathon A. Leipsic, MD, FRCPC: receives research support from Edwards Lifesciences Corporation, Inc., Medtronic and is a consultant/advisor for Circle Cardiovascular Imaging Inc. and HeartFlow, Inc.

Harold Litt, MD, PhD: receives research support from Siemens Medical Solutions USA, Inc.

Santiago Martínez-Jiménez, MD: receives royalties from Elsevier

Constantino S. Peña, MD: is a consultant/advisor and serves on a speakers' bureau for BD, Boston Scientific Corporation, and Avanos Corporate; serves on a speakers' bureau for Penumbra, Inc., Cook, and Abbott; and is a consultant/advisor for W. L. Gore & Associates, Inc.

UNAPPROVED/OFF-LABEL USE DISCLOSURE

The EOCME requires CME faculty to disclose to the participants:

1. When products or procedures being discussed are off-label, unlabelled, experimental, and/or investigational (not US Food and Drug Administration [FDA] approved); and
2. Any limitations on the information presented, such as data that are preliminary or that represent ongoing research, interim analyses, and/or unsupported opinions. Faculty may discuss information about pharmaceutical agents that is outside of

FDA-approved labelling. This information is intended solely for CME and is not intended to promote off-label use of these medications. If you have any questions, contact the medical affairs department of the manufacturer for the most recent prescribing information.

TO ENROLL

To enroll in the *Radiologic Clinics of North America* Continuing Medical Education program, call customer service at 1-800-654-2452 or sign up online at http://www.theclinics.com/home/cme. The CME program is available to subscribers for an additional annual fee of USD 327.60.

METHOD OF PARTICIPATION

In order to claim credit, participants must complete the following:
1. Complete enrolment as indicated above.
2. Read the activity.
3. Complete the CME Test and Evaluation. Participants must achieve a score of 70% on the test. All CME Tests and Evaluations must be completed online.

CME INQUIRIES/SPECIAL NEEDS

For all CME inquiries or special needs, please contact elsevierCME@elsevier.com.

RADIOLOGIC CLINICS OF NORTH AMERICA

RELATED SERIES

Magnetic Resonance Imaging Clinics
Neuroimaging Clinics
PET Clinics

THE CLINICS ARE AVAILABLE ONLINE!
Access your subscription at:
www.theclinics.com

Preface
Cardiovascular Computed Tomography

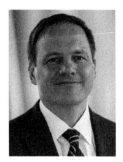   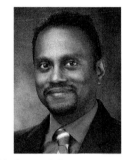

Suhny Abbara, MD, FACR, FSCCT   Prabhakar Rajiah, MBBS, MD, FRCR

Editors

Cardiac computed tomography (CT) has had a tremendous impact on the fields of cardiac and vascular medicine, which has accelerated in the past decade. This has been in part due to technical developments of CT scanner hardware and software and postprocessing software, which have been unprecedented in pace, as well as evolution and advancement of the evidence, the pace of which has skyrocketed in past years. There are now well over a dozen prospective randomized controlled trials showing the utility of cardiac CT. Therefore, we feel that dedicating an issue of *Radiologic Clinics of North America* to cardiac CT is both timely and important.

We have aimed to cover a wide variety of the most essential applications of cardiac CT. We were fortunate to draw upon a cadre of the most experienced and accomplished authors in their respective fields. I am deeply grateful to each lead author and their respective teams for their expertise and the many hours they have put into creating these articles. Thank you!

This issue of *Radiologic Clinics of North America* will span the topics of calcium scoring and coronary CT angiography with a focus on how and when to do it on a review of the state of the evidence. Transcatheter aortic and mitral valve replacements have matured as a new alternative treatment to open heart surgery. This development has been enabled and aided by cardiac CT procedure planning, and therefore, an article is dedicated to the cardiac CT planning for these interventions. We have included articles that focus on specific disease entities or conditions, such as cardiac masses, nonischemic cardiomyopathies, pericardial disease, congenital heart and congenital aortic disease, cardiac valves, postsurgical findings of the thorax, and cardiac trauma. In addition, there are articles that are dedicated to the sequelae of atherosclerosis, namely acute coronary and aortic syndromes, acute myocardial infarction, and the wide spectrum of imaging findings and complications that can be seen with chronic myocardial infarction.

We truly hope that the readers will enjoy reviewing these articles as much as we have, and that this issue will be a useful resource for interpreting cardiac CT examinations.

Respectfully,

Suhny Abbara, MD, FACR, FSCCT
Cardiothoracic Imaging
Department of Radiology
UT Southwestern Medical Center
Florence Building (E6.122B)
5323 Harry Hines Boulevard
Dallas, TX 75390, USA

Prabhakar Rajiah, MBBS, MD, FRCR
Cardiothoracic Imaging
Department of Radiology
UT Southwestern Medical Center
5323 Harry Hines Boulevard
E6.122G, Mailstop 9316
Dallas, TX 75390, USA

E-mail addresses:
Suhny.Abbara@UTSouthwestern.edu (S. Abbara)
Prabhakar.rajiah@utsouthwestern.edu (P. Rajiah)

Radiol Clin N Am 57 (2019) xv
https://doi.org/10.1016/j.rcl.2018.09.010
0033-8389/19/© 2018 Published by Elsevier Inc.

radiologic.theclinics.com

Calcium Scoring for Cardiovascular Computed Tomography: How, When and Why?

John Jeffrey Carr, MD, MSc

KEYWORDS

- Coronary artery calcium • Calcium score • Atherosclerosis • Cardiovascular disease • Prevention
- Computed tomography • Cardiac

KEY POINTS

- Individuals with any coronary artery calcium (scores greater than zero) have progressed from early to advanced coronary atheroma. Individuals with advance coronary atheroma are at risk for plaque rupture and acute myocardial infarction.
- The total calcium score or Agatston score is a robust measure of the amount of calcified plaque an individual has and is a good estimate of total coronary plaque burden, calcified and non-calcified.
- For adults less than 60 years of age the presence of any calcified plaque by a dedicated cardiac CT exam or as an unsuspected finding on a conventional chest CT exam substantially increases their 10-year risk of atherosclerotic cardiovascular disease. The individual with coronary artery calcium under age 60 years is at or above the threshold of risk where evidence-based risk factor reduction efforts are warranted.
- The absence of coronary artery calcium, or total calcium score of zero, indicates a less than 1% chance of developing cardiovascular disease over the next decade of life.

INTRODUCTION

Cardiovascular disease (CVD), specifically ischemic heart disease, is the number one cause of death and healthy years of life lost in the United States.[1] CVD is also the largest cause of death globally with developing countries accounting for more than 60% of the global burden of heart disease.[2] Primary prevention of CVD through strategies to reduce risk factors, include healthy lifestyle choices and when necessary use of targeted therapies, is essential to addressing this epidemic. The 2013 American Heart Association/American College of Cardiology Guidelines on CVD risk set an absolute risk for clinical disease of 7.5% or greater over 10 years as a level where therapy with cholesterol-lowering statin medications has a substantial benefit.[3,4] The application of these guidelines in the United States results in nearly one-half of the adult population over

40 years of age potentially eligible for statin therapy and a call from many across the scientific and broader community for a more targeted approach.[5,6] Coronary artery calcium (CAC) score measured by computed tomography (CT) is an imaging biomarker with substantial data supporting it as the most informative of available nontraditional markers of atherosclerotic CVD (ASCVD).[3,7–9]

Coronary atherosclerosis is responsible for the vast majority of ASCVD. The early lesions of atherosclerosis begin during childhood and substantial disease burden has been documented in young adults at autopsy for non-CVD deaths.[10] The pathologic transition from early to advanced atherosclerotic lesions indicates the potential for plaque rupture, plaque erosion, and coronary thrombosis with the potential for sudden death and clinically evident disease occurring through multiple pathways.[11] The presence of CT-detectable calcified plaque indicates the

Departments of Radiology, Biomedical Informatics, and Cardiovascular Medicine, Vanderbilt University Medical Center, 2525 West End Avenue, Suite 300-B, Nashville, TN 37203-8281, USA
E-mail address: j.jeffrey.carr@vumc.org

Radiol Clin N Am 57 (2019) 1–12
https://doi.org/10.1016/j.rcl.2018.09.002
0033-8389/19/© 2018 Elsevier Inc. All rights reserved.

radiologic.theclinics.com

presence of advanced macroscopic fibrocalcified plaque in the coronary arteries. Thus an individual with CT-identified CAC crosses a threshold from having CVD risk factors to documented subclinical coronary artery disease. The CAC score is also a direct measure of the amount of calcified atheroma and is highly correlated with total coronary atheroma that includes the measured calcified plaque and unmeasured non-calcified plaque.[12] In the next sections, the steps necessary to perform a CAC CT study, calculate a calcium score, and interpret results are discussed.

KEY POINTS CONCERNING CORONARY ARTERY CALCIUM

- Coronary artery calcification by CT indicates the presence of advanced atherosclerotic plaques in the coronary arteries.
- Calcified plaques are a part of atherogenesis and may represent an attempt at healing of the vessel wall after plaque rupture, hemorrhage, or erosion with the probability of noncalcified lesions, at adjacent or distant locations in the coronary arteries.
- Coronary calcification was identified as a noninvasive risk marker CVD with fluoroscopy of the heart.[13]
- The CAC score quantifies the amount of calcified plaque and is a good estimate for total coronary plaque, calcified and noncalcified.[9,12]
- The presence of any CAC by CT indicates a substantial increase in the risk of clinical coronary heart disease and ASCVD, which includes both cerebrovascular (stroke) and coronary heart disease (acute myocardial infarction).[14–16]
- Established prevention strategies that combine lifestyle changes and medications (statins) have the ability to decrease the risk of ASCVD substantially.[3,4]

ANATOMY AND IMAGING TECHNIQUE

The anatomy of the coronary arteries with noncontrast cardiac CT can be divided into the landmarks necessary for performing the scan and then measuring CAC. The imaging technique consists of scout topograms in the frontal and lateral projections. Targeting the heart, an axial scan series is performed with ECG gating to compensate for and decrease coronary motion. The CAC scan series is a set of axial cross-sectional images of the coronary arteries without intravenous contrast media or the need for premedication to control the heart rate. The axial set of images is then analyzed using a computer workstation to measure the amount of calcified plaque present in the epicardial coronary arteries, reported as the total calcium score, which is also known as the Agatston score.[9,17]

ANATOMY: KEY POINTS

- The carina of the trachea: the superior landmark for starting the scan is a location 1 to 2 cm above the carina to insure including the entire left anterior descending (LAD) coronary artery (Fig. 1).
- The aortic root, at 3-o'-clock: the left lateral border of the aortic root, near the origin of the left coronary artery at approximately 03:00 on the clock face can be used for setting the center of image for reconstruction of the heart. The technologist can use this location to set the superior-inferior and left-right offsets for a targeted display field of view including the heart and coronary arteries.
- The interventricular septum: the plane that divides the right and left sided chambers; the LAD coronary artery is the origin of the septal perforating arteries. Thus, the plane dividing the right and left ventricles can help to locate the LAD on noncontrast CT (Fig. 2).

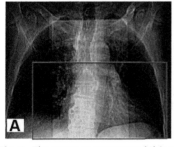 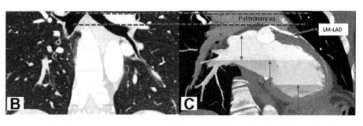

Fig. 1. The scout or topogram (A) is used by the computed tomography (CT) operator to prescribe the scan range with the superior landmark being 1 to 2 cm above the carina of the trachea and the inferior landmark the inferior border of the heart (red box). Coronal oblique reformats posteriorly at the level of the carina with lung window settings (B) and more anteriorly at the level of the left main origin (C) from coronary CT angiography study. The left main commonly courses superiorly before angling inferior as the left anterior descending (LAD). Note how the entire left coronary artery course is below the pulmonary arteries that are anatomically related to the tracheal bifurcation. The double arrowhead lines demonstrate the 4 cm prospective ECG gated acquisitions sets of slices in this 64 channel CT scanner (64 slices × 0.65 mm slices = 40 mm detector width). LM, left main.

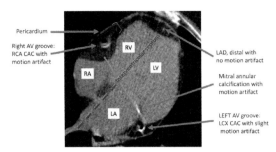

Fig. 2. The right atrium (RA), right ventricle (RV), left atrium (LA), and left ventricle (LV) are labeled. Minor motion artifactual streaking is present in calcification of the RCA, LCX, and mitral annulus. The pericardium is identified by the blue arrow and the epicardial space deep to the pericardium contains epicardial fat and the coronary arteries and is noted by the red bracket. Mitral annular calcification is deep to the epicardium and epicardial space. This location differentiates mitral annular from LCX calcification. CAC, coronary artery calcium.

- The atrioventricular groove, right (coronary sulcus): the right atrioventricular groove contains the right coronary artery and the atrioventricular plane (green line) divides the atria from the ventricles. The atrioventricular grooves contain epicardial adipose tissue that provides intrinsic contrast between the coronary arteries and surrounding fat.
- The atrioventricular groove, left (coronary sulcus): the left atrioventricular groove contains the left circumflex (LCX) coronary artery as well as the great coronary vein. The great coronary vein is usually larger than the LCX and returns blood to the coronary sinus and then right atrium.

PRESCRIBING AND PERFORMING THE SCAN

The scan range for performing a CAC scan is limited to the heart and coronary arteries. By limiting the scan range to the anatomy of interest, the length of the scan in the head–foot direction (z-axis) is minimized. This factor also benefits the patient by reducing the scan time, breath hold time, and radiation exposure. Anatomically, the left main coronary artery originates from an ostium in the left coronary sinus of the aortic root. The left main coronary is of variable length before it branches to form the LAD and circumflex coronary arteries (LCX). Anatomically, the left coronary is immediately inferior to the pulmonary arteries (see Fig. 1). The oblique angulation of the aortic valve results in the left main/proximal LAD initially coursing superiorly (cephalad) before angling inferiorly (caudal) with the LAD continuing in the interventricular plane. The course of the LAD is in close proximity to the interventricular septum secondary

to the origin of the septal perforating arteries from the LAD. When prescribing the axial scan superior start location, the CT technologist should set the superior slice 1 to 2 cm above the location of the carina of the trachea as visualized on the frontal scout topogram (see Fig. 1). This step will ensure that the superior most segment of the LAD is included in the scan volume. The 1 to 2 cm above the carina provides a margin for breath-hold and patient movement between the scout and axial scan. The scan range should continue inferiorly through the heart, which varies in length based on size and orientation in the thorax. The lateral scout topogram can be helpful in identifying the inferior aspect of the heart.

STANDARDIZED COMPUTED TOMOGRAPHY SCANNING PROTOCOL FOR CORONARY ARTERY CALCIUM SCORE DETERMINATION

- The scan range extends from 1 to 2 cm above the carina of the trachea through diaphragmatic aspect of the heart.
- The scan obtained during suspended inspiration to reduce respiratory and voluntary patient movement during the scan.
- Use 120 KVp. Note that imaging with 100 KVp can significantly decrease radiation exposure; however, it requires a different calibration to prevent a shift of the CAC score.
- Use a 2.5- to 3.0-mm slice thickness.
- Filtered backprojection reconstruction: the use of iterative reconstruction methods allows further reduction in radiation exposure; however, a shift in CT numbers will require calibration.
- Half-scan reconstruction algorithm optimized to maximize temporal resolution and freeze coronary motion is sometimes referred to as a dedicated cardiac mode or partial scan mode.
- Prospective ECG gating with image acquisition in late diastole, 70% to 80% of the R-R interval.
- Low radiation exposure, with a 0.5- to 1.8-mSv effective dose
- Reconstruction of the images with a display field of view of 350 mm or smaller based on the size of the heart to maximize spatial resolution for measuring CAC.

The imaging goal when performing a CAC scan is to obtain a contiguous set of axial slices, 2.5 to 3.0 mm thick, through the heart including the epicardial coronary arteries. The cephalic to caudal distance of the heart varies between individuals; however, the range is about 12 to 15 cm resulting in 40 to 50 slices of 3.0 mm in thickness.

The epicardial coronary arteries course on the external surface of the heart in the epicardial space deep to the pericardium and surrounded by epicardial adipose tissue (see **Fig. 2**). The fat surrounding the coronary arteries provides the intrinsic contrast that allows identification of the coronary arteries even in the absence of calcifications or intravascular contrast media. Coronary motion can create artifacts that blur the vessel and any associated calcified plaques resulting in measurement error in any derived CAC score (**Fig. 3**). To compensate for coronary motion, ECG gating is used to limit the scan acquisition to a consistent window during the cardiac cycle where coronary artery motion is minimized in late diastole, 70% to 75% of the R-R interval. Manufactures vary in how they define the scan acquisitions window, with some using the leading edge and others the center of the temporal window of the views used to reconstruct a given image. It is important to understand the approach used by your specific model of CT scanner to allow you to optimize image quality with respect to cardiac gating (**Fig. 4**).

Prospective ECG gating was used with the original electron-beam CT (EBCT) and remains widely implemented on current multi-channel CT systems. In prospective ECG gating, an axial as opposed to helical scan acquisition mode is used. In the axial scan mode, the table is stationary during scan acquisition and the X-ray on time is triggered by the patient's ECG waveform at a pre-specified time during the cardiac cycle, typically late diastole or 75% of the R-R interval. In this approach, the ECG triggers the scan acquisition and a block of slices is obtained at the first location. For a 4-channel and 64-channel CT scanner this acquisition would result in 4 (4 × 2.5 mm = 20 mm) and 16 slices (16 × 2.5 mm = 40 mm), respectively. The table would move to the next location during the subsequent heartbeat and acquire the second block of 4 or 16 slices, respectively, during the third cardiac cycle (see **Fig. 4**). The "scan then move" sequence for sets of two heart beats repeats until scan range is successfully covered. The x-ray tube pulses and produces x-rays only during the specified time in late diastole, resulting in short scan times and very low radiation exposure. The advantage of the 64-channel CT scanner is that each step-and-shoot acquisition covers the wider 4 cm detector width compared with only 2 cm on the 4-slice scanner. The current generation of whole organ wide detector scanners has detectors 16 cm wide allowing the entire heart to be imaged in a single rotation. Wider detectors decrease, or in the case of whole heart coverage detectors, eliminate the seams and overlaps that occur when variations occur between heartbeats during the scan (**Fig. 1C**).

Since the introduction of the electron beam and single-slice spiral CT in the 1980s, there have been rapid advancements in cardiac CT technology. Cardiac CT systems are now capable of temporal resolution of 50 to 100 milliseconds, with whole heart coverage, and substantial improvements in image quality while reducing radiation exposure. Coronary CT angiography is the primary application driving the technological development; however, these advances have resulted in a dramatic

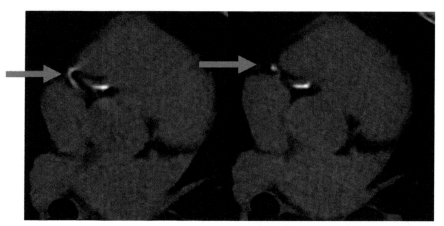

Fig. 3. Right coronary artery (RCA) motion artifact (blue arrow). The image on the left demonstrates mismapping of the calcified plaque in the proximal RCA creating a characteristic streak or "hook-shaped" motion artifact. The image to the right is the same scan with the reconstructed image shifted 5% of the R-R interval earlier in the cardiac cycle. The calcified plaque in the RCA is a more defined focus of calcification in the vessel wall. Motion unsharpness and the associated artifactual streaking of the plaque increase the area of the plaque and decreases the density. In the Agatston scoring method (see text) the lesion score is calculated by multiplying the calcified plaque area by the highest density pixel value in the calcified lesion. This type of artifact increases the area and lowers the density of a given lesion.

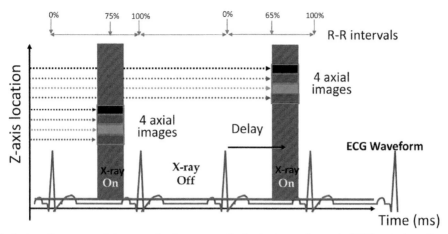

Fig. 4. This timing diagram explains aspects of a prospectively electrocardiograph (ECG)-gated cardiac computed tomography (CT) acquisition. The ECG QRS wave signal electrical systole and the R-R interval. For a heart rate of 60 bpm, the R-R interval is 1 seconds or 1000 milliseconds. If the gantry speed is 0.4 seconds (400 ms) then the minimum half-scan tube on time is 200 milliseconds. If the scanner prescribes the cardiac phase based on the center of the collected views used to reconstruct the image a 75% cardiac phase is center at 750 milliseconds after the QRS and the x-ray turns on at 650 milliseconds and off at 850 milliseconds. The use of an expanded tube on time, commonly referred to as "padding," allows the user to reconstruct multiple adjacent phases at the expense of slightly increased radiation exposure. During the third heartbeat, the CT couch increments the table to the next location. As an example only, during the third heartbeat if a different scanner was used that specifies the cardiac phase based on the tube on time, a cardiac phase of 65% would result in the tube coming on at 650 milliseconds and turning off at 850 milliseconds identical to the first heartbeat, but the resulting cardiac phases would be labeled 75% and 65% of the R-R interval, respectively.

improvement in the image quality for CAC through improved spatial resolution, reduced image noise and improved coronary motion compensation. The various CT vendors have taken several approaches to coronary imaging based on developing faster gantry speeds, wider and more efficient detectors, powerful X-ray tubes and dual-source systems. The measurement of calcified plaque by noncontrast CT and calcium score has been demonstrated to be remarkably robust in the setting of substantial technological advancement.

CORONARY ARTERY CALCIUM SCORE

The seminal work on the CAC score was published by Drs Agatston, Janowitz, Hildner, Zusmer, Viamonte, and Detrano in 1990 where they described a method to acquire axial CT images and quantify the amount of calcifications defining a total coronary calcium score.[9] Their methodology for calculating the calcium score, with only minor modification, remains the standard for clinical practice and medical decision making nearly 3 decades later. The ability to image the coronary arteries was possible based on the development of an ultrafast cardiac CT scanner using an electron gun and focusing rings to sweep a tungsten target ring to create x-rays as opposed to a conventional x-ray tube. The EBCT design, Imatron C-100

ultrafast CT scanner, was able to freeze cardiac motion with a 100-millisecond temporal resolution and image the coronary arteries with 3-mm, thin slices. Limitations of the EBCT included a limited ability to increase technique for larger patients, resulting in substantial image noise. To measure the CAC score, a set of 20 contiguous 3-mm-thick slices was acquired using prospective ECG gating in late diastole (80% of the R-R interval). Each image was acquired with a temporal resolution of 100 milliseconds during a breath-hold of 30 to 45 seconds using prospective ECG gating. To measure CAC, they set a threshold for calcific lesion to 130 CT numbers or more (also known as Hounsfield units) and an area of 1 mm^2 or greater. For each calcified lesion meeting the criteria, the area of the lesion and brightest pixel was determined. A lesion score was calculated by multiplying the area of lesion by the density weighting factor based on highest CT number in each lesion. Then for each epicardial vessel, the number of lesions per vessel is summed to create a vessel score and the sum of all vessel scores results in the "total coronary calcium score."

TOTAL CALCIUM SCORE (AKA AGATSTON SCORE, CORONARY ARTERY CALCIUM SCORE)

Criteria for scoring CAC

- Calcification identified in an epicardial coronary artery
- Calcified lesion with pixels measuring 130 CT numbers or greater (aka Hounsfield units) and a calcified lesion area of 1 mm^2 or greater

Calculate the calcified lesion score

- Measure lesion area in mm^2 by summing pixels meeting the criteria
- Identify the highest CT number pixel in a given lesion
- Based on the brightest lesion pixel, determine the density weighting factor by the following ranges of brightest pixel CT numbers:
  ○ 130 to 199; then weighting factor = 1
  ○ 200 to 299, then weighting factor = 2
  ○ 300 to 399; then weighting factor = 3
  ○ 400 or greater; then weighting factor = 4
- The sum of the lesion scores for each vessel is the vessel subscore
- The sum of the vessel scores is the total calcium score, also known as the Agatston score

PERFORMING THE ANALYSIS FOR CORONARY ARTERY CALCIUM SCORE

The images are loaded into a workstation that has a CAC scoring program (**Fig. 5**). These programs, if used for clinical practice, are medical devices approved by the US Food and Drug Administration. Most programs provide the facility with the ability to print a custom report for the patient or

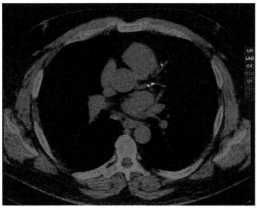

Fig. 5. Calcium scoring program display at the level of the left main coronary artery with color-coding turned on (*magenta*) for potentially scoreable lesions of 130 Hounsfield units or greater and an area of 1 mm^2 or greater. A legend for the color coding of the vessels is located vertically along the right sided margin. Calcified plaques in the ramus and LAD are color coded yellow. The ribs, scapula, vertebra, and a calcified right infrahilar node are all color coded magenta. The individual using the program to score coronary artery calcium simply clicks on magenta lesions that are located along the course of the respective coronary arteries.

referring provider. The image analyst should review the set of images to determine if the scan coverage was adequate and to review for any image artifacts. An initial review of the scan for noncoronary calcifications that can be present in the aortic root, aortic valve, mitral annulus, and along the pericardium or within the myocardium can help to prevent errors in scoring CAC. Most programs have the ability to toggle ON and OFF color coding of calcifications through the image that meet the criteria for CAC and this can be very useful when trying to differentiate calcium in the wall of the aorta versus proximal left main or right coronary artery (RCA) (**Fig. 6**). Next, from the origin of the left coronary artery the user should trace the course of the left main and the LAD follow the course of the vessel to the cardiac apex. If calcifications are seen, then the lesion is selected using the onscreen cursor and color coded to the vessel segment. The process is repeated for the LCX and RCA with each CAC plaque identified color coded to the appropriate vessel. Once completed, a CAC score table is created of the vessel subscores (left main, LAD, LCX and RCA) as well as the total calcium score.

Potential errors in calculating the CAC score can falsely increase or decrease the score. Erroneously elevated scores are related to scoring calcified structures that are not coronary arteries such as the mitral annulus, aortic root, and aortic valve leaflets. Intracoronary stents and surgical clips are commonly metallic and should not be scored as calcified plaque (**Fig. 7**). Any automated feature that grows lesions should be carefully supervised and reviewed by the user. It is not uncommon for these algorithms to expand scoring to calcifications related to the aortic root and mitral annulus and, in some situations, ribs, vertebra, or calcified lymph nodes may be erroneously included. In most cases, this misclassification can be rapidly removed by the user and alternative tools used to select only the calcifications related to the coronary arteries.

TIPS AND PITFALLS FOR MEASURING THE CALCIUM SCORE

- Because the aortic wall and root commonly calcify, carefully evaluate the coronary ostia and proximal right and left coronary arteries and make sure that calcification included as part of the CAC score are truly in the coronary arteries and not in the wall of the aorta (see **Fig. 6**).
- Mitral annular calcifications are a common pitfall for being misscored as CAC. The mitral annulus follows the same course and is deep to the adjacent circumflex artery in the left atrioventricular groove. If there is a vessel-specific score in the circumflex artery and no

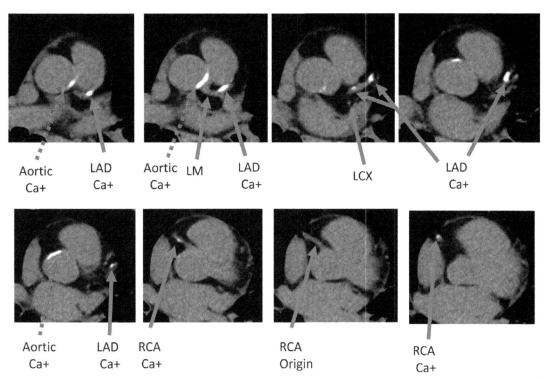

Fig. 6. A set of 8 contiguous slices through the origins of the left and right coronary arteries from the respective coronary sinuses of the aortic root. Aortic wall calcifications are present adjacent to the origin of the left main (LM) and right coronary artery (RCA). Aortic calcifications should not be included in measures of coronary artery calcium (CAC). LAD, left anterior descending; LCX, left circumflex.

or very little plaque in the other coronary vessels, then the possibility of mitral annular calcification being mistakenly scored as LCX CAC should be considered. The mitral annulus is deep to the epicardium, whereas the circumflex artery is more superficial and located in the epicardial space and surrounded by epicardial adipose tissue (see **Fig. 2**).

- CAC scoring programs typically include a calcified plaque connectivity algorithm and that region grows once a single point of CAC lesion is identified by the user. When using this function, it is essential to carefully review your work because the region grow functionality can incorporate adjacent non-coronary structures such as the aortic valve,

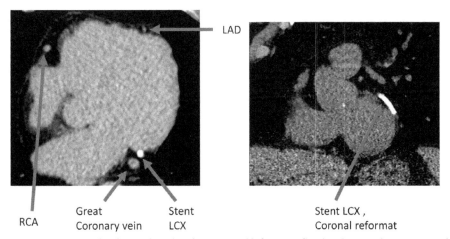

Fig. 7. An intracoronary stent has been placed in the proximal left circumflex (LCX). Note the presence of the great coronary vein in the left atrioventricular groove and its larger size. The left anterior descending (LAD) and right coronary artery (RCA) can both be seen deep to the pericardium and surrounded by epicardial adipose tissue.

mitral annulus, and even calcified mediastinal lymph nodes and adjacent ribs.

- Obese individuals and individuals unable to elevate their arms over their head can have images with degraded image quality and increased image noise. In severe cases image noise can exceed the 130 CT number threshold creating fields of pixels exceeding 130 CT numbers.
- Patient-related clothing, undergarments, and piercings can create metallic streak artifacts that degrade image quality. Underwire bras, body piercing over the chest, and metallic clothing should be removed if possible before the study (**Fig. 8**)
- Prospective ECG gating with cardiac CT results in blocks of slices acquired during different heartbeats. Malalignment of these blocks should be recognized by the interpreting provider to avoid diagnostic errors (**Fig. 9**).

THE HISTORICAL DEVELOPMENT OF THE COMPUTED TOMOGRAPHY TECHNOLOGY AND THE CORONARY ARTERY CALCIUM SCORE

The development of spiral CT, single channel CT, and then multidetector CT ushered in a period of rapid innovation for conventional spiral CT designs. One of the early efforts to use conventional CT scanners used a novel dual slice spiral CT.[18] The improved coverage with acquiring 2 slices at once allowed for the heart to be covered in a single reasonable 15- to 25-second breath-hold. The lack of cardiac gating and relatively low temporal resolution results in motion artifacts, but the work demonstrated the feasibility of using conventional CT scanners to measure coronary calcium and the feasibility of a multislice acquisition. The

development in the late 1990s of more powerful x-ray tubes coupled with subsecond gantry speeds provided the capability for the initial comparison of single slice spiral CT scanners to EBCT. The 0.8-second full rotation of the gantry translates into a half-scan reconstruction temporal resolution of 0.4 seconds or 400 milliseconds, or more conservatively 500 milliseconds if accounting for the fan angle. The temporal resolution was 4-fold greater than the 100 milliseconds temporal resolution of EBCT systems; however, the single slice spiral CT scanners had advantages in reduced image noise, higher spatial resolution, and greater stability for measuring CT numbers. These early attempts demonstrated the feasibility of using spiral CT with ECG gating to image the coronary arteries and calculate the CAC score using the Agatston and novel methods with excellent correlation and agreement in measuring calcified plaque.[19,20] The development of 64-slice CT scanners by multiple vendors resulted in cardiac CT scanners with even more robust imaging capability and broader use with characteristics and interscan variability comparable with EBCT.[21] The advent of spiral CT for CAC expanded the ability for researchers to study CAC as a biomarker of CVD risk. The National Heart Lung and Blood Institute–funded Multi-Ethnic Study of Atherosclerosis (MESA) provided a structure to standardized the measurement of CAC for multiple population-based studies as well as in clinical practice.[22] These advances put the technology into the hands of additional clinical research teams that are responsible for the expansive knowledge base of peer-reviewed publications exceeding 1250 articles.[23] More recent technological advances include the use of iterative reconstruction to

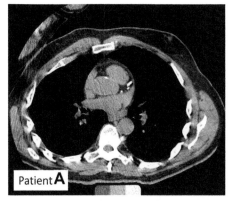
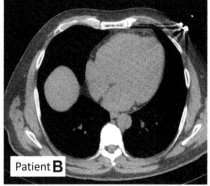

Fig. 8. Patient A was unable to position right arm over his head resulting in subtle streak artifact manifest as dark bands through the ascending aorta, left atrium, and descending aorta. Also note the hook artifacts at the edges of each rib indicating respiratory motion artifacts. Patient B was scanned with metallic nipple rings resulting large artifacts in the region of the LAD. A common metallic artifact is underwire bra. The importance of removing metallic clothing and jewelry is increasingly critical as we continue to reduce radiation exposure.

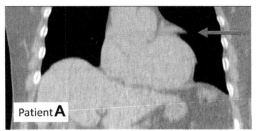 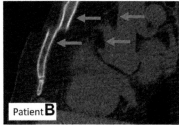

Fig. 9. Slab artifacts: coronary artery calcium computed tomography scans performed with prospective electrocardiographic gating and axial scan mode are prone to artifacts related to alignment of the slabs that are acquired at different times and during different heartbeats. Review of the entire stack of images in the coronary and sagittal planes often makes these artifact more obvious. Artifacts related to variations in cardiac phase impact the appearance of the heart alone (patient A, coronal reformat), whereas patient respiratory or voluntary motions will include the surround soft tissues (patient B, sagittal reformat).

further reduce radiation exposure and low kVp imaging.[24–26] Although both techniques hold significant promise for further reduction in radiation exposure, they achieve this at the expense of altering the brightness of calcification and necessitating the need for robust calibration.[23]

ALTERNATIVE SCORING METHODS FOR CORONARY ARTERY CALCIUM

The Agatston scoring method has several features that tend to increase score variability. Specifically, the lesion weighting factor is based on the brightest single pixel in a given calcified plaque, a feature that increases variability. Alternative methods have been evaluated to measure CAC plaque volume, mass, slice interpolation volume, density score, and various approaches to calibration.[20,27,28] These efforts have been shown in some cases to decrease variability and improve precision in measurement of calcified plaque. The advances in CT technology at 64 slices and beyond made it apparent that CAC was easily visible on routine CT examinations and visual assessment of the CAC score on non–ECG-gated chest CT scans has shown excellent correlation with the total calcium score.[29] The ability of CT scans to identify and measure CAC is robust in that the images are highly sensitive to the presence and amount of CAC. Comparing the CAC score with weight may be helpful in this regard. An individual's weight is one of several established predictors for developing CVD. A person's "weight" can be measured using a low-cost personal scale, a high-cost medical grade scale or an individual skilled in guessing weight. Measurement error will vary for each method; however, all three will be able to differentiate between a person weighing 100, 300 or 400 lbs (45.4, 136, or 181.4 kg) and be able to quantify CVD risk. In all cases, the measurement tool will be able to appropriately classify the person on the spectrum from normal to obese. Likewise, the amount of calcified plaque present makes the CAC score robust to categorizing individuals at various thresholds of plaque burden such as proposed in the Coronary Artery Calcium Data and Reporting System.[17] The Coronary Artery Calcium Data and Reporting System provides a standardize approach for guiding management with both dedicated CT Scans where the CAC score is calculated as well as routine CT examinations that include the heart where CAC can be visually estimated (Table 1). The Coronary Artery Calcium Data and Reporting System provides guidance for standardization reporting of CAC that should improve understanding of the results for health care providers and patients.

INTERPRETATION GUIDELINES FOR CORONARY ARTERY CALCIUM EXAMINATIONS

- Best practices for reporting diagnostic tests showed be followed describing the patient, examination performed, technical parameters, and radiation exposure.
- The total calcium score (Agatston scoring method) should be provided.
- The percentile for the individuals age, gender, and ethnicity should be provided based on established cohorts relative to the population being studied if available.
- The National Institute of Health's MESA study supports online access to CAC tools that includes: the MESA Risk Score Calculator, CAC Score Reference Values (including percentiles by ethnicity), and Arterial Age Calculator.[30]
- The report should indicate the presence or absence of CAC in the major epicardial coronary arteries (left main, LAD, LCX, and RCA).
- Additional findings related to the heart and surrounding structures that are visible around the heart.

Table 1
Coronary artery calcium data and reporting system CAC-DRS

CAC Score (Agatston)	Visual Score Estimate (V0 to V3)	Vessels with CAC (N1 to N4)	Cardiovascular Risk
0	V0 absent	None	Very low
1–99	V1 limited	N1-N2, rarely N3 or N4	Increased
100–299	V2 Moderate	≥ N1	Moderately increased
≥300	V3 High	≥ N1	Moderate to severely increased

The CAC-DRS provides a framework for standardized reporting of CAC scores between dedicated scans for the measurement of CAC and the qualitative reporting of calcified plaque using a visual scoring system. When visual scoring is used the reader estimates plaque burden as absent, limited, moderate or high plaque burden (V0-V3) and then reports the number of major epicardial coronary arteries with any CAC (left main, left anterior descending, left circumflex, and right coronary artery) as N1 to N4 as appropriate.
Abbreviations: CAC, coronary artery calcium; CAC-DRS, Coronary Artery Calcium Data and Reporting System.

- Any coronary calcium, including single foci of CAC, indicates significantly increased ASCVD risk over the next 10 to 15 years.[14,15] This information may be particularly useful when CAC is identified on conventional CT scans using a visual scoring approach.
- The American Heart Association/American College of Cardiology 2013 Guidelines recommend revising upward an individual's ASCVD risk estimate based on a CAC score of 300 or greater or the 75th percentile or greater for age, sex, and ethnicity.[3] Practically, the 75th percentile and not the 300 score threshold will drive management for individuals less than 65 years of age. For women 50 years of age or less, regardless of ethnicity, the presence of any CAC will place her well above the 75th percentile and at significantly increased ASCVD risk. For a 50-year-old man, the presence of calcium score of 1 places them at the 59th, 73rd, 64th, and 69th percentiles for White, Black, Chinese, and Hispanic race/ethnicity, respectively. Practically, the presence of any CAC identified on a chest CT would be greater than a score of 1 and place a man 50 years or younger at the 75th percentile or greater.
- Absence of CAC indicates a less than 1% risk at 10 years of clinical ASCVD.

WHAT THE REFERRING PHYSICIAN NEEDS TO KNOW

- The presence of any CAC by CT indicates the presence of coronary artery disease, specifically advanced coronary plaque and, thus, significantly increased risk for developing clinical ASCVD over the next 10 to 15 years.
- CAC identified in individuals before the age of 50 years is associated with increased risk of clinical coronary heart disease and scores of greater than 100 are associated with increase all-cause mortality.[15]
- Any calcified plaque in middle-aged adults (<60 years of age) is associated with a substantially increased risk of clinical heart disease over the next 10 to 15 years and a calcium score of greater than 100 is associated with a 1-in-5 chance of death over the next 10 to 15 years.
- A calcium score of zero is associated with a less than 1% ten-year cardiovascular risk.
- CAC adds significantly to traditional risk factors for predicting cardiovascular risk and can be useful in select patients at intermediate 10-year ASCVD risk (5%–15%) for raising or lowering predicted ASCVD risk and to inform statin therapy decisions through shared decision making between patient and health care providers.[7]
- Current prevention guidelines for ASCVD recommend shared decision making and consideration of statin therapy for individuals with a greater than 7.5% ten-year risk based on traditional risk factors using the pooled cohort risk equation.[3,4,7]
- Individuals with family history of early onset ASCVD, human immunodeficiency virus infection, or other conditions that put them at increased ASCVD not adequately evaluated in population-based risk calculators may benefit from CT CAC scoring.[23]

SUMMARY

The CAC is a robust imaging biomarker of ASCVD risk supported by a robust evidence base of more than 1250 publications generated over 50 years dating back early work with cinefluoroscpy. CAC is calcified plaque in the coronary arteries and whether identified formally on a CT scan specifically for CAC scoring scan or as an unsuspected finding on a CT angiography study performed for pulmonary emboli, the value to the individual of this knowledge is substantial. For most adults under age 70 years, the presence of even limited amounts of CAC (scores <100) will in most cases increase their 10-year risk to above the threshold where a discussion of the benefits of statin therapy is indicated.[3] Current guidelines balances the individual's absolute risk of ASCVD and the potential risk reduction from treatment against the potential negative consequences of therapy. Unfortunately, randomized trials of ASCVD screening strategies linked to prevention measures have not been performed and logistically and financially would be extremely challenging. As pointed out in the 2013 American Heart Association/American College of Cardiology Guidelines, neither traditional CVD risk scores (Framingham Risk Score and Pooled Cohort Equation) or CT calcium score have randomized trials to document improved clinical outcomes. The 2018 US Preventive Services Task Force systematic review found insufficient evidence to support universal incorporation of the CAC into population screening for ASCVD.[31,32] The accompanying editorial by Drs Wilkins and Lloyd-Jones correctly state, "At present, direct evidence is limited to determine whether the use of CAC screening to reclassify risk for patients and intermediate risk results in overall reductions in morality and CVD events, but there is no evidence to suggest that event rates would be worse with such a strategy. Avoidance of statin therapy in the majority of intermediate-risk patient who have a CAC score of 0 also could be desirable."[7] They state the evidence is strong that CAC score reclassifies the large number of patients falling in the intermediate category of risk into low- and high-risk groups, providing valuable information for shared decision making between patients and providers. They in alignment with the recent Expert Consensus Statement from the SCCT, which recommends a selective and serial testing approach based on office-based assessment of traditional risk factors followed by selective use of the CAC score in patients found to be at intermediate ASCVD absolute (5%–15% ten-year risk) when clinical decision making may be impacted as to statin therapy.

In conclusion, the CAC score is currently the most established and well-researched biomarker of risk for reclassifying individuals who, with office-based testing, are found to be at intermediate risk for ASCVD. A gap in our knowledge is a large-scale primary prevention screening trial that couples a strategy to identify individuals at increased risk and target them for guideline-based preventions strategies that include statin therapy. To be of sufficient power, such a trial would require a large number of people and extended follow-up for clinical events, but would have the potential to more accurately target statin therapy to reduce CVD events and decrease the off-target harms and cost of statin therapy in individuals unlikely to benefit from the therapy. As health care providers, we are entrusted with advising our patients based on the best available although commonly incomplete evidence. Fortunately for our patients, the evidence is clear that individuals with CAC are at significantly increased risk of clinical ASCVD. Likewise, individuals without CT evidence of CAC are at extremely low 10-year risk of ASCVD (<1%). The CAC score is a powerful tool to foster patient-centered care and advance shared decision making and engagement of individuals in their lifestyle and health care choices.

ACKNOWLEDGMENTS

This manuscript was supported by intramural funding provided by Vanderbilt University Medical Center and grant R01-HL098445 from the National Heart, Lung, and Blood Institute (NHLBI) to Vanderbilt University Medical Center and Wake Forest University Medical Center.

REFERENCES

1. Mokdad AH, Ballestros K, Echko M, et al. The state of US health, 1990-2016: burden of diseases, injuries, and risk factors among US states. JAMA 2018;319(14):1444–72.

2. Mackay J, Mensah G. The atlas of heart disease and stroke. In: WHO, editor. WHO; 2004. Available at: http://www.who.int/cardiovascular_diseases/resources/atlas/en/.

3. Goff DC Jr, Lloyd-Jones DM, Bennett G, et al. 2013 ACC/AHA guideline on the assessment of cardiovascular risk: a report of the American College of Cardiology/American Heart Association Task Force on practice guidelines. Circulation 2014; 129(25 Suppl 2):S49 73.

4. Stone NJ, Robinson JG, Lichtenstein AH, et al. 2013 ACC/AHA guideline on the treatment of blood cholesterol to reduce atherosclerotic cardiovascular risk in adults: a report of the American College of Cardiology/American Heart Association Task Force on practice guidelines. Circulation 2014;129(25 Suppl 2):S1–45.

5. Pencina MJ, Navar-Boggan AM, D'Agostino RB Sr, et al. Application of new cholesterol guidelines to a population-based sample. N Engl J Med 2014; 370(15):1422–31.

6. Saint Louis C. Guidelines may double statin use. The New York Times 2014;24:2014.

7. Wilkins JT, Lloyd-Jones DM. USPSTF recommendations for assessment of cardiovascular risk with nontraditional risk factors: finding the right tests for the right patients. JAMA 2018;320(3):242–4.

8. Yeboah J, McClelland RL, Polonsky TS, et al. Comparison of novel risk markers for improvement in cardiovascular risk assessment in intermediate-risk individuals. JAMA 2012;308(8):788–95.

9. Agatston AS, Janowitz WR, Hildner FJ, et al. Quantification of coronary artery calcium using ultrafast computed tomography. J Am Coll Cardiol 1990; 15(4):827–32.

10. Strong JP, Malcom GT, McMahan CA, et al. Prevalence and extent of atherosclerosis in adolescents and young adults: implications for prevention from the Pathobiological Determinants of Atherosclerosis in Youth Study. JAMA 1999;281(8):727–35.

11. Virmani R, Kolodgie FD, Burke AP, et al. Lessons from sudden coronary death : a comprehensive morphological classification scheme for atherosclerotic lesions. Arterioscler Thromb Vasc Biol 2000;20(5):1262–75.

12. Rumberger JA, Simons DB, Fitzpatrick LA, et al. Coronary artery calcium area by electron-beam computed tomography and coronary atherosclerotic plaque area. A histopathologic correlative study [see comments]. Circulation 1995;92(8):2157–62.

13. Lieber A, Jorgens J. Cinefluorography of coronary artery calcification. Correlation with clinical arteriosclerotic heart disease and autopsy findings. Am J Roentgenol Radium Ther Nucl Med 1961;86:1063–72.

14. Budoff MJ, Young R, Burke G, et al. Ten-year association of coronary artery calcium with atherosclerotic cardiovascular disease (ASCVD) events: the multi-ethnic study of atherosclerosis (MESA). Eur Heart J 2018;39(25):2401–8.

15. Carr JJ, Jacobs DR Jr, Terry JG, et al. Association of coronary artery calcium in adults aged 32 to 46 years with incident coronary heart disease and death. JAMA Cardiol 2017;2(4):391–9.

16. Detrano R, Guerci AD, Carr JJ, et al. Coronary calcium as a predictor of coronary events in four racial or ethnic groups. N Engl J Med 2008;358(13):1336–45.

17. Hecht HS, Blaha MJ, Kazerooni EA, et al. CAC-DRS: coronary artery calcium data and reporting system. an expert consensus document of the society of cardiovascular computed tomography (SCCT). J Cardiovasc Comput Tomogr 2018;12(3):185–91.

18. Shemesh J, Apter S, Rozenman J, et al. Calcification of coronary arteries: detection and quantification with double-helix CT. Radiology 1995;197(3):779–83.

19. Carr J, Burke G. Subclinical cardiovascular disease and atherosclerosis are not inevitable consequences of aging. J Am Geriatr Soc 2000;48(3):342–3.

20. Becker CR, Kleffel T, Crispin A, et al. Coronary artery calcium measurement: agreement of multirow detector and electron beam CT. AJR Am J Roentgenol 2001;176(5):1295–8.

21. Budoff MJ, McClelland RL, Chung H, et al. Reproducibility of coronary artery calcified plaque with cardiac 64-MDCT: the multi-ethnic study of atherosclerosis. Am J Roentgenol 2009;192(3):613–7.

22. Carr JJ, Nelson JC, Wong ND, et al. Calcified coronary artery plaque measurement with cardiac CT in population-based studies: standardized protocol of Multi-Ethnic Study of Atherosclerosis (MESA) and Coronary Artery Risk Development in Young Adults (CARDIA) study. Radiology 2005;234(1):35–43.

23. Hecht H, Blaha MJ, Berman DS, et al. Clinical indications for coronary artery calcium scoring in asymptomatic patients: expert consensus statement from the Society of Cardiovascular Computed Tomography. J Cardiovasc Comput Tomogr 2017; 11(2):157–68.

24. Kurata A, Dharampal A, Dedic A, et al. Impact of iterative reconstruction on CT coronary calcium quantification. Eur Radiol 2013;23(12):3246–52.

25. Messerli M, Rengier F, Desbiolles L, et al. Impact of advanced modeled iterative reconstruction on coronary artery calcium quantification. Acad Radiol 2016;23(12):1506–12.

26. Nakazato R, Dey D, Gutstein A, et al. Coronary artery calcium scoring using a reduced tube voltage and radiation dose protocol with dual-source computed tomography. J Cardiovasc Comput Tomogr 2009;3(6):394–400.

27. Callister TQ, Cooil B, Raya SP, et al. Coronary artery disease: improved reproducibility of calcium scoring with an electron-beam CT volumetric method. Radiology 1998;208(3):807–14.

28. McCollough CH, Ulzheimer S, Halliburton SS, et al. Coronary artery calcium: a multi-institutional, multi-manufacturer international standard for quantification at cardiac CT. Radiology 2007;243(2):527–38.

29. Chiles C, Duan F, Gladish GW, et al. Association of coronary artery calcification and mortality in the national lung screening trial: a comparison of three scoring methods. Radiology 2015;276(1):82–90.

30. (MESA) M-ESoA. MESA CAC Tools and Calculators. 2018; MESA Risk Score, CAC Score Reference values and arterial age calculators. 2018, Available at: https://www.mesa-nhlbi.org/CAC-Tools.aspx. Accessed September 11, 2018.

31. US Preventive Services Task Force, Curry SJ, Krist AH, et al. Risk assessment for cardiovascular disease with nontraditional risk factors: US preventive services task force recommendation statement. JAMA 2018;320(3):272–80.

32. Lin JS, Evans CV, Johnson E, et al. Nontraditional risk factors in cardiovascular disease risk assessment: updated evidence report and systematic review for the US preventive services task force. JAMA 2018;320(3):281–97.

Technical Aspects, Interpretation, and Body of Evidence for Coronary Computed Tomography Angiography

Jan-Erik Scholtz, MD[a,b], Sandeep Hedgire, MD[a],
Brian B. Ghoshhajra, MD, MBA[a,*]

KEYWORDS

- Coronary CT angiography • Coronary interpretation • Emergency department • Coronary stenosis

KEY POINTS

- Coronary computed tomography angiography has high sensitivity for the detection of coronary stenosis and excellent negative predictive value to rule out stenosis.
- Due to rapid technical developments, images of excellent quality are obtained with rare artifacts and low radiation doses.
- Recently established and updated guidelines provide guidance through coronary interpretation with structured and consistent reporting.

INTRODUCTION

Heart disease is the leading cause of death in the United States, accounting for approximately 23% of all deaths.[1] Acute chest discomfort as a main symptom of coronary artery disease (CAD) is a major reason for hospital admission, and accounted for 6.3 million of 130 million emergency department (ED) visits in the United States in 2013.[2] However, nearly 75% of patients with chest discomfort are diagnosed with noncardiac or nonischemic cardiac problems.[3]

CAD has a wide range of presentations, spanning from classic signs and symptoms of ischemic heart disease to sudden death and acute coronary syndrome (ACS) despite low pretest probability for CAD. Randomized controlled trials have shown coronary computed tomography angiography (CTA) to be an excellent tool in ruling out CAD in low-risk patients[4–7] and efficacious to reduce length of hospital stay and decrease rates of normal invasive coronary angiograms (ICA) compared with alternative standard of care testing. Coronary CTA allows for the quick and comprehensive noninvasive anatomic quantification of coronary arteries with high sensitivity and specificity for the detection of CAD.[8,9] Initial studies have shown that patients at higher risk, including patients with a history of CAD, a growing population in the United States due to improved medical care, may also benefit from coronary CTA as the initial noninvasive imaging test.[10]

In this review article, we discuss the technical aspects of coronary CTA, and give a

[a] Cardiac MR PET CT Program, Department of Radiology (Cardiovascular Imaging), Division of Cardiology, Massachusetts General Hospital, Harvard Medical School, 165 Cambridge Street, Suite 400, Boston, MA 02114-2750, USA; [b] Department for Diagnostic and Interventional Radiology, University Hospital Frankfurt, Theodor-Stern-Kai 7, Frankfurt 60590, Germany
* Corresponding author.
E-mail address: bghoshhajra@mgh.harvard.edu

Radiol Clin N Am 57 (2019) 13–23
https://doi.org/10.1016/j.rcl.2018.08.010

comprehensive overview of coronary CTA interpretation and reporting, as well as the supporting body of evidence.

TECHNICAL ASPECTS

Cardiac CTA studies should be performed or supervised by a physician trained in cardiovascular imaging. His or her competency should include the ability to perform coronary CTA with low radiation following the ALARA ("As Low As Reasonably Achievable") principle.

Although a 64-slice detector is considered the minimum requirement for coronary CTA,[11] newer generation scanners have wide z-axis coverage of up to 320 slices to allow shorter scan times and can offer imaging of the complete heart within a single heartbeat. In dual-source CT, scanners are equipped with 2 X-ray tubes in 90-degree position to each other, which provides temporal resolution up to 75 ms. All CT vendors have introduced new scanner equipment and modern postprocessing techniques that support technologists and physicians in their daily clinical practice. The risk of slab-to-slab and motion artifacts is reduced. Many of the dose-saving techniques can run automatically or semiautomatically and tailor the scan parameters to the patient habitus, examined body region and indication, and provide excellent image quality with low radiation.

In comparison with single-photon emission computed tomography (SPECT) with estimated effective doses of approximately 10 mSv, effective doses in coronary CTA have decreased from the initial 21 mSv to typical ranges between 1.5 and 5.0 mSv.[12–14] On modern scanners, tailored scan protocols allow radiation doses below 1.0 mSv[15–17] in some cases; however, patient characteristics such as body weight and the type of CT system used have relevant influence on radiation exposure.

Although standard tube potentials are 100 to 120 kVp, new scanners automatically select tube potential in a range between 70 and 150 kVp in 10-kVp steps based on the body habitus. In comparison with tube potential, which is selected manually or automatically before the CTA, based on the scout and is constant throughout the scan, automatic tube current modulation is a well-established dose-saving technique that adapts tube current in real-time throughout the scan. Independent of any other dose-reduction method, a potent way to optimize radiation is to limit the z-range to the indication/examined organs (ie, only image the heart rather than the entire chest). Caution is necessary in patients with prior coronary revascularization; coronary artery

bypass grafts often have arterial origins more cranial than the heart-only scan range and, thus, the scan field needs to be widened in the z-range usually up to the junction of the first rib and clavicle. Shielding of radiation-sensitive organs is controversial when discussed in the literature. We recommend displacement of the breast tissue cranial to the scan range as an alternative that results in less radiation, as soft tissue is then outside of the scan range[18] (**Fig. 1**). In obese patients, it may be advantageous to adapt automatic selected scan parameters, as the automatic software may increase radiation excessively. Current scanners display the estimated radiation exposure before the scan and, thus, effects of manual adjustments of scan parameters can be directly predicted.

Medications typically given during coronary CTA are beta-blockers for heart rate control and nitroglycerin for coronary vasodilation. With most

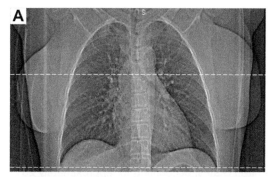
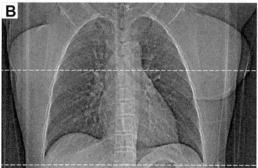

Fig. 1. Pre breast displacement. (*A*) Coronary CTA scout radiograph showing most part of mobile breast tissue lying in the z-axis of scan range. (*B*) Post breast displacement. Breast displacement with patient positioning belt in place moves most part of mobile breast tissue out of the scan range. (*From* Vadvala H, Kim P, Mayrhofer T, et al. Coronary CTA using scout-based automated tube potential and current selection algorithm, with breast displacement results in lower radiation exposure in females compared to males. Cardiovasc Diagn Ther 2014;4(6):472; with permission.)

equipment, a heart rate of 60 to 65 beats per minute is required for optimal image quality at the lowest possible radiation doses. However, scans at higher heart rates are possible due to improvement of temporal resolution. Thus, beta-blocker administration before coronary CTA may not be necessary, for instance, when using dual-source CT hardware.[19,20] Default scan mode in most coronary CTA programs is the prospectively electrocardiogram (ECG)-triggered axial acquisition.[11] The X-ray tube is activated only during a prespecified phase of the cardiac cycle, usually in a period of minimal motion during end-systole and diastole. End-systolic phases are often superior in patients with higher heart rates.[21] A too narrow time window should be avoided, as this would leave no flexibility to select additional phases in case of motion artifacts. By using "padding," a wider acquisition window over a longer interval of the cardiac cycle is possible to avoid nondiagnostic scans.[19] In retrospectively ECG-gated spiral acquisition, images are acquired throughout the entire cardiac cycle while the table moves slowly forward (**Fig. 2**). Although diagnostic accuracy is similar to prospectively ECG-triggered scans, radiation dose is higher.[22] Therefore, retrospective ECG-gating should be mainly used in studies that require evaluation of cardiac function or valves, in patients with tachycardia, or tachyarrhythmia. On dual-source CT platforms, an additional, high-pitch helical prospectively triggered mode is available that allows scans with seamless z-sampling of a single cardiac phase at pitch values of 3.4. These scans are triggered during early diastole and completed within 1 cardiac cycle allowing very low radiation doses. As only 1 phase during the cardiac cycle is acquired, this mode should be used only in patients in whom excellent image quality is expected (regular heart rate <60 beats per minute, body mass index <30 kg/m^2).

Atrial Fibrillation

Patients with atrial fibrillation are commonly scanned with retrospective ECG-gating with an optimal reconstruction phase at end-diastole.[23] Prospectively ECG-triggered acquisitions, particularly with additional phases, and arrhythmia rejection, have been shown to offer robust, simple, and low-radiation-dose alternatives to traditional retrospective ECG-gating in the setting of arrhythmia.[24,25]

Injection Protocols

Dual-head power injectors allow administration of iodine, saline, and a mixture of both. Thus, biphasic and triphasic injection protocols can

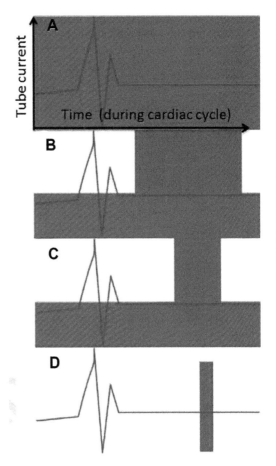

Fig. 2. Scan mode and ECG modulation. Retrospective ECG-gated acquisition was initially the conventional technique for CCTA, where the full tube current (shaded *red*) is maintained throughout the entire cardiac cycle (*A*). With ECG tube current modulation, the tube current is reduced during systole to lower the amount of radiation dose (*B*). Further radiation reduction could be achieved by limiting the duration of full tube current to either the end-systole or the late-diastole (*C*) windows. Prospectively ECG-triggered acquisition (*D*) results in a lower radiation dose than retrospective ECG-gated acquisition (*A–C*) by turning the tube current completely off for data acquisition outside the desirable phases. Note that for retrospectively ECG-gated modes (*A–C*), helical-mode acquisitions are performed with up to 80% z-axis overlap between rotations, whereas in prospectively ECG-triggered modes, the z-axis overlap between acquisitions is approximately 10% (or, in "single-heartbeat" modes, nonexistent), which further reduces radiation exposure. (*From* Chan AKW, Ferencik M, Abbara S, et al. Low radiation coronary CT. Curr Cardiovasc Imaging Rep 2014;7(9):9284; with permission.)

achieve high contrast in the coronary arteries, ascending aorta, and left cardiac chambers, while the right cardiac chambers are less-intense contrasted, but still allow evaluation of cardiac chambers. High iodine concentration contrast agents are preferred to achieve greater contrast-to-noise ratios. A total volume of 50 to 120 mL should be injected at high rates of 5 to 7 mL/s, preferably through the right antecubital vein. For timing the start of the scan, either bolus tracking or a test bolus are acceptable.

Post Processing

Iterative reconstruction algorithms have been introduced by all major vendors. More than 50% noise reduction is achievable compared with standard filtered back projection reconstruction.[26] Thus, CTA examinations with lower tube potential and, thus, lower radiation exposure are possible, with at least equal or lower noise levels, similar or better contrast profiles, and, generally, improved image quality compared with standard 120 kVp acquisition with filtered back projection image reconstruction.[20,21]

The reconstructed field of view should be reduced to include only the heart to maximize spatial resolution. Axial images should be reconstructed with thinnest available slice thickness (0.5–0.6 mm) and most vendors recommend a slice increment of 50% of the slice width. A semi-sharp reconstruction kernel should be used for most patients. Multiple phases should be reconstructed to find the best phase for coronary artery evaluation (if available), which may be at different time points for right and left coronary arteries. An even smaller field of view (8 cm) may be reconstructed for evaluation of coronary stents and in-stent restenosis.[26] An additional large field of view should be reconstructed to allow evaluation of extracardiac structures such as pulmonary nodules.[27–29]

Coronary Computed Tomography Angiography in Pediatric Patients

Most common indications for coronary CTA in pediatric patients are anomalies of origin, course, and termination of the coronary arteries. Other indications include diagnosis or follow-up of Kawasaki disease or other causes of aneurysm such as Behçet disease. Rare indications are Williams syndrome, imaging of fistula, and patients before and after tetralogy of Fallot surgical repair.

Pediatric patients generally have higher heart rate at rest. A weight-based approach to beta blockade should be used, but patients may still have high heart rates. If pediatric patients are not able to follow breathing instructions, CTA under general anesthesia should be considered to avoid unnecessary radiation exposure. Contrast can be given at lower flow rates as low as 1 mL/s through a small-gauge intravenous cannula. For routine coronary imaging, 1 mL/kg contrast is in generally sufficient, whereas complex anatomy may require a higher-contrast load (2 mL/kg).

INTERPRETATION OF CORONARY COMPUTED TOMOGRAPHY ANGIOGRAPHY

After finishing the CTA acquisition, images should directly be reviewed for image quality and artifacts.[26] Due to improvements of the hardware with increased spatial and temporal resolution, step artifacts are becoming less common. Common artifacts are breathing artifacts, which ideally can be avoided by correct breath training before the CTA. We recommend ruling out slow filling versus nonenhancement of the left atrial appendage with an additional delayed acquisition, as this may mimic a thrombus. The benefit of an image quality check while the patient is still on the scanner table is the possibility to directly repeat the scan if necessary. Artifacts and image quality should be mentioned in the report, including mentioning the coronary segment with limited interpretation.

For reliable interpretation of coronary CTA, knowledge of normal cardiac anatomy and physiology, as well as coronary arterial abnormalities is essential. This allows accurate interpretation of the pathologic findings and their potential effect in context with the clinical presentation. This includes knowledge of coronary atherosclerosis and its effects on myocardial physiology, congenital cardiac anomalies and postsurgical cardiac changes.

Due to the complexity of the cardiac anatomy, interpretation should be routinely performed on a 3-dimensional workstation to allow necessary postprocessing including curved multiplanar reformations of the coronary arteries, multiplanar reformation for detailed evaluation of coronary stenosis and cardiac chambers and valves, or volume/rendering technique for congenital anatomy and physiology.

The Society of Cardiovascular Computed Tomography established guidelines for the interpretation and reporting of coronary CTA in 2009 and updated these in 2014.[30,31] It includes a detailed list of required, optional, and recommended elements of coronary CTA reports (**Table 1**).

Noncontrast CT imaging is required for the detection of calcifications of the coronary arteries and allows preliminary interpretation of the cardiac anatomy. Calcium scoring software identifies pixels that exceed 130 Hounsfield Units to calculate Agatston Score, a risk stratification for major adverse cardiac events. Although the absence of

Table 1
Elements of a coronary computed tomography angiography report

Parameter	Examples	SCCT Guidelines[a]
Clinical data		
General	Indication	Required
Demographics	Name, referring clinician…	
Prior cardiac imaging	CT, nuclear testing, none	Recommended
Procedure data		
Description	Test type (eg, CCTA)	Required
Equipment	Scanner type, no. of detectors	Recommended
Acquisition	Scan mode, ECG-synchronization, dual-energy	Recommended
Medication	Beta-blocker, nitroglycerin Type and volume of contrast	Required Required
Complication		Required
Results		
Technical quality	Overall quality "Standardized" nomenclature for overall quality	Required
Coronary		
Calcium scoring		Required
Coronary anatomy	Dominance, anomalies, aneurysm, myocardial bridge	Required
Stenosis location and severity		Required
Standardized nomenclature for stenosis grading	% or nomenclature	Recommended
Standardized nomenclature for coronary segmentation		Recommended
Uninterpretable segments		Required
Prior cardiac procedures	Operation…	Required
Noncoronary cardiac	Vessels, cardiac chambers, myocardium, valves	Required
Noncardiac	Lung, mediastinum, bony structures	Required
Other	Devices, foreign material, none	Required
Impression		Required
Recommendation		Optional

Abbreviations: CCTA, coronary computed tomography angiography; CT, computed tomography; ECG, electrocardiogram; SCCT, Society of Cardiovascular Computed Tomography.
[a] Based on the Guidelines for the interpretation and reporting of coronary CT angiography from the SCCT Guidelines Committee.[31]

calcium in the coronary arteries does not necessarily indicate normal coronary anatomy without stenosis, some sites advocate the option to skip CTA if an extensive amount of calcium is evident on the noncontrast scan, with increased likelihood of a nonevaluable segment due to calcium blooming artifact. We do not advocate that approach, because many thresholds have been proposed for CTA cancellation, and we often note many scans have high or complete diagnostic yield despite high calcium burden.

Initial coronary CTA interpretation should start with evaluation of the origin, course, and terminus of the coronary arteries. The Society of Cardiovascular Computed Tomography (SCCT) introduced an 18-segment coronary artery model to guide evaluation of the main coronary vessels and their branches.[31] Subsequently, coronary stenosis should be evaluated and stenosis grades should be estimated in concordance with the 2014 SCCT reporting guidelines to provide structured and consistent coronary artery stenosis reports[31] (**Table 2**). Coronary CTA has high accuracy for detecting coronary artery stenosis with a sensitivity above 90% and specificity in the lower 80% range[13] (**Fig. 3**). For quantification of luminal

Table 2
Worst coronary stenosis and CAD-RADS classification

Maximal Stenosis	CAD-RADS
0%	0
1%–24%	1
25%–49%	2
50%–69%	3
A: 70%–99%	4
B: Left main >50% or obstructive 3-vessel disease (70%–99%)	A or B
100%	5
Nondiagnostic	N

Abbreviation: CADS-RADS, Coronary Artery Disease–Reporting and Data System.

stenosis and plaque extent, dedicated software is available. Further, the SCCT recently introduced Coronary Artery Disease–Reporting and Data System (CAD-RADS) classification that aims to classify the CTA-based stenosis results and to integrate this classification into clinical patient management.[32,33] Due to its novelty, the impact of CAD-RADS on CTA-based patient management and outcome is so far unknown. In the clinical practice, stenoses are commonly overestimated rather than underestimated.[34]

Generally, coronary plaques are classified into calcified, partially calcified and noncalcified plaques. To categorize a plaque as high risk, at least 2 of 4 of the following characteristics should be present: spotty calcification, lipid-rich (low attenuation) plaque, positive remodeling, and napkin-ring sign.

Although initial evaluation of coronary origin and course can be done via axial views, multiplanar and curved multiplanar reformations allow a quick overview of coronary stenosis. For detailed stenosis quantification, multiplanar reformatted images are recommended.

Further, there are other reasons for caliber fluctuation of the coronary artery beside arteriosclerotic plaques. This includes patients with aneurysm or dissection after trauma, patients with Takayasu disease, Kawasaki disease, systemic lupus erythematosus, polyarthritis nodose, or other vasculopathies including fibromuscular dysplasia. Although coronary vasospasm is proven by diagnostic ICA, patients with cocaine-induced vasospasm may present to coronary CTA as the initial imaging test through the ED. In patients of young age, origin and course of the coronary arteries should be interpreted carefully

to delineate a "benign" from a potentially significant anomalous interarterial and intramural course.

As the population ages and medical treatments extend lifespans, there is a growing population of patients presenting with prior coronary revascularization. Although stents with a luminal diameter of greater than 2.5 mm can be reliably evaluated for perfusion or restenosis, stents with smaller luminal diameter may be limited in their evaluation. In contrast, coronary bypass grafts can be safely evaluated by CTA. Caution has to be exercised during scanning as the scan range has to be widened over the complete thorax. Chronic total occlusion can be identified by coronary CTA and may augment diagnostic ICA via the detection of calcification and other features.

A complete structured coronary CTA report should further include evaluation of noncoronary cardiac and extracardiac structures, as incidental findings are common in elderly patients and may be the reason for initial presentation or makes further follow-up necessary.[27,35,36]

BODY OF EVIDENCE

Diagnostic accuracy of coronary CTA in stable patients with suspected CAD has been tested in numerous single-center studies and summarized in meta-analyses showing sensitivity ranges of 98% to 99% and specificity between 82% and 89% with a high diagnostic accuracy (area under the curve [AUC] between 0.97 and 0.99) for detection of CAD.[9,37,38] Severe coronary calcification leads to decreased diagnostic accuracy due to lower specificity.[39]

In a meta-analysis evaluating 11 retrospective studies of greater than 1500 patients, pooled sensitivity for coronary CTA versus exercise electrocardiography and SPECT was 98% versus 67% and 99% versus 73%, respectively. Specificity of coronary CTA was 82% versus 46% for exercise electrocardiography, and 71% versus 48% for SPECT.[40] A review comparing diagnostic performance of coronary CTA and stress testing showed sensitivity of 96% and 66%, respectively.[41] In the CORE320 study, comparison of coronary CTA and SPECT revealed diagnostic accuracy with AUC values of 0.91 and 0.69, respectively.[42] In the SCOT-HEART study, coronary CTA plus standard of care and standard of care alone were prospectively compared in stable patients with chest pain.[43] At 6 weeks, addition of coronary CTA resulted in a reclassification of CAD diagnosis in 27% of the patients (compared with 1% in standard of care) and resulted in a 38% reduction in myocardial infarctions after 1.7 years.

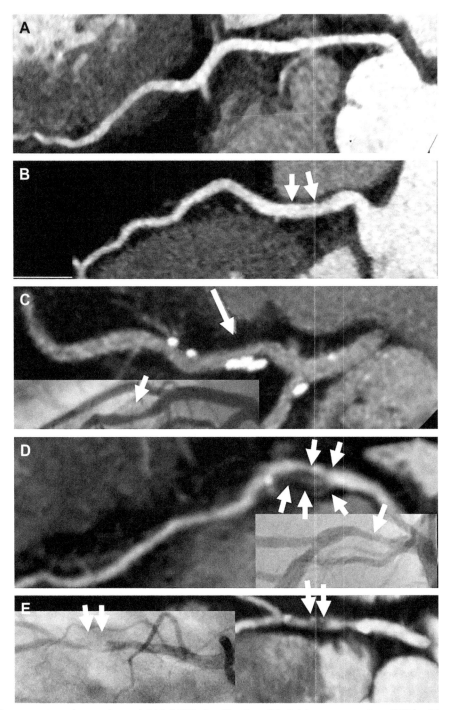

Fig. 3. Coronary stenosis severity and CAD-RADS classification. (*A*) right coronary artery (RCA) without stenosis (0%) and no stenosis at any other coronary vessel / CAD-RADS 0; (*B*) Soft plaque with minimal luminal narrowing (1%–24%) of the RCA (*arrows*) / CAD-RADS 1. (*C*) Mid left anterior descending (LAD) with mild luminal narrowing (25%–49%) (*arrows*) and ICA correlation (*arrows*) / CAD-RADS 2. (*D*) Proximal LAD with up to moderate coronary stenosis (50%–69%) (*arrows*) and ICA correlation (*arrows*) / CAD-RADS 3. (*E*) Distal RCA with severe stenosis (70%–99%) (*arrows*) and ICA correlation (*arrows*) / CAD-RADS 4A.

In the PROMISE study, event rates were not different after 2 years in patients with suspected randomized to CAD coronary CTA (3.3%) or stress testing (3.0%).[6]

Implementation of coronary CTA in the ED setting for patients with acute chest pain has been proven to allow efficient management of these patients with fast discharge of patients after ruling-out significant coronary stenosis (<50% diameter luminal narrowing), while missed ACS was below the acceptable rate of 1%.[19]

FUTURE TRENDS
Computed Tomography Fractional Flow Reserve

Fractional flow reserve (FFR) is a technique used in ICA to measure pressure differences across a coronary stenosis to determine the likelihood that the stenosis results in myocardial ischemia.[44] Noninvasive computed tomography-derived FFR (FFR-CT) is a novel technique based on computational fluid dynamics modeling to estimate functional data from a purely anatomic data set.[45] It is a potentially powerful tool with the option of further extension providing virtual stenting and treatment planning to determine optimal strategies for revascularization or optimal medical treatment.[46,47] It is recommended to use this adjunct in patients whose coronary arteries are likely to be minimally diseased or normal.[48] The diagnostic accuracy of FFR-CT varies markedly across the spectrum of disease and is well summarized in the review of Cook and colleagues.[48] So far, there is a lack of knowledge about the additional value of FFR-CT over plain coronary CTA. Although normal and up to mild stenosis on the one end of the spectrum, and severe stenosis on the other end, are detected with certainty by an experienced cardiovascular-trained radiologist, moderate stenosis may benefit from additional FFR-CT. A retrospective study suggested that FFR-CTA with a typically used cut point of 0.80 was a better predictor of revascularization or major adverse cardiac events than severe stenosis on CTA.[49] The additional cost of FFR-CT needs to be carefully weighted to the expected additional value.

Dual-Energy Computed Tomography

Dual-energy CT (DECT) is a novel technique that allows tissue decomposition and characterization. Although single-energy CT is performed with polychromatic energy levels of photons set to 120 kVp, 2 polychromatic data sets, typically with 80 and 140 kVp, are acquired in DECT. There are several vender-specific techniques; how those 2 data sets are generated, which can be acquired by single-source CT with rapid voltage switching in a single gantry rotation, tube voltage switching between sequential gantry rotation, or use of dual-layer detector, or by dual-source CT where the scanner is equipped with 2 X-ray tubes.[50] These 2 acquired data sets allow for quantification of tissue decomposition, which is clinically used to detect and quantify gout or characterization of kidney stones or distinguish between iodine and calcium.[51,52] In comparison with single-energy CT, it has been shown that DECT provides better tissue characterization with enhanced visualization of myocardial perfusion defects.[53,54] It allows the mapping of iodine distribution in the myocardium as a quantitative marker for perfusion and blood volume. Furthermore, postprocessing of those 2 data sets allows the generation of virtual monochromatic images, which are analogous to conventional single-energy CT images, but provides images with reduced beam-hardening and blooming artifacts.[55] This can be used to evaluate the lumen in coronary stents and the degree of luminal stenosis in heavily calcified plaques more precisely.[56] Novel postprocessing techniques may allow calcium subtraction, avoiding stenosis overestimation by calcium blooming. Further, evaluation of myocardium can be improved, as beam-hardening artifacts, for example, from high-contrast aortic lumen or pacemaker leads, are reduced.[54] The combination of coronary CTA with DECT myocardial perfusion imaging has been shown to improve the specificity of CTA for significant coronary stenosis while sensitivity was still high. These studies suggest that myocardial perfusion imaging with DECT may decrease the number of false-positive results on coronary CTA.[57]

SUMMARY

Coronary CTA has become a viable imaging modality for patients with acute chest pain as well as stable outpatients with high diagnostic accuracy to exclude CAD and rule out significant coronary artery stenosis. Due to rapid technical developments, semiautomatic and automatic tools support the imaging team to provide excellent diagnostic images with rare artifacts at a low radiation level. Recently established and updated guidelines provide guidance for interpretation and consistent and structured reporting.

REFERENCES

1. Centers for Disease Control and Prevention. Underlying cause of death 1999–2010 help. Available at: http://wonder.cdc.gov/wonder/help/ucd.html. Accessed September 16, 2018.
2. Rui P, Kang K, Albert M. National Hospital Ambulatory Medical Care Survey: 2013 EmergNational hospital ambulatory medical care survey: 2013 emergency department summary tables. Centers for Disease Control and Prevention; 2013.

Available at: http://www.cdc.gov/nchs/data/ahcd/nhamcs_emergency/2013_ed_web_tables.pdf.

3. Kohn MA, Kwan E, Gupta M, et al. Prevalence of acute myocardial infarction and other serious diagnoses in patients presenting to an urban emergency department with chest pain. J Emerg Med 2005; 29(4):383–90.

4. Raff GL, Hoffmann U, Udelson JE. Trials of imaging use in the emergency department for acute chest pain. JACC Cardiovasc Imaging 2017;10(3):338–49.

5. Litt HI, Gatsonis C, Snyder B, et al. CT angiography for safe discharge of patients with possible acute coronary syndromes. N Engl J Med 2012;366: 1393–403.

6. Hoffmann U, Truong QA, Schoenfeld DA, et al. Coronary CT angiography versus standard evaluation in acute chest pain. N Engl J Med 2012;367:299–308.

7. Douglas PS, Hoffmann U, Patel MR, et al. Outcomes of anatomical versus functional testing for coronary artery disease. N Engl J Med 2015; 372(14):1291–300.

8. Amsterdam EA, Wenger NK, Brindis RG, et al. 2014 AHA/ACC guideline for the management of patients with Non–ST-elevation acute coronary syndromes: a report of the American College of Cardiology/American Heart Association Task Force on Practice Guidelines. J Am Coll Cardiol 2014;130:e344–426.

9. Mowatt G, Cook JA, Hillis GS, et al. 64-Slice computed tomography angiography in the diagnosis and assessment of coronary artery disease: systematic review and meta-analysis. Heart 2008; 94(11):1386–93.

10. Scholtz J-E, Addison D, Bittner DO, et al. Diagnostic performance of coronary CTA in intermediate-to-high-risk patients for suspected acute coronary syndrome. JACC Cardiovasc Imaging 2018;11(9): 1369–71.

11. Abbara S, Blanke P, Maroules CD, et al. SCCT guidelines for the performance and acquisition of coronary computed tomographic angiography: a report of the Society of Cardiovascular Computed Tomography Guidelines Committee: endorsed by the North American Society for Cardiovascular Imaging (NASCI). J Cardiovasc Comput Tomogr 2016;10(6):435–49.

12. Chinnaiyan KM, Boura JA, DePetris A, et al. Progressive radiation dose reduction from coronary computed tomography angiography in a statewide collaborative quality improvement program: results from the Advanced Cardiovascular Imaging Consortium. Circ Cardiovasc Imaging 2013;6(5):646–54.

13. Achenbach S. Coronary CT angiography—future directions. Cardiovasc Diagn Ther 2017;7(5):432–8.

14. Arbab-Zadeh A, Di Carli MF, Cerci R, et al. Accuracy of computed tomographic angiography and single-photon emission computed tomography-acquired myocardial perfusion imaging for the diagnosis of coronary artery disease. Circ Cardiovasc Imaging 2015;8(10):e003533.

15. Hell MM, Bittner D, Schuhbaeck A, et al. Prospectively ECG-triggered high-pitch coronary angiography with third-generation dual-source CT at 70 kVp tube voltage: feasibility, image quality, radiation dose, and effect of iterative reconstruction. J Cardiovasc Comput Tomogr 2014;8:418–25.

16. Schuhbaeck A, Achenbach S, Layritz C, et al. Image quality of ultra-low radiation exposure coronary CT angiography with an effective dose <0.1 mSv using high-pitch spiral acquisition and raw data-based iterative reconstruction. Eur Radiol 2013;23(3): 597–606.

17. Achenbach S, Marwan M, Ropers D, et al. Coronary computed tomography angiography with a consistent dose below 1 mSv using prospectively electrocardiogram-triggered high-pitch spiral acquisition. Eur Heart J 2010;31(3):340–6.

18. Vadvala H, Kim P, Mayrhofer T, et al. Coronary CTA using scout-based automated tube potential and current selection algorithm, with breast displacement results in lower radiation exposure in females compared to males. Cardiovasc Diagn Ther 2014; 4(6):470–9.

19. Ghoshhajra BB, Takx RAP, Staziaki PV, et al. Clinical implementation of an emergency department coronary computed tomographic angiography protocol for triage of patients with suspected acute coronary syndrome. Eur Radiol 2017;27(7): 2784–93.

20. Meyersohn NM, Szilveszter B, Staziaki PV, et al. Coronary CT angiography in the emergency department utilizing second and third generation dual source CT. J Cardiovasc Comput Tomogr 2017;11(4): 249–57.

21. Scholtz J-E, Ghoshhajra B. Advances in cardiac CT contrast injection and acquisition protocols. Cardiovasc Diagn Ther 2017;7(5):439–51.

22. Menke J, Unterberg-Buchwald C, Staab W, et al. Head-to-head comparison of prospectively triggered vs retrospectively gated coronary computed tomography angiography: meta-analysis of diagnostic accuracy, image quality, and radiation dose. Am Heart J 2013;165(2):154–63.e3.

23. Oda S, Honda K, Yoshimura A, et al. 256-slice coronary computed tomographic angiography in patients with atrial fibrillation: optimal reconstruction phase and image quality. Eur Radiol 2016;26: 55–63.

24. Lee AM, Beaudoin J, Engel LC, et al. Assessment of image quality and radiation dose of prospectively ECG-triggered adaptive dual-source coronary computed tomography angiography (cCTA) with arrhythmia rejection algorithm in systole versus diastole: a retrospective cohort study. Int J Cardiovasc Imaging 2013;29:1361–70.

25. Lee AM, Engel L-C, Hui GC, et al. Coronary computed tomography angiography at 140 kV versus 120 kV: assessment of image quality and radiation exposure in overweight and moderately obese patients. Acta Radiol 2014;55:554–62.

26. Ghekiere O, Salgado R, Buls N, et al. Image quality in coronary CT angiography: challenges and technical solutions. Br J Radiol 2017;90(1072): 20160567.

27. Scholtz J-E, Lu MT, Hedgire S, et al. Incidental pulmonary nodules in emergent coronary CT angiography for suspected acute coronary syndrome: impact of revised 2017 Fleischner Society guidelines. J Cardiovasc Comput Tomogr 2018;12(1): 28–33.

28. Koonce J, Schoepf JU, Nguyen SA, et al. Extra-cardiac findings at cardiac CT: experience with 1,764 patients. Eur Radiol 2009;19:570–6.

29. Venkatesh V, You JJ, Landry DJ, et al. Extracardiac findings in cardiac computed tomographic angiography in patients at low to intermediate risk for coronary artery disease. Can Assoc Radiol J 2010;61(5): 286–90.

30. Raff GL, Abidov A, Achenbach S, et al. SCCT guidelines for the interpretation and reporting of coronary computed tomographic angiography. J Cardiovasc Comput Tomogr 2009;3:122–36.

31. Leipsic J, Abbara S, Achenbach S, et al. SCCT guidelines for the interpretation and reporting of coronary CT angiography: a report of the Society of Cardiovascular Computed Tomography Guidelines Committee. J Cardiovasc Comput Tomogr 2014; 8(5):342–58.

32. Cury RC, Abbara S, Achenbach S, et al. CAD-RADS(TM) coronary artery disease—reporting and data system. An expert consensus document of the Society of Cardiovascular Computed Tomography (SCCT), the American College of Radiology (ACR) and the North American Society for Cardiovascular Imaging. J Cardiovasc Comput Tomogr 2016;10:269–81.

33. Foldyna B, Szilveszter B, Scholtz J-E, et al. CAD-RADS–a new clinical decision support tool for coronary computed tomography angiography. Eur Radiol 2018;28(4):1365–72.

34. Lu MT, Meyersohn NM, Mayrhofer T, et al. Central core laboratory versus site interpretation of coronary CT angiography: agreement and association with cardiovascular events in the PROMISE trial. Radiology 2018;287(1):87–95.

35. Schietinger BJ, Bozlar U, Hagspiel KD, et al. The prevalence of extracardiac findings by multidetector computed tomography before atrial fibrillation ablation. Am Heart J 2008;155(2):254–9.

36. Magnacca M, Poddighe R, Casolo G, et al. Prevalence of cardiac and extracardiac incidental findings in the evaluation of coronary artery disease by multidetector computed tomography. G Ital Cardiol (Rome) 2016;17(5):363–9.

37. Paech DC, Weston AR. A systematic review of the clinical effectiveness of 64-slice or higher computed tomography angiography as an alternative to invasive coronary angiography in the investigation of suspected coronary artery disease. BMC Cardiovasc Disord 2011;11:32.

38. von Ballmoos MW, Haring B, Juillerat P, et al. Meta-analysis: diagnostic performance of low-radiation-dose coronary computed tomography angiography. Ann Intern Med 2011;154(6):413.

39. Arbab-Zadeh A, Miller JM, Rochitte CE, et al. Diagnostic accuracy of computed tomography coronary angiography according to pre-test probability of coronary artery disease and severity of coronary arterial calcification. The CORE-64 (Coronary Artery Evaluation Using 64-Row Multidetector Computed Tomography Angiography) international multicenter study. J Am Coll Cardiol 2012;59(4): 379–87.

40. Nielsen LH, Ortner N, Norgaard BL, et al. The diagnostic accuracy and outcomes after coronary computed tomography angiography vs. conventional functional testing in patients with stable angina pectoris: a systematic review and meta-analysis. Eur Heart J Cardiovasc Imaging 2014;15(9): 961–71.

41. Arbab-Zadeh A. Stress testing and non-invasive coronary angiography in patients with suspected coronary artery disease: time for a new paradigm. Heart Int 2012;7(1):e2.

42. Rochitte CE, George RT, Chen MY, et al. Computed tomography angiography and perfusion to assess coronary artery stenosis causing perfusion defects by single photon emission computed tomography: the CORE320 study. Eur Heart J 2014;35(17): 1120–30.

43. SCOT-HEART investigators. CT coronary angiography in patients with suspected angina due to coronary heart disease (SCOT-HEART): an open-label, parallel-group, multicentre trial. Lancet 2015;385: 2383–91.

44. Tonino PAL, De Bruyne B, Pijls NHJ, et al. Fractional flow reserve versus angiography for guiding percutaneous coronary intervention. N Engl J Med 2009; 360(3):213–24.

45. Taylor CA, Fonte TA, Min JK. Computational fluid dynamics applied to cardiac computed tomography for noninvasive quantification of fractional flow reserve: scientific basis. J Am Coll Cardiol 2013; 61(22):2233–41.

46. Kim K-H, Doh J-H, Koo B-K, et al. A novel noninvasive technology for treatment planning using virtual coronary stenting and computed tomography-derived computed fractional flow reserve. JACC Cardiovasc Interv 2014;7(1):72–8.

47. Hecht HS. The game changer? J Am Coll Cardiol 2014;63(12):1156–8.

48. Cook CM, Petraco R, Shun-Shin MJ, et al. Diagnostic accuracy of computed tomography–derived fractional flow reserve. JAMA Cardiol 2017;2(7):803.

49. Lu MT, Ferencik M, Roberts RS, et al. Noninvasive FFR derived from coronary CT angiography: management and outcomes in the PROMISE trial. JACC Cardiovasc Imaging 2017;10(11):1350–8.

50. Danad I, Fayad ZA, Willemink MJ, et al. New applications of cardiac computed tomography: dual-energy, spectral, and molecular CT imaging. JACC Cardiovasc Imaging 2015;8(6):710–23.

51. Graser A, Johnson TRC, Chandarana H, et al. Dual energy CT: preliminary observations and potential clinical applications in the abdomen. Eur Radiol 2009;19(1):13–23.

52. Bongartz T, Glazebrook KN, Kavros SJ, et al. Dual-energy CT for the diagnosis of gout: an accuracy and diagnostic yield study. Ann Rheum Dis 2015; 74(6):1072–7.

53. So A, Hsieh J, Narayanan S, et al. Dual-energy CT and its potential use for quantitative myocardial CT perfusion. J Cardiovasc Comput Tomogr 2012;6(5): 308–17.

54. Bucher AM, Wichmann JL, Schoepf UJ, et al. Quantitative evaluation of beam-hardening artefact correction in dual-energy CT myocardial perfusion imaging. Eur Radiol 2016;26:3215–22.

55. Sandfort V, Palanisamy S, Symons R, et al. Optimized energy of spectral CT for infarct imaging: experimental validation with human validation. J Cardiovasc Comput Tomogr 2017;11(3):171–8.

56. Mangold S, De Cecco CN, Schoepf UJ, et al. A noise-optimized virtual monochromatic reconstruction algorithm improves stent visualization and diagnostic accuracy for detection of in-stent re-stenosis in lower extremity run-off CT angiography. Eur Radiol 2016;26(12):4380–9.

57. De Santis D, Jin KN, Schoepf UJ, et al. Heavily calcified coronary arteries: advanced calcium subtraction improves luminal visualization and diagnostic confidence in dual-energy coronary computed tomography angiography. Invest Radiol 2018;53(2): 103–9.

Acute Coronary and Acute Aortic Syndromes

Avanti Gulhane, MD, DNB[a], Harold Litt, MD, PhD[b],*

KEYWORDS

• Acute • Myocardial ischemia • Dissection • Intramural hematoma • Penetrating ulcer

KEY POINTS

• Computed tomography (CT) is an appropriate method for safe and rapid triage of patients presenting with acute chest pain to the emergency department as acute coronary syndrome (ACS) (particularly patients at low to intermediate risk) or acute aortic syndromes (AASs).
• Technical advances in CT have led to improved image quality for evaluation of suspected ACS or AAS.
• Knowledge of aortic dissection and its variants is important for accurate diagnosis.

INTRODUCTION

Acute chest pain is the leading cause for emergency department (ED) visits in United States for those older than 65 years and the third leading cause overall.[1] Acute coronary syndrome (ACS) refers to any constellation of clinical symptoms compatible with acute myocardial ischemia, including stable anginal pain of transmural myocardial infarction (MI) with electrocardiogram (ECG) ST-segment elevation (STEMI) or non-STEMI (NSTEMI). Unstable angina pectoris (UA) has clinical symptoms of ACS without serum biomarker elevation and transient ECG changes of ischemia but a positive stress test and moderate to severe coronary stenosis. Prinzmetal angina is characterized by severe spasm of epicardial coronary arteries without any precipitating factor and may present as NSTEMI/UA. The typical chest pain of ACS is described as substernal tightness, pressure, squeezing, or heaviness with or without pain radiating to the neck or arm. Other symptoms such as dyspnea, nausea, vomiting, palpitations, or sudden cardiac arrest can also be observed.[2]

Acute aortic syndrome (AAS) is a constellation of clinically indistinguishable aortic diseases including acute aortic dissection (AAD), penetrating atherosclerotic ulcer (PAU), and intramural hematoma (IMH).[3] AAS is much less frequent than ACS, with only one AAS for every 130 patients with chest pain due to ACS. Conditions requiring urgent intervention such as unstable aortic aneurysms, inflammatory diseases of the aorta, and traumatic rupture are also an expression of AAS.[4] The incidence of AAD is 2.6 to 3.5 cases per 100,000 person-years,[3] with PAU representing 2.3% to 11% and IMH 10% to 30% of all AAS.[5] The nature of pain in AAS is classically described as sharp, tearing, ripping, migrating, or pulsating.[3,6] Other signs and symptoms include syncope, neurologic deficit, pulse deficit between the extremities, acute heart failure, myocardial ischemia, lower extremity ischemia, abdominal pain, and shock. Hypertension is a common risk factor for AAD, and a high clinical suspicion of Marfan syndrome is present in younger patients. A bicuspid aortic valve or a history of aortic surgery should also raise the suspicion of AAD.[7]

Disclosure Statement: H. Litt receives grant funding from Siemens Healthineers for unrelated CT projects.
a Cardiovascular Imaging, Department of Radiology, Perelman School of Medicine, University of Pennsylvania, 1 Silverstein, 3400 Spruce Street, Philadelphia, PA 19104, USA; b Cardiothoracic Imaging Division, Department of Radiology, Perelman School of Medicine, University of Pennsylvania, 1 Silverstein, 3400 Spruce Street, Philadelphia, PA 19104, USA
* Corresponding author.
E-mail address: Harold.litt@uphs.upenn.edu

radiologic.theclinics.com

Several criteria have been proposed to rule out ACS, including TIMI risk score, Goldman criteria, the ACC/AHA Guidelines for Management of UA and NSTEMI likelihood of ACS categories, and the HEART score; however, studies demonstrate their unreliability in excluding ACS.[8,9] Advances in multidetector-row computed tomography (MDCT), coupled with ECG gating for noninvasive imaging of the aorta and coronary vasculature, allows visualization of coronary vessels to at least third-order branches.[10] Safe and rapid triage of patients presenting with acute chest pain to the ED, particularly at low to intermediate risk for ACS, remains a major challenge and cardiac MDCT has emerged as potentially valuable diagnostic tool with high negative predictive value, easy availability,[8,11–13] 35% relative reduction in length of stay, and 20% reduction in hospital costs when CCTA is used instead of exercise treadmill ECG-based care for triage of ACS.[11] CCTA may play a role in reducing unnecessary catheter angiography in these patients,[10] although increased downstream testing in older patients and more cardioprotective medications being prescribed has been shown in multiple studies.[14,15] Contrast-enhanced, cardiac-gated multidetector CT is nearly 100% sensitive and specific for evaluating AAS.[7]

NORMAL ANATOMY OF THE AORTA AND CORONARY ARTERIES

In suspected AAS, careful evaluation is needed of the aortic root, extending from the level of the aortic valve to the sinotubular junction, including the annulus and sinuses of Valsalva (SV). The aortic annulus is the junction of the proximal ascending aorta with the left ventricular outflow tract. The normal aorta dilates at the level of the sinuses, tapering at the sinotubular junction to within 2 to 3 mm of the annular size. The loss of the normal "waist" of the aorta at the sinotubular junction is a predictor of future aortic events. The descending aorta begins just distal to the origin of the left subclavian artery at a point termed the "aortic isthmus." This isthmus is particularly vulnerable to deceleration forces during trauma because the relatively mobile ascending aorta and arch become fixed to the thoracic cage at this site. As a result, most descending aortic dissections and intramural hematomas have their origin at the isthmus.[16]

Coronary Arteries

It is pertinent to know the normal course, segmental anatomy, and branches of the coronary arteries with their regional supply for evaluating ACS. The trifurcation of left main coronary artery (LMCA) into left anterior descending coronary artery (LAD), left circumflex coronary artery (LCX), and the Ramus intermedius is a common variant, without any associated additional risk for ACS. Coronary dominance is determined by the artery supplying the posterior wall of left ventricle (LV) and giving rise to the posterior descending coronary artery (PDA) and posterolateral branch (PLB). The coronary system is called codominant when right coronary artery (RCA) gives rise to PDA and LCX gives rise to posterolateral branches.[17] Anatomic anomalies carrying an increased risk of ACS include single coronary artery; congenital hypoplastic, stenotic, or atretic LMCA; LMCA originating from the pulmonary artery; anomalous origin of LMCA from right SV (**Fig. 1**); and RCA from left SV with an interarterial course and coronary fistulae.[18] Myocardial bridging of an epicardial coronary artery with greater than 70% systolic compression, abnormal diastolic filling time, or arrhythmia should be considered as a potential cause of ACS.[18]

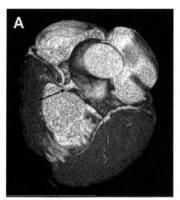 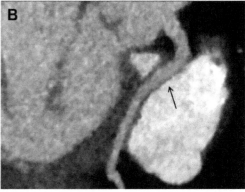

Fig. 1. A 52-year-old woman with complaints of progressive shortness of breath. CCTA ([A] VR and [B] MPR) shows anomalous coronary circulation with a single coronary artery arising from the right SV, anomalous origin of the LMCA from RCA (*arrows*), with intraarterial and intramuscular course. Patient was managed surgically. MPR, multiplanar reconstruction; VR, volume rendering.

IMAGING TECHNIQUES

ECG gating and synchronization allows data acquisition and image reconstruction at specific points in the cardiac cycle, optimizing image quality in ACS as well as AAS.

Acute Coronary Syndrome

Coronary artery calcium scoring
Mean Agatston scores and coronary calcium volume scores are widely used for cardiovascular risk stratification. Increasing coronary artery calcium (CAC) is generally predictive of a higher likelihood of ACS and obstructive coronary artery disease (CAD).[19] In patients presenting to the ED with low to intermediate pretest probability of ACS, a zero CAC score has an excellent negative predictive value (NPV) to rule out ACS.[20] But in patients at high risk for ACS, a calcium score of 0 may still be associated with myocardial ischemia on provocative testing.[21,22] An unenhanced acquisition may allow optimization of the contrast-enhanced acquisition to reduce radiation doses, but its value in the ED is uncertain because the effective dose of a CAC acquisition is similar to CCTA doses obtained with modern scanners using low peak kilovoltage (kVp) technique.[8]

Coronary computed tomography angiography
Prospective ECG triggering with scanning and reconstruction performed during late diastole is routinely used. It requires a well-controlled heart rate, generally less than 65 bpm for accurate evaluation of ACS,[23] and achieves almost 4-fold reduction in radiation doses (1–5 mSv) as compared with retrospective gating.[24,25] The high spatial and temporal resolution needed for CCTA requires a scanner with minimum of 64 detector rows and appropriate software. CCTA can achieve a spatial resolution of 0.3 to 0.4 mm. The overall temporal resolution of current cardiac MDCT varies from 100 to 200 ms, with dual source CT scanners (DSCT) reaching true temporal resolution of between 66 and 83 ms potentially obviating the need for beta blockers for slowing the heart rate.[10]

Technical advancements
Newer techniques such as adaptive delay; "padding," that is, minor lengthening of the X-ray tube on time to capture additional data on either side of the optimal cardiac phase; gated reconstruction algorithms; and softer spatial resolution kernels have greatly improved diagnostic quality of CCTA acquisitions.[10,25] Strategies such as X-ray beam filtration, beam collimation, automatic pitch adaptation, ECG-controlled tube current modulation, iterative reconstruction, low kVp imaging, high-pitch (3.2–3.4) acquisition with DSCT, and new detectors with low inherent noise can reduce radiation doses significantly (up to 80% at lower heart rates).[10,12,23–27] Diagnostic image quality has been reported with low kVp imaging using 70 to 100 kVp, instead of the usual 120kVp, improving the contrast-to-noise ratio and reducing iodine load to the patient.[25] Edge-enhancing image filters can separate high-density calcification from intraluminal iodinated contrast material, providing calcium-free angiograms and reducing overestimation of luminal stenosis due to blooming artifact.[28]

Improved patient outcomes have been reported when coronary revascularization is guided by a fractional flow reserve (FFR) compared with degree of anatomic stenosis.[29] FFR can be calculated from CT angiograms (**Figs. 2** and **3**) with high diagnostic accuracy to exclude hemodynamically significant CAD, thus improving clinical outcomes in patients with suspected ACS.[30,31]

DSCT can assess myocardial perfusion defects in ACS by reconstructing iodine color maps from dynamic first-pass myocardial perfusion, with results comparable to MR imaging/single-photon emission CT (SPECT).[32] Static myocardial perfusion imaging obtains a single image of myocardial attenuation during first-pass perfusion giving a snapshot of iodine distribution, whereas attenuation followed over several consecutive time points constitutes dynamic myocardial perfusion imaging. A cutoff value of 75 to 78 mL/100 mL/min has been reported for the detection of hemodynamically significant stenosis.[29]

Acute Aortic Syndrome

The sensitivity and specificity of ECG-gated CT for acute aortic abnormalities have been reported to be 100%. ECG gating and beta blockade improves assessment of the aortic root including the coronary artery origins and the valve apparatus, helps visualization of subtle aortic lesions such as limited intimal tears that might be missed without gating, and in those cases in which pulsation artifacts mimic aortic lesions or do not allow their exclusion. Faster scanners can reduce pulsation artifacts even without gating. For centers with a low prevalence of patients with AAS, a dedicated gated protocol should still be available following an inconclusive nongated study. Reconstructing time-resolved datasets can display dynamic changes in the position of a dissection flap, the size of a true or false lumen, and provide insight into the hemodynamic consequences of a given pathology.[6]

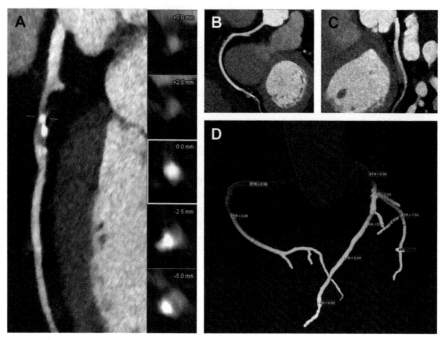

Fig. 2. A 59-year-old woman with a history of HTN with atypical chest pain, abnormal ECG, initial troponin negative (0.010 ng/mL). CAC: 36. CCTA (% R-R: 71): (*A*) MPR revealed 70% stenosis of mid-LAD due to calcified plaque. (*B*) Normal RCA. (*C*) Normal LCX. (*D*) FFR on CCTA by cFFR (Siemens Healthineers) shows normal FFR value. Cardiac catheterization identified eccentric 60% stenosis in the mid-LAD that was investigated with invasive FFR. The resting pressure gradient across the LAD stenosis was 0.97 and with adenosine 0.91. Medical management was deemed appropriate.

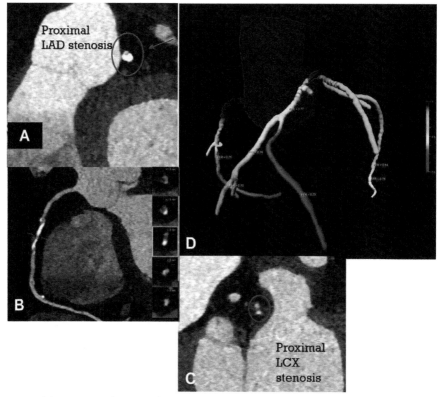

Fig. 3. A 51-year-old woman with acute chest pain and H/o HT and hypercholesterolemia. Nuclear stress test: negative for ischemia. CCTA: (*A*) 80% stenosis of the proximal to mid-LAD (*circle*); (*B*) 70% stenosis of the mid-RCA by calcified plaque; (*C*) 50% stenosis of the mid-LCX by noncalcified plaque (*circle*); (*D*) FFRCT showing ischemia in all LAD, LCX, as well as RCA. Catheter angiography confirmed CCTA results and CABG done.

Dual source computed tomography scanners for acute aortic syndrome

Simulated low keV monoenergetic datasets derived from dual-energy data significantly improve attenuation of aorta with improved contrast-to-noise ratio.[33] Material-specific imaging with DSCT yields virtual noncontrast images eliminating the need for precontrast acquisitions. This enables differentiation of amorphous calcifications from intramural hematoma or intimal calcifications in dissection. In traumatic rupture, virtual unenhanced differentiation of high attenuation hematoma from actively extravasating iodine is possible. Angiographic-like images of the aorta can be obtained by subtracting the virtual noncontrast images from the contrast-rich 80-kVp images.[32–34]

IMAGING PROTOCOLS

A dedicated workflow is needed in order to achieve high-quality CCTA and aortic studies.[6]

Acute Coronary Syndrome

Proper patient selection (**Table 1**) is necessary because CCTA may lead to higher cardiac catheterization and revascularization procedures

Table 1
Summary of imaging protocol for acute coronary syndrome

Appropriate indications	*Absolute contraindications*
• Clinically suspected ACS but ECG negative or indeterminate for myocardial ischemia	• Definite ACSs
	• GFR <30 unless on chronic dialysis, or evidence of ATN
• Early hsTrop negative, or equivocal initial troponin or single troponin elevation without additional evidence of ACS	• Previous anaphylaxis after iodinated contrast administration or contrast allergy after adequate steroid/antihistamine preparation
	• Pregnancy
• Low to intermediate pretest likelihood by risk stratification tools	*Relative contraindications*
	• Renal insufficiency
• Equivocal or inadequate previous functional testing during index ED or within previous 6 mo	• Multiple myeloma
	• Untreated hyperthyroidism
	• Cardiac rhythm disturbances

Scan protocol

On arrival:
• Secure IV line
• Secure ECG gating
• Breath-hold test to monitor heart rate
• Administer oral or IV metoprolol if HR is >60bpm, BP >90 mm Hg systolic
• Sublingual nitroglycerin (400–800 µg) when BP >100 mm Hg
FOV: midpulmonary artery to diaphragm
Non-contrast CT: prospective ECG-triggered, low-dose scan for coronary calcium assessment.
Contrast-enhanced CT:
   Tube current: automated current adjustment mode
   Tube potential: automated adjustment or 100 kVp if BMI <30 kg/m² and 120 kVp if BMI >30 kg/m²
   i. Prospective ECG-triggered axial scan if:
     • Regular heart rate <65 bpm during breath-hold after beta-blockade
     • No cardiac arrhythmias or premature beats before or during test breath-hold
     • <400 Agatston score (may depend on scanner technology used)
   ii. Retrospective ECG-gated helical scan if:
     • Heart rates higher than prospective-triggered target range
     • Significantly irregular rhythm.
   iii. High-pitch helical scan if:
     • HR<60 bpm and BMI <30 kg/m²
Image reconstruction with approximately 50% overlap:
• Typically two data sets, one in mid-diastole (65%–80%) and one in end systole (35%–45%) if retrospective technique was used
• 10% increments (10 phases) for single source CT scanners or 5% increments (20 phases) for dual-source CT scanners with a reduced pixel matrix of 256 × 256 for volume assessment

Abbreviations: ATN, acute tubular necrosis; BMI, body mass index; BP, blood pressure; FOV, field of view; GFR, glomerular filtration rate; HR, heart rate; hsTrop, high-sensitive troponin; IV, intravenous.
  Data from Refs.[6,8,12,21,23]

without concomitant improvement in the odds of experiencing an MI.[21,35,36]

Patient preparation

After securing ECG gating and intravenous access, a breath-hold test is performed to monitor the heart rate to decide on the need for beta-blockers and usage of prospective versus retrospective gating. Oral or intravenous doses of metoprolol can be administered for heart rate control. For patients with contraindications to beta-blockers, calcium channel blockers, preferably diltiazem, is an alternative.[8] Sublingual nitroglycerin (400–800 μg when blood pressure >100 mm Hg) is used to dilate the coronaries, improving contrast-to-noise ratio and vessel visualization.[6,12] Contraindications to nitroglycerin include recent phosphodiesterase inhibitor therapy (for erectile dysfunction or pulmonary hypertension), hypotension, and critical aortic stenosis.[8]

SCAN PROTOCOL
Acute Aortic Syndrome

The standard protocol for evaluating AAS should include a precontrast CT to recognize the presence of IMH and high-density blood in the vicinity, indicating aortic rupture.[6] Low-dose technique accompanied by thick collimation can reduce total radiation dose with the scan range of noncontrast CT restricted from the lung apex to upper abdomen. Contrast-enhanced CT is then preformed from the thoracic inlet to femoral head to exclude involvement of major aortic arch branches as well as the iliac arteries. In general, a body weight–adapted iodine concentration accounting for flow rate of 1.0 to 1.6 g per second is sufficient to opacify the entire aorta in most patients. A 64-slice MDCT allows scanning the entire aorta with submillimeter collimation within a single breath-hold, thus making high-resolution 3-dimensional reconstruction and other postprocessing displays possible.[37,38]

Combined triple-rule-out protocol

Triple-rule-out CT in the ED setting seems relevant for patients in whom clinical evaluation does not suggest a most likely cause of chest pain among ACS, AAS, and acute pulmonary embolism (Fig. 4). An optimized TRO protocol provides excellent image quality for aortic, coronary, and pulmonary arterial evaluation while minimizing contrast agent and radiation dose. Patients with high CAC score are not suitable for TRO-CT. Prospective ECG-gated scanning is performed in a single breath-hold, starting 1–2 cm above the aortic arch up to the base of the heart. The contrast bolus should be appropriate to provide uniform enhancement of the pulmonary and coronary arteries as well as the aorta, requiring some adjustment from a typical coronary CT protocol.[39]

IMAGING FINDINGS/PATHOLOGY
Acute Coronary Syndrome

European Society of Cardiology/ACCF/AHA/World Heart Federation Task Force for the Universal Definition of Myocardial Infarction defines STEMI, NSTEMI, and UA as follows: (1) STEMI: a new ST elevation at the J point in at least 2 contiguous leads of greater than or equal to 2 mm (0.2 mV) in men or greater than or equal to 1.5 mm (0.15 mV) in women in leads V2–V3 and/or of greater than or equal to 1 mm (0.1 mV) in other contiguous chest leads or the limb leads in the absence of LV hypertrophy or left bundle branch block[40]; (2) NSTEMI: a new finding of ST-

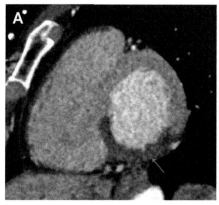 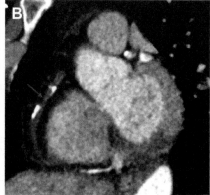

Fig. 4. A 58-year-old man presented to the ED for strokelike symptoms. Clinical suspicion was AAD. ECG showed STE and q waves in II, III, and avF, with depression in avL. Initial troponin negative. TRO-CT demonstrated transmural perfusion defect in RCA territory (A) with a total RCA occlusion (B) (arrows).

segment depression of greater than 1 mm or T-wave inversion of at least 3 mm in at least 2 anatomically contiguous leads and elevated serial levels of troponin I; (3) UA: clinical symptoms that suggest ACS, such as typical chest discomfort or the equivalent, with an unstable pattern of chest pain (at rest, new onset, or crescendo angina), optimally with a markedly positive stress test (SPECT, echo, or treadmill testing) and/or an invasive coronary angiogram demonstrating a greater than 50% epicardial coronary stenosis.[6,41] The underlying mechanism of ACS is partial or complete luminal thrombosis of an epicardial coronary artery, with or without vasospasm, due to coronary plaque enlargement, instability, and rupture or erosion.[42] Completely obstructive CAD occurs in STEMI causing MI; NSTEMI has partially obstructing lesions causing myocardial ischemia/cell death, therefore causing elevated troponins and; UA is a result of myocardial ischemia without cell death and normal troponins.

In the report, information is provided about the imaging sequences performed, contrast agent used, overall contrast/beta-blocker/nitrate administered, and the overall radiation dose.[23]

Coronary artery stenosis is reported as follows:

1. Rate overall image quality as interpretable/uninterpretable, specify nonevaluable segments/arteries and reason
2. Arterial distribution (right or left dominant, codominant)
3. Presence of coronary atherosclerotic plaque, its morphology and composition (none, calcified, noncalcified, both) according to American Heart Association (AHA) classification per vessel and optionally per 15-segment AHA model or 18-segment SCCT (Society of Cardiovascular Computed Tomography) model.

Coronary artery disease reporting and data system

The CAD reporting and data system (CAD-RADS) was devised to standardize reporting of CCTA on per patient level for the highest grade of coronary stenosis and to facilitate communication amongst clinicians. For patients presenting with acute chest pain, negative first troponin, negative or nondiagnostic ECG, and low to intermediate risk (TIMI risk score <4), CAD-RADS interpretation is as follows[43]:

1. CAD-RADS 0: (0% stenosis)—ACS highly unlikely. No further evaluation is required, need to consider other causes.
2. CAD-RADS 1: (1%–24% stenosis)—ACS highly unlikely. Consider evaluation of non-ACS cause, if normal troponin and no ECG changes (Fig. 5).

3. CAD-RADS 2: (25%–49% stenosis)—ACS unlikely. Consider evaluation of non-ACS cause, if normal troponin and no ECG changes. If clinical suspicion of ACS is high or if high-risk plaque features are noted, then consider hospital admission with cardiology consultation.
4. CAD-RADS 3: (50%–69% stenosis)—ACS possible. Consider hospital admission, cardiology consultation, functional testing, and/or invasive coronary angiography (ICA). Other treatments should be considered if presence of hemodynamically significant lesion.
5. CAD-RADS 4: (A: 70%–99% stenosis) or (B: left main >50% or 3-vessel obstructive (70%) disease)—ACS likely. Hospital admission, cardiology consultation, further evaluation with ICA, and revascularization to be done as deemed appropriate (Fig. 6).
6. CAD-RADS 5: (100% total occlusion)—ACS very likely. Expedited ICA is considered on a timely basis and revascularization if appropriate in case of acute occlusion.
7. CAD-RADS N: Nondiagnostic study, ACS cannot be excluded, needs additional or alternative evaluation.

Outpatient follow-up for preventive therapy and risk factor modification is recommended for CAD-RADS 1 and 2 categories. In addition to these, antiischemic therapy is recommended for CAD-RADS 3, 4, and 5 categories. CAD-RADS categories are complemented by modifiers to indicate the presence of stents (S), grafts (G), and vulnerable plaque (V).[43]

The absence of plaque and significant arterial stenosis on CTA excludes ACS (sensitivity 100%), whereas only half of the patients with obstructive CAD on CTA have ACSs.[6]

Culprit lesions

Plaques showing ruptured fibrous caps or voluminous necrotic cores covered by thin and inflamed fibrous caps are potential substrate for ACS and termed culprit lesions (see Fig. 2).[44] These lesions may subsequently rupture or induce expansive remodeling of the vascular segment and are responsible for most MIs without significant coronary luminal stenosis before the event.[45] On CCTA, morphologic characteristics of culprit lesions include positive remodeling, low-attenuation plaque (<30 HU) (Fig. 7), spotty calcification, the napkin-ring sign,[43] ulceration, intramural dye penetration, and overhanging edges. Positive remodeling is defined as increase in diameter of the vessel at the plaque site by at least 10% than the reference segment proximal to the lesion in a normal-appearing vessel segment (remodeling

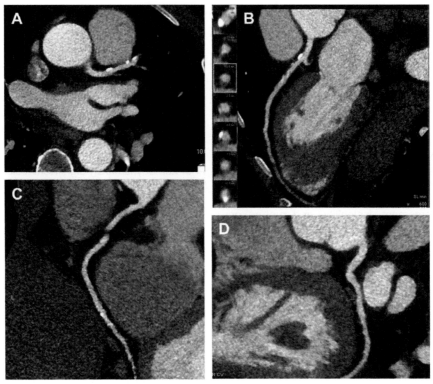

Fig. 5. A 58-year-old man with hypertension and hyperlipidemia presented to the ED with acute stabbing chest pain. HEART risk score: 3, low risk. ECG: nonspecific ST abnormality with ST elevation in lateral leads. Initial troponin negative. Prospective gated CCTA was performed at 70% phase (end diastole). Total CAC score is 168. (*A*) Axial view. (*B*) MPR of LMCA and LAD showing eccentric calcifications without significant stenosis. (*C*) MPR RCA: slab artifact in mid-RCA, otherwise normal. (*D*) MPR LCX: normal. CCTA ruled out ACS.

index >1.1). Spotty calcification is defined as 3 mm calcifications on curved multiplanar reformation images occupying only 1 side on cross-sectional images.[44] Napkin-ring sign is said to be present when a ring of high attenuation (not exceeding 130 HU) exists around a coronary artery plaque.[46] This can be attributed to intraplaque vasa vasorum enhancement, hemorrhage, or thrombus with peripheral enhancement or microcalcifications in the plaque.[46] When present together, culprit lesions are associated with high positive predictive value (95%) for ACS.

Left ventricle evaluation

LV is assessed qualitatively based on the AHA 17-segment model in a retrospective gated acquisition for[6]

1. Regional wall motion abnormality, graded as hypokinetic, akinetic, dyskinetic, or aneurysmal and to be present in at least 2 contiguous myocardial segments or in 1 segment visualized in 2 different views to be considered a true-positive finding.

2. Regional subendocardial or transmural hypoattenuation/enhancement of the myocardium in a coronary distribution, suspicious for ischemia or infarction (**Fig. 8**).

3. Location of regional dysfunction must match the stenosis location.

4. Global LV function is graded as normal, mildly, moderately, or severely impaired.

The presence of resting myocardial enhancement defects on CTA has a sensitivity and specificity of about 90% to identify patients with MI.[6,47,48]

Noncardiac findings

Assessment should include aortic dissection, pulmonary embolism, pulmonary nodules, pneumonia, pneumothorax, pericardial effusion, hiatal hernia, and rib fractures.

Acute Aortic Syndrome

Classic dissection

AAD shows a double-barrel lumen, consisting of a true lumen and a false lumen separated by a

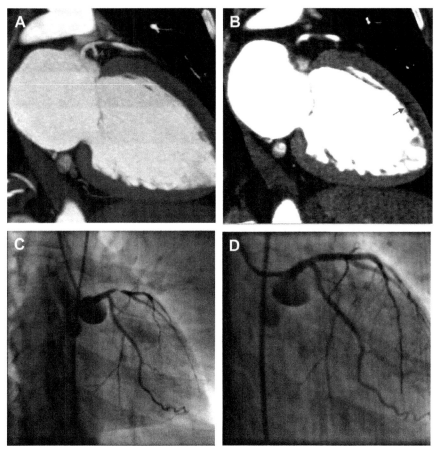

Fig. 6. A 50-year-old man with chest pain, first troponin negative. CCTA (*A*) demonstrates severe stenosis of proximal LAD with subendocardial perfusion defect (*arrows*). (*B*) Cardiac catheterization (*C*) confirmed CCTA findings, with subsequent PTCA to LAD (*D*).

dissection or intimal flap, with a primary intimal tear usually clearly visualized.[38,49] The fundamental pathophysiology of AAD is noninflammatory loss of vascular smooth muscle cells and elastolysis of the medial layer of the aortic wall components.[49,50] The most common comorbid condition is severe arterial hypertension.[49] Other predisposing factors are aortic disease (eg, bicuspid aortic valve, aortic coarctation, aneurysm), connective tissue diseases (eg, Marfan and Ehler–Danlos syndrome), trauma, cocaine abuse, and pregnancy.[37] Loss of transmural pressure and elastic recoil across the dissection flap causes loss of response of the true lumen to absolute aortic pressures leading to its collapse, whereas expansion of the false lumen is due to reduced elastic recoil on its elastin-poor thin outer wall. The dissection may remain patent as a false lumen thrombosis;

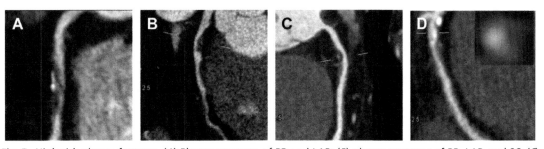

Fig. 7. High-risk plaque features. (*A*) Plaque presence of PR and LAP; (*B*) plaque presence of PR, LAP, and SC; (*C*) plaque presence of SC; (*D*) napkin-ring sign plaque.

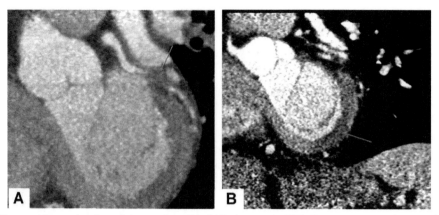

Fig. 8. A 65-year-old man developed chest pain at World Series game. CCTA shows a near total LCX occlusion with a perfusion defect in LV basal lateral wall (*arrows*).

recommunicate with the true lumen through fenestrations; or rupture into the pericardial, pleural, or peritoneal cavities.[38]

The DeBakey classification system categorizes AAD on the basis of the origin of the intimal tear and the extent of the dissection: Type I: originates in the ascending aorta and propagates distally to include at least the aortic arch and typically the descending aorta; Type II: originates in and is confined to the ascending aorta; Type III: originates in the descending aorta and propagates most often distally; Type IIIa: limited to the descending thoracic aorta; and Type IIIb: extending below the diaphragm. The Stanford classification system divides AAD into 2 categories, those that involve the ascending aorta and those that do not—Type A (**Fig. 9**): all dissections involving the ascending aorta regardless of the site of origin and Type B (**Fig. 10**): all dissections that do not involve the ascending aorta.[16]

The intimomedial flap in type A dissection is right anterolateral in the ascending aorta, posterosuperior along the convexity in the arch, left posterolateral to the true lumen in descending thoracic aorta, and anteriorly or posteriorly in the aorta below the diaphragm.[38] Although smaller lumen size and dense contrast opacification are characteristic of the true lumen, there are several other important signs that can help to differentiate the true from false lumina. False lumens are larger, less opacified with contrast, and may show a "beak sign" (**Fig. 11A**) manifested as an acute angle between the intimomedial flap and outer false lumen on axial CT images.[37,51] The cobweb sign is typical of the false lumen and corresponds to strands from incompletely torn connective tissue of the aortic media.[37,51] The intimomedial rupture sign refers to the discontinuous ends of the intimomedial flap at the site of entry tear that

point toward false lumen and indicates the direction of blood flow through entry tear from true to false lumen.[37] Intimal calcification occurs along the wall of the true lumen or true lumen side of the intimomedial flap[37] (see **Fig. 11A**). Intimointimal intussusception in case of a circumferential flap seems as a "windsock" (**Fig. 12**).[38] The "Mercedes-Benz sign" refers to appearance of the flap in rare cases of secondary dissection in one of the channels forming 3 channels in total.[38] Intraluminal thrombus is more frequently encountered in the false lumen,[37] when the primary intimal tear is more distal (eg, in the descending aorta).[49] In CT, stagnating blood in the false lumen is isodense, whereas clotted blood is hyperdense relative to flowing blood within the true lumen in noncontrast CT.[49]

The size of the false lumen diameter is a predictor for aortic rupture.[37] Details about origins of branch vessels relative to true versus false lumen and also side branch involvement is helpful before percutaneous repair (**Fig. 11B**).[37] Extension of a dissection into the aortic root suggests possible dysfunction of the aortic valve.[16] Presence of a pericardial effusion suggests possible proximal extension of type A dissection and the danger of imminent rupture. Rupture can be identified as irregularity of the aortic wall with extravasation of contrast material.[38] The frequent involvement of left-sided branches in AAD leads to higher risk of ischemia of the left kidney.[16]

MDCT can recognize the nature of obstruction/perfusion depending on different configurations of the flap involving a branch visceral artery including (1) perfusion through the false lumen, (2) uncertain perfusion with proximal/upstream dynamic obstruction of true lumen, (3) dynamic obstruction of flow with the flap prolapsing into the ostium of the branch, (4) fixed obstruction

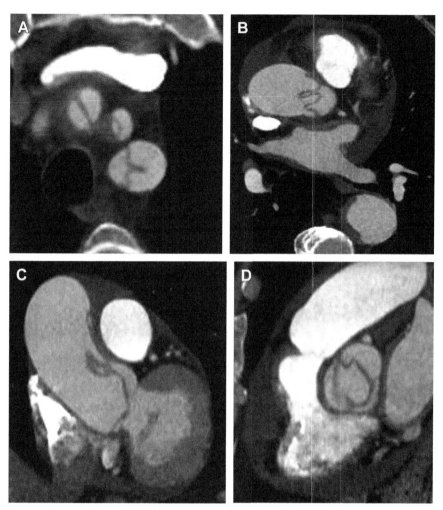

Fig. 9. An 83-year-old man who presented to the ED with transient memory loss, back pain, and numbness from waist to bilateral toes. CTA: Type A dissection extending into arch vessels (*A*) and aortic root (*B–D*) causing aortic regurgitation.

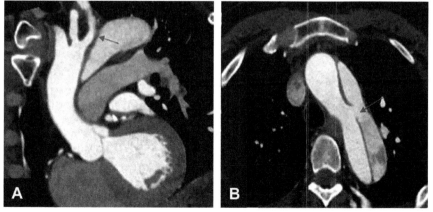

Fig. 10. A 57-year-old man, active cocaine and heroin user, who presented to the ED with substernal nonradiating chest pain and left lower extremity pain. His ECG showed ST elevations in V3, V4, with TWI in precordial leads. Gated CTA showing Type B dissection with entry tear in the midaortic arch distal to left subclavian artery at the isthmus (*arrow in A*), with the intimal flap showing fenestration (*arrow in B*). TWI, T-wave inversion.

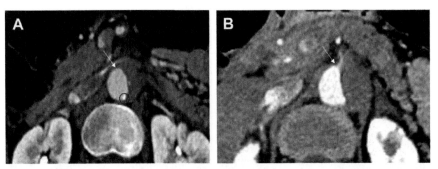

Fig. 11. Gated CTA. (A) Beak sign (arrow) and displaced intimal calcifications (circle) in Type B dissection. (B) Critical stenosis of celiac artery by the intimal flap.

when the intimal dissection stops at a bifurcation, and (5) mixed obstruction.[16]

In complicated Stanford type B dissection, assessment is made for presence of a sufficient landing zone without excessive aortic tortuosity (ie, proximal neck of more than 5 mm distal to left subclavian artery) and adequate vascular access (ie, iliac arterial diameter larger than 8 mm) for endovascular stent-graft repair, which is an emerging therapeutic option.[37] Diameter expansion more than 1 cm per year or a diameter of 5.5 cm or more with refractory pain and malperfusion is an

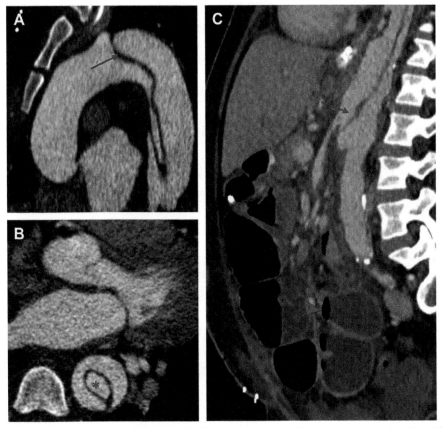

Fig. 12. A 50-year-old woman with poorly controlled HTN and multiple TIAs, who presented to ED with 2 days of intractable nausea, vomiting, and abdominal pain. She was hypertensive with systolic blood pressure as high as 260 mm Hg. She underwent exploratory laparotomy and was found to have extensive ischemic bowel, which was managed surgically. Gated CTA. (A) Type B dissection distal to origin of left subclavian artery (arrow). (B) Circumferential dissection flap (asterisk). (C) The dissection flap extends into the superior mesenteric artery (arrow) with compression of the true lumen proximally. Dilated bowel loops are noted (arrowhead). Patient subsequently underwent TEVAR. HTN, hypertension; TIA, transient ischemic attack.

indication for surgical intervention or TEVAR in chronic type B dissections.[50,52]

Intramural hematoma

IMH arising due to hemorrhage of the vasa vaso-rum of the aorta is now regarded a non-specific imaging finding in a spectrum of unrelated aortic conditions such as PAU, iatrogenic ADs, traumatic injuries and rupturing aneurysms (**Fig. 13**).[49] There is an increasingly reported overlap between classic aortic dissection (AD) and IMH and many consider that the hematoma results from micro-scopic tears in the aortic intima. Thus, complete thrombosis of the false lumen resulting in the im-aging features of IMH is the extreme within this spectrum.[49] Focal IMH has also been reported in association with PAU.[49] The term "dissection variant IMH" is used for a thrombosed AD that has no complete flow channel but tiny communi-cations between the true and false lumen commonly exist and clearly show differentiation from other aortic diseases with hemorrhagic con-tent within the aortic wall.[49]

Nonenhanced CT identifies intramural hema-toma as a hyperdense, crescent-shaped lesion within the aortic wall, originally defined to have no demonstrable intimal flap or radiologically apparent intimal tear; however, small communica-tions between the true and false lumen can be detected. On initial imaging, small "ulcerlike pro-jections"—defined as a localized blood-filled pouch protruding from the true lumen into the thrombosed false lumen of the aorta—can be observed, considered to represent the site of an intimal disruption and is therefore a possible indi-cator of the formation of a flow channel between the true and thrombosed false lumen, which later evolves into classic AD. Thickness of IMH greater than 11 mm is associated with progression of IMH to frank aortic dissection.[37]

Penetrating atherosclerotic ulcer

PAU is a deep ulcerated plaque that penetrates from the pathologically thickened intima through the in-ternal elastic lamina into the medial layer of the aorta (**Fig. 14**). PAU is a sign of advanced atherosclerosis and therefore a manifestation of a diseased intima (and not the media). The lesion may penetrate even beyond the media and extend through to the adventitia, producing a periaortic pseudoaneurysm and even transmural aortic rupture.[49]

On imaging, PAUs commonly show a "crater-like ulceration" of the thickened aortic wall, which is different from the linear or crescent shape of primary intimal tear in dissection variant IMH.[16] These patients invariably demonstrate extensive atheroma and calcification throughout the aorta, often with an irregular surface and more than one ulcerlike lesion.[49,51] It is important to distin-guish between nonpenetrating atheromatous ul-cers (ie, ulcerated plaque confined to the calcified thickened intima), chronic healed pene-trating ulcers (which are reendothelialized and not an acute threat), and those lesions that acutely penetrate the aortic wall with a high risk of complications such as perforation and rupture.[16,37]

The key distinguishing features of acute lesions are intramural blood and periaortic stranding, which can help identify a culprit lesion. In the setting of acute aortic pain, a CT scan without IMH or peri-aortic stranding near an identifiable ulcerlike lesion does not exclude an acute aortic condition, hence follow-up imaging is recommended.[16]

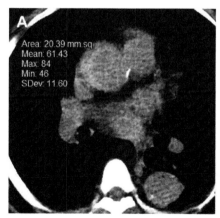 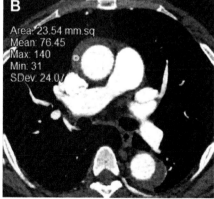

Fig. 13. A 66-year-old woman with H/o CKD, systemic hypertension, hyperlipidemia presented to the ED with chest, back, and upper abdominal discomfort. CTA ([A] non-contrast and [B] contrast-enhanced study) showing acute aortic intramural hematoma extending from the root to descending thoracic aorta. CKD, chronic kidney disease.

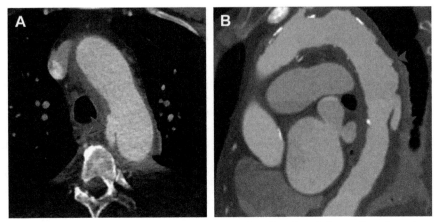

Fig. 14. Gated CTA showing multiple PAU in the arch (*arrowhead in A*) and descending thoracic aorta (*arrowheads in B*).

Unstable aneurysms

Pathologically, an aneurysm is characterized by dilation of the aorta due to loss of elastin and smooth muscle cells in all layers of the aortic wall and involves the entire circumference.[49] The risk of rupture is significantly higher for aneurysms greater than 5.5 cm in diameter. Rapid increase in the size of the thoracic aortic aneurysm (ie, aortic diameter increase more than 1 cm per year) also strongly correlates with aortic rupture.[37] On imaging, unstable aneurysms can show high-attenuating crescent ("crescent sign") in the wall, discontinuous calcification in a circumferentially calcified aorta, aorta conforming to the neighboring vertebral body ("draped" aorta), an eccentric nipple shape to the aorta, periaortic stranding, periaortic or mediastinal hematoma, hemorrhagic pleural fluid, or frank rupture with blood beyond the confines of the aortic wall.[7,16]

Limited dissection of the aorta (limited intimal tear)

With similar predisposing factors as cystic medial necrosis,[6] limited intimal tear is a complex primary intimal tear extending from the intima into part or all of the media but without development of a separate flow channel in the media with an "eccentric one-sided bulge" on imaging (**Fig. 15**).[49]

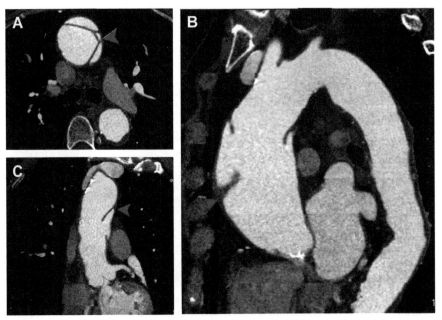

Fig. 15. Gated CTA showing AAD variant: limited intimal tear: (*A*) axial, (*B*) sagittal, and (C) coronal reformations showing dilated ascending aorta with multiple intimal flaps (*arrowheads*) but no false lumen.

DIAGNOSTIC CRITERIA
Acute Coronary Syndrome

In the ED, diagnostic tools for assessing and managing patients who may have ACS are clinical history, ECG results, levels of cardiac markers, and the results of stress testing (**Box 1**).[53]

The third universal definition includes identification of an intracoronary thrombus by angiography or imaging evidence of new loss of viable myocardium or a new regional wall motion abnormality as independent criteria for the diagnosis of MI.[53] On imaging, a normal CCTA effectively rules out ACS in patients with a low to intermediate probability of CAD. In high-risk patients, total occlusion of a coronary vessel on CCTA makes ACS very likely. ACS is likely to be present in those having 70% to 99% stenosis or left main greater than 50% or 3-vessel obstructive (70%) disease. Culprit lesions, identified on CCTA, are prognostic indicators linked to increased risk of MI.[43]

For the evaluation of potential UA/NSTEMI, high CAC is a good predictor of future coronary events.[19]

Acute Aortic Syndrome

Reports of newer-generation multidetector helical CT scanners show sensitivities of up to 100% and specificities of 98% to 99% for detection of AAS. The diagnostic algorithm proposed in Thoracic Artery Disease National Guidelines is highly sensitive (95.7%) for the detection of acute AD at initial presentation. The aortic dissection detection risk score (ADD-RS) is a tool allowing standardized assessment of the pretest probability of AAS. ADD-RS of 0 to 3 is calculated on the basis of the number of risk categories (high-risk predisposing conditions, high-risk pain features, high-risk examination features) identified in a patient.[54] Integration of ADD-RS with D-dimer may be considered to standardize diagnostic rule-out of AAS (**Table 2**).[55]

DIFFERENTIAL DIAGNOSIS
Acute Coronary Syndrome/Acute Aortic Syndrome

- Pulmonary embolism has clinical features similar to ACS, including chest pain, ECG changes, and elevated cardiac biomarkers. On CT pulmonary angiography, acute emboli are seen as intravascular filling defects with or without corresponding pulmonary parenchymal changes of infarction (**Table 3**).[56]
- Cardiac tamponade with classic signs of sinus tachycardia, elevated jugular venous pressure, and pulsus paradoxus can be confused with ACS. On imaging, pericardial effusion, enlargement of the superior vena cava/inferior vena cava (IVC) with contrast reflux within the IVC/hepatic veins/azygous vein and flattened right ventricle is seen.
- Conditions that can mimic a dissection flap are mural thrombus in a fusiform aneurysm; pericardial recess; periaortic fibrosis or mediastinal, pulmonary, or retroperitoneal tumors; anemia with apparent high attenuation of the aortic wall; and vascular structures around the aorta.[38,57]

PEARLS, PITFALLS, AND VARIANTS
Pearls

- A zero CAC score has an excellent NPV to rule out ACS in most patients presenting to the ED with low to intermediate pretest probability of ACS and can be safely discharged.[20,58]
- Plaque characterization for presence of culprit lesions (positive remodeling, LAP, spotty calcification, and napkin-ring sign) with assessment of degree of luminal stenosis confers high diagnostic accuracy of CCTA in patients with low to intermediate risk for ACS presenting in the ED.[59]
- CTA-derived FFR can exclude hemodynamically significant CAD with high diagnostic accuracy and improve clinical outcomes in patients with suspected ACS.[30]
- The presence of a true and a false lumen separated by a dissection flap with a primary intimal tear on CTA is diagnostic of AAD.[38,49]

Box 1
Diagnostic criteria for acute coronary syndrome

Definite ACS

If ST segment elevation present

No ST segment elevation, but ST and T segment changes present with ongoing chest pain, positive cardiac biomarkers, and hemodynamic abnormalities

No ST segment elevation, nondiagnostic findings on ECG, normal initial serum cardiac biomarkers, but recurrent pain and positive findings on follow-up for greater than 12 hours from symptom onset

No ST segment elevation, nondiagnostic findings on ECG, normal initial serum cardiac biomarkers, no recurrent pain, and negative findings on follow-up for greater than 12 hours from symptom onset, but stress study to provoke ischemia is positive (consider evaluation of LV function if ischemia is present).

From Thygesen K, Alpert JS, Jaffe AS, et al. Third universal definition of myocardial infarction. Circulation 2012;126(16):2022; with permission.

Table 2
Diagnostic criteria for acute aortic syndrome

High-risk clinical features

Predisposing conditions (Category 1)	Symptoms (Category 2)	Signs (Category 3)

1. Marfan syndrome
2. Family H/o aortic disease
3. Known aortic valve disease
4. Recent aortic manipulation
5. Known thoracic aortic aneurysm
	Chest, back, or abdominal pain described as
	• Abrupt in onset
	• Severe in intensity
	• Ripping or tearing
		1. Evidence of perfusion deficit
		  • Pulse deficit
		  • Systolic BP differential
		  • Focal neurologic deficit
		2. Murmur of aortic insufficiency
		3. Hypotension or shock state

Risk-based diagnostic evaluation

ADD risk score 0 (no high-risk feature present)	ADD risk score 1 (any single high-risk category present)	ADD risk score 2–3 (2 or 3 high-risk categories present)
Expedited aortic imaging (CT/MR imaging or TEE if clinically unstable) If: • No alternative diagnosis identified • Unexplained hypotension Or • Widened mediastinum on chest radiograph • D-dimer >500 ng/ml	Expedited Aortic imaging (CT/MR imaging or TEE if clinically unstable) If: No strong suggestion of alternate diagnosis: • On history or physical examination • Or chest radiograph Or ECG inconsistent with STEMI	Immediate surgical consultation and expedited aortic imaging is diagnostic

Abbreviaiton: TEE, transesophageal echocardiogram.
Data from Thygesen K, Alpert JS, Jaffe AS, et al. Third universal definition of myocardial infarction. Circulation. 2012;126(16):2020–2035.

Table 3
Differential diagnosis for acute coronary syndrome and acute aortic syndrome

ACS	AAS
1. Pulmonary embolism	1. ACS
2. Aortic dissection or leaking aneurysm	2. Pulmonary embolism
3. Pericarditis or myocarditis	3. Mural thrombus in a fusiform aneurysm
4. Cardiac tamponade	4. Periaortic fibrosis
5. Aortic stenosis and/or regurgitation	5. Mediastinal, pulmonary, or retroperitoneal tumors
6. Pancreatitis, cholecystitis, esophagitis/peptic ulcer disease	6. Anemia with apparent high attenuation of the aortic wall
7. Costochondritis, rib fractures	7. Pericardial recess
8. Anxiety, asthma	8. Vascular structures around the aorta such as the aortic sinus, left brachiocephalic vein, and left superior intercostal vein

Data from Rogers AM, Hermann LK, Booher AM, et al. Sensitivity of the aortic dissection detection risk score, a novel guideline-based tool for identification of acute aortic dissection at initial presentation: results from the international registry of acute aortic dissection. Circulation. 2011;123(20):2213–2218 and Nazerian P, Mueller C, Soeiro AM, et al. Diagnostic Accuracy of the Aortic Dissection Detection Risk Score Plus D-Dimer for Acute Aortic Syndromes: The ADvISED Prospective Multicenter Study. Circulation. 2018;137(3):250–258.

- Presence of a hyperdense, crescent-shaped lesion within the aortic wall without an intimal flap is diagnostic of IMH, and a craterlike ulceration of the thickened aortic wall with extensive calcifications throughout the aorta accurately identifies PAU.[16,49,51]

Pitfalls

- Blooming artifacts due to calcifications leading to overestimation of luminal stenosis.[10]
- Motion artifacts resulting in errors in diagnosis at heart rates above 70 bpm in ACS as well as AAS.[60]
- Thrombosed false lumen can be mistaken for an aortic aneurysm with mural thrombus.[44]

- Neointimal calcifications can mimic displaced intimal calcifications on unenhanced CT leading to erroneous diagnosis of AAD.

Variants

- Cystic medial necrosis with an abnormal aortic medial layer is a common pathologic variant occurring from severe hypertension, normal aging, familial aortic diseases, vasculitis, and connective tissue diseases.[6]
- IMH is considered as a variant or a precursor of AD and many have regarded IMH as synonymous with a "thrombosed type" or "noncommunicating" AD.[49]

WHAT THE REFERRING PHYSICIANS NEED TO KNOW
For Acute Coronary Syndrome

- Calcium score for risk stratification[61]
- CAD-RADS category
- Presence of culprit lesions
- Findings of LV dysfunction

For Acute Aortic Dissection

- Stanford type A versus type B with site of origin of intimal flap
- Extension of intimal flap to aortic valve or coronary ostia, aortic branch vessels.
- Evidence of organ ischemia
- Any direct or indirect signs of rupture

For Intramural Hematoma

- Site and extent of involvement
- An opinion concerning cause of IMH (ie, trauma, PAU)
- Signs of rupture or aneurysmal dilation of aorta

For Penetrating Atherosclerotic Ulcer

- Location especially if multiple ulcers are present
- Presence and extent of associated IMH
- Description of any saccular aneurysm or pseudoaneurysm
- Signs of rupture/leaking
- Information to aid potential endovascular therapy

SUMMARY

Advances in CTA, with rapid utilization in the ED, are playing a major role in deciding management of patients with ACS and AAS. Optimization of the CTA technique and up-to-date knowledge of the imaging capabilities can further improve the diagnostic accuracy of CTA in vast majority of patients presenting to the ED with the diagnosis of ACS or AAS.

REFERENCES

1. CDC. National hospital ambulatory medical care survey: emergency department summary tables. Bethesda (MD): National Center for Health Statistics by Centers for Disease Control and Prevention; 2014.
2. Hsc J, White C. Acute coronary syndrome. In: Ho V, Reddy G, editors. Cardiovascular imaging, vol. 1. Philadelphia: Saunders/Elsevier; 2011. p. 715–25.
3. Corvera JS. Acute aortic syndrome. Ann Cardiothorac Surg 2016;5(3):188–93.
4. Apostolakis E, Papakonstantinou NA, Baikoussis NG, et al. Imaging of acute aortic syndrome: advantages, disadvantages and pitfalls. Hellenic J Cardiol 2015; 56:169–80.
5. Lansman SL, Saunders PC, Malekan R, et al. Acute aortic syndrome. J Thorac Cardiovasc Surg 2010; 140(6 Suppl):S92–7.
6. Fleischmann D, Hoffmann U. CT evaluation of chest pain: acute coronary syndrome and acute aortic syndrome. In: Hodler J, Kubik-Huch RA, von Schulthess GK, et al, editors. Diseases of the chest and heart, vols. 2015–2018. Milano (Italy): Springer; 2015. p. 119–28.
7. Smith AD, Schoenhagen P. CT imaging for acute aortic syndrome. Cleve Clin J Med 2008;75(1):7–9, 12, 15–17 passim.
8. Lee NJ, Litt H. Cardiac CT angiography for evaluation of acute chest pain. Int J Cardiovasc Imaging 2016;32(1):101–12.
9. Korley FK, Gatsonis C, Snyder BS, et al. Clinical risk factors alone are inadequate for predicting significant coronary artery disease. J Cardiovasc Comput Tomogr 2017;11(4):309–16.
10. Hassan A, Nazir SA, Alkadhi H. Technical challenges of coronary CT angiography: today and tomorrow. Eur J Radiol 2011;79(2):161–71.
11. Hamilton-Craig C, Fifoot A, Hansen M, et al. Diagnostic performance and cost of CT angiography versus stress ECG–a randomized prospective study of suspected acute coronary syndrome chest pain in the emergency department (CT-COMPARE). Int J Cardiol 2014;177(3):867–73.
12. Raff GL, Chinnaiyan KM, Cury RC, et al. SCCT guidelines on the use of coronary computed tomographic angiography for patients presenting with acute chest pain to the emergency department: a report of the Society of Cardiovascular Computed Tomography Guidelines Committee. J Cardiovasc Comput Tomogr 2014;8(4):254–71.
13. Litt HI, Gatsonis C, Snyder B, et al. CT angiography for safe discharge of patients with possible acute coronary syndromes. N Engl J Med 2012;366(15): 1393–403.
14. Bamberg F, Mayrhofer T, Ferencik M, et al. Age- and sex-based resource utilisation and costs in patients with acute chest pain undergoing cardiac CT angiography: pooled evidence from ROMICAT II and ACRIN-PA trials. Eur Radiol 2018;28(2):851–60.
15. Chang AM, Litt HI, Snyder BS, et al. Impact of coronary computed tomography angiography findings on initiation of cardioprotective medications. Circulation 2017;136(22):2195–7.
16. Baliga RR, Nienaber CA, Bossone E, et al. The role of imaging in aortic dissection and related syndromes. JACC Cardiovasc Imaging 2014;7(4): 406–24.
17. Stojanovska J, Patel S. Coronary anatomy. In: Ho V, Reddy G, editors. Cardiovascular imaging, vol. I. Philadelphia: Saunders/Elsevier; 2011. p. 38–55.
18. Altin C, Kanyilmaz S, Koc S, et al. Coronary anatomy, anatomic variations and anomalies: a retrospective coronary angiography study. Singapore Med J 2015;56(6):339–45.
19. Bittner DO, Mayrhofer T, Bamberg F, et al. Impact of coronary calcification on clinical management in patients with acute chest pain. Circ Cardiovasc Imaging 2017;10(5) [pii:e005893].
20. Hinzpeter R, Higashigaito K, Morsbach F, et al. Coronary artery calcium scoring for ruling-out acute coronary syndrome in chest pain CT. Am J Emerg Med 2017;35(10):1565–7.
21. Rybicki FJ, Udelson JE, Peacock WF, et al. 2015 ACR/ACC/AHA/AATS/ACEP/ASNC/NASCI/SAEM/SCCT/SCMR/SCPC/SNMMI/STR/STS appropriate utilization of cardiovascular imaging in emergency department patients with chest pain: a joint document of the American College of Radiology Appropriateness Criteria Committee and the American College of Cardiology Appropriate Use Criteria Task Force. J Am Coll Cardiol 2016;67(7):853–79.
22. Schenker MP, Dorbala S, Hong EC, et al. Interrelation of coronary calcification, myocardial ischemia, and outcomes in patients with intermediate likelihood of coronary artery disease: a combined positron emission tomography/computed tomography study. Circulation 2008;117(13):1693–700.
23. Hausleiter J, Meyer T, Hermann F, et al. Estimated radiation dose associated with cardiac CT angiography. JAMA 2009;301(5):500–7.
24. den Harder AM, Willemink MJ, de Jong PA, et al. New horizons in cardiac CT. Clin Radiol 2016;71(8):758–67.
25. Roobottom CA, Mitchell G, Morgan-Hughes G. Radiation-reduction strategies in cardiac computed tomographic angiography. Clin Radiol 2010;65(11): 859–67.
26. Leschka S, Stolzmann P, Schmid FT, et al. Low kilovoltage cardiac dual-source CT: attenuation, noise, and radiation dose. Eur Radiol 2008;18(9):1809–17.

27. Hedgire SS, Baliyan V, Ghoshhajra BB, et al. Recent advances in cardiac computed tomography dose reduction strategies: a review of scientific evidence and technical developments. J Med Imaging (Bellingham) 2017;4(3):031211.

28. Raupach R, Bruder H, Krauss B, et al. Reduction of the blooming effect for calcified plaques in ct angiographic examinations by means of dual-energy CT. Radiological Society of North America 2006 Scientific Assembly and Annual Meeting, November 26 - December 1, 2006 ,Chicago IL. 2017. Available at: http://archive.rsna.org/2006/4433566.html. Accessed September 1, 2018.

29. De Cecco CN, Varga-Szemes A, Meinel FG, et al. Beyond stenosis detection: computed tomography approaches for determining the functional relevance of coronary artery disease. Radiol Clin North Am 2015;53(2):317–34.

30. Leipsic J, Yang TH, Thompson A, et al. CT angiography (CTA) and diagnostic performance of noninvasive fractional flow reserve: results from the Determination of Fractional Flow Reserve by Anatomic CTA (DeFACTO) study. AJR Am J Roentgenol 2014;202(5):989–94.

31. Renker M, Schoepf UJ, Wang R, et al. Comparison of diagnostic value of a novel noninvasive coronary computed tomography angiography method versus standard coronary angiography for assessing fractional flow reserve. Am J Cardiol 2014;114(9):1303–8.

32. Aran S, Daftari Besheli L, Karcaaltincaba M, et al. Applications of dual-energy CT in emergency radiology. AJR Am J Roentgenol 2014;202(4):W314–24.

33. Vlahos I, Chung R, Nair A, et al. Dual-energy CT: vascular applications. AJR Am J Roentgenol 2012;199(5 Suppl):S87–97.

34. Vlahos I, Godoy MC, Naidich DP. Dual-energy computed tomography imaging of the aorta. J Thorac Imaging 2010;25(4):289–300.

35. Lee NJ, Litt H. Cardiac CT in the emergency department: contrasting evidence from registries and randomized controlled trials. Curr Cardiol Rep 2018;20(4):24.

36. Woodard PK, McWilliams SR, Raptis DA, et al. R-SCAN: cardiac CT angiography for acute chest pain. J Am Coll Radiol 2017;14(9):1212–4.

37. Yoo SM, Lee HY, White CS. MDCT evaluation of acute aortic syndrome. Radiol Clin North Am 2010;48(1):67–83.

38. McMahon MA, Squirrell CA. Multidetector CT of aortic dissection: a pictorial review. Radiographics 2010;30(2):445–60.

39. Halpern EJ. Triple-rule-out CT angiography for evaluation of acute chest pain and possible acute coronary syndrome. Radiology 2009;252(2):332–45.

40. O'Gara PT, Kushner FG, Ascheim DD, et al. 2013 ACCF/AHA guideline for the management of ST-elevation myocardial infarction: a report of the American College of Cardiology Foundation/American Heart Association Task Force on Practice Guidelines. Circulation 2013;127(4):e362–425.

41. Amsterdam EA, Wenger NK, Brindis RG, et al. 2014 AHA/ACC guideline for the management of patients with non-ST-elevation acute coronary syndromes: a report of the American College of Cardiology/American Heart Association Task Force on Practice Guidelines. Circulation 2014;130(25):e344–426.

42. Stone GW, Maehara A, Lansky AJ, et al. A prospective natural-history study of coronary atherosclerosis. N Engl J Med 2011;364(3):226–35.

43. Cury RC, Abbara S, Achenbach S, et al. CAD-RADS(TM) coronary artery disease - reporting and data system. An expert consensus document of the Society of Cardiovascular Computed Tomography (SCCT), the American College of Radiology (ACR) and the North American Society for Cardiovascular Imaging (NASCI). Endorsed by the American College of Cardiology. J Cardiovasc Comput Tomogr 2016;10(4):269–81.

44. Motoyama S, Sarai M, Harigaya H, et al. Computed tomographic angiography characteristics of atherosclerotic plaques subsequently resulting in acute coronary syndrome. J Am Coll Cardiol 2009;54(1):49–57.

45. Pflederer T, Marwan M, Schepis T, et al. Characterization of culprit lesions in acute coronary syndromes using coronary dual-source CT angiography. Atherosclerosis 2010;211(2):437–44.

46. Otsuka K, Fukuda S, Tanaka A, et al. Napkin-ring sign on coronary CT angiography for the prediction of acute coronary syndrome. JACC Cardiovasc Imaging 2013;6(4):448–57.

47. Nagao M, Matsuoka H, Kawakami H, et al. Myocardial ischemia in acute coronary syndrome: assessment using 64-MDCT. AJR Am J Roentgenol 2009;193(4):1097–106.

48. Nagao M, Matsuoka H, Kawakami H, et al. Quantification of myocardial perfusion by contrast-enhanced 64-MDCT: characterization of ischemic myocardium. AJR Am J Roentgenol 2008;191(1):19–25.

49. Ueda T, Chin A, Petrovitch I, et al. A pictorial review of acute aortic syndrome: discriminating and overlapping features as revealed by ECG-gated multidetector-row CT angiography. Insights Imaging 2012;3(6):561–71.

50. Nienaber CA, Clough RE. Management of acute aortic dissection. Lancet 2015;385(9970):800–11.

51. Maddu KK, Shuaib W, Telleria J, et al. Nontraumatic acute aortic emergencies: part 1, acute aortic syndrome. AJR Am J Roentgenol 2014;202(3):656–65.

52. Maddu KK, Telleria J, Shuaib W, et al. Nontraumatic acute aortic emergencies: part 2, pre- and postsurgical complications related to aortic aneurysm in the

emergency clinical setting. AJR Am J Roentgenol 2014;202(3):666–74.

53. Thygesen K, Alpert JS, Jaffe AS, et al. Third universal definition of myocardial infarction. Circulation 2012;126(16):2020–35.

54. Rogers AM, Hermann LK, Booher AM, et al. Sensitivity of the aortic dissection detection risk score, a novel guideline-based tool for identification of acute aortic dissection at initial presentation: results from the international registry of acute aortic dissection. Circulation 2011;123(20):2213–8.

55. Nazerian P, Mueller C, Soeiro AM, et al. Diagnostic accuracy of the aortic dissection detection risk score plus D-dimer for acute aortic syndromes: the ADvISED prospective multicenter study. Circulation 2018;137(3):250–8.

56. Husainy MA, Gopalan D, Pakkal M, et al. Mimics of acute coronary syndrome on MDCT. Emerg Radiol 2013;20(3):235–42.

57. Terpenning S, White CS. Imaging pitfalls, normal anatomy, and anatomical variants that can simulate disease on cardiac imaging as demonstrated on multidetector computed tomography. Acta Radiol Short Rep 2015;4(1). 2047981614562443.

58. De Filippo M, Capasso R. Coronary computed tomography angiography (CCTA) and cardiac magnetic resonance (CMR) imaging in the assessment of patients presenting with chest pain suspected for acute coronary syndrome. Ann Transl Med 2016;4(13):255.

59. Munnur RK, Cameron JD, Ko BS, et al. Cardiac CT: atherosclerosis to acute coronary syndrome. Cardiovasc Diagn Ther 2014;4(6):430–48.

60. Mowatt G, Cummins E, Waugh N, et al. Systematic review of the clinical effectiveness and cost-effectiveness of 64-slice or higher computed tomography angiography as an alternative to invasive coronary angiography in the investigation of coronary artery disease. Health Technol Assess 2008;12(17). iii–iv, x–143.

61. Kim T, Litt H. Acute aortic syndrome. In: Ho V, Reddy G, editors. Cardiovascular imaging, vol. 1. Philadelphia: Saunders/Elsevier; 2011. p. 1288–305.

Acute Myocardial Infarct

Alastair Moore, MD[a],*, Harold Goerne, MD[b,c], Prabhakar Rajiah, MBBS, MD[a],
Yuki Tanabe, MD[a], Sachin Saboo, MD[a], Suhny Abbara, MD[a]

KEYWORDS

- Acute MI • Complications of acute MI • Cardiac CT • Dual-energy CT • Acute MI on cardiac CT
- Acute MI on CT

KEY POINTS

- Appropriate selection for cardiac computed tomography (CT) is paramount because patients with definite acute coronary syndrome (ACS) should be referred urgently to coronary angiography for intervention, and cardiac computed tomography (CT) is likely to delay definitive therapy.
- The imaging findings of acute myocardial infarction (MI) may be detected not only on cardiac tailored examinations but also incidentally on routine chest CT obtained for the exclusion of other causes of chest pain.
- MI occurs first within the subendocardium and progresses with time toward the epicardium, eventually becoming transmural in extent; acute MI manifests on CT by relative hypoperfusion in a vascular territory commonly with regional wall motion abnormalities and maintained myocardial thickness.
- The mechanical complications of acute MI, such as left ventricular free wall rupture, cardiac tamponade, and ventricular septal defect, are associated with high mortality and are important sequelae for the radiologist to recognize.

INTRODUCTION

Myocardial infarction (MI) is myocardial necrosis caused by myocardial ischemia, an imbalance between oxygen supply and myocardial demand. It is part of the clinical presentation of acute coronary syndrome (ACS), which is a broader term encompassing ST-segment elevation MI (STEMI), non-STEMI, and unstable angina pectoris.[1] ACS is estimated to occur in more than 750,000 people every year with more than two-thirds presenting with non-STEMI.[1] Coronary artery disease–related deaths account for more than 370,000 deaths a year in the United States.[2] The average age at presentation is 68 years with men presenting 50% more frequently than women.[1]

Patients presenting with STEMI are urgently referred to the coronary angiography suite for prompt treatment and typically do not undergo preprocedural imaging; however, those presenting with ACS not related to STEMI are apt to undergo further testing to exclude acute MI. Cardiac computed tomography (CT), and specifically coronary CT angiography (CTA), plays in important role in the diagnostic work-up of certain patients presenting with ACS and is becoming more ubiquitous in emergency departments.

The diagnosis of acute MI requires a change in cardiac biomarkers with at least one value higher than the 99th percentile of the upper reference value. It also requires ischemic symptoms, new electrocardiogram (ECG) changes (ST-T abnormality, left bundle branch block, or pathologic Q waves), new nonviable myocardium on imaging, regional wall motion abnormality on imaging, or intracoronary or stent thrombus on angiography or at autopsy. The diagnosis may be made posthumously without a change in biomarkers if there were symptoms of myocardial ischemia and ECG

a Department of Radiology, Cardiothoracic Imaging, UT Southwestern Medical Center, 5323 Harry Hines Boulevard, Dallas, TX 75390-8896, USA; b Department of Radiology, Cardiovascular Imaging Service, IMSS Western National Medical Center, Belisario Dominguez 1000, Guadalajara, Jalisco 44340, Mexico; c Cardiovascular Imaging Service, Imaging and Diagnosis Center (CID), Av. Americas 2016, Guadalajara, Jalisco 44610, Mexico
* Corresponding author. Department of Radiology, Cardiothoracic Imaging, UT Southwestern Medical Center, E6.120 B, 5323 Harry Hines Boulevard, Dallas, TX 75390-8896.
E-mail address: alastair.j.e.moore@gmail.com

Radiol Clin N Am 57 (2019) 45–55
https://doi.org/10.1016/j.rcl.2018.08.006

changes when death occurred, before biomarkers could be obtained or would be expected to rise. There are also specific criteria for the diagnosis of percutaneous coronary intervention–related MI and coronary artery bypass grafting–related MI that require a higher threshold for cardiac biomarkers. Acute MI is divided into subcategories based on its cause. Type 1 is MI secondary to atherosclerotic plaque disruption leading to intraluminal thrombosis. Type 2 is MI caused by myocardial ischemia that is not secondary to atherosclerotic plaque. Type 3 is MI that results in death when biomarkers are unavailable. Type 4a is MI related to percutaneous coronary intervention. Type 4b is MI secondary to stent thrombosis. Type 5 is MI related to coronary artery bypass grafting.[3]

Chronic MI is diagnosed when a patient's presentation not consistent with acute MI, and noncardiac causes have been excluded. It also requires pathologic Q waves on ECG, nonviable myocardium on imaging that fails to contract, or findings of prior MI by pathology.[3]

Infarction is not the only potential outcome of consequence following an episode of myocardial ischemia, and two entities are worth mentioning that may be encountered by the radiologist. The first, myocardial stunning, refers to reduced regional ventricular contraction following the resolution of a brief acute ischemic event. There is no infarcted tissue, and the motion abnormality persists despite adequate perfusion for hours or days following the event. The second entity is hibernating myocardium. This refers to myocardium with chronically reduced contractility in the presence of chronically diminished myocardial perfusion. It probably results from myocardial cells entering a state of low metabolism, and if the causative factor resulting in the reduced blood flow is removed (ie, with coronary bypass), ventricular function is normalized.[4,5] In these scenarios, cardiomyocytes can regain normal contractility and are therefore referred to as "viable" (as are normal cardiomyocytes). To clarify, the term "viable" may also refer to a cardiac segment, even if it contains some infarcted cardiomyocytes. A viable cardiac segment with diminished contractility contains enough viable cardiomyocytes that it is likely to regain function following revascularization. Imaging plays a crucial role in predicting which patients will benefit from revascularization (discussed later).

PATHOPHYSIOLOGY OF MYOCARDIAL INFARCT

Within the first 30 minutes following coronary occlusion, oxygen-deprived cardiomyocytes switch from aerobic to anaerobic metabolism resulting in a cascade of cellular abnormalities that, if allowed to progress, result in irreversible cellular damage and myocardial necrosis (infarct). Depletion of ATP results in a loss of membrane potential, cellular swelling, and eventually impaired integrity of the cell membrane from calcium influx and other molecular imbalances. The result is a region of MI, the full extent of which is usually complete within 6 hours. This infarcted myocardium is surrounded by at-risk (ischemic) myocardium whose damage may be reversible with reperfusion, if performed within the first 6 hours. Perfusion to the affected myocardium may also cause irreversible damage to myocytes as a result of further influx of intracellular calcium and the introduction of oxygen free radicals.[6] Myocardial blood flow, in the presence of coronary occlusion, is reduced more significantly in the subendocardium (toward the ventricular lumen) than in the subepicardium. Consequently, MI occurs first within the subendocardium and progresses with time toward the epicardium, eventually becoming transmural in extent. Originally described in dogs in the late 1970s, this is dubbed the "wavefront of myocardial necrosis."[7]

After approximately 2 months, debris, inflammatory cells, and edema are replaced by scar tissue resulting in a decrease in size of the infarcted tissue and myocardial thinning.[8] Although the mechanism is unclear, healed myocardium frequently contains adipose tissue, an entity termed "fatty metaplasia."[9,10] The calcium that accumulates during acute MI remains unabsorbed and is identified in the chronically infarcted tissue.[11]

MANAGEMENT OF ACUTE CORONARY SYNDROME

ACS requires a systematic approach for accurate and timely diagnosis and treatment, and the role of CT is only one facet of a complex algorithm.

The Society of Cardiovascular Computed Tomography has outlined a multidisciplinary approach to patients presenting with acute chest pain and has rendered recommendations on the specific use of CT. Discussed in more detail elsewhere in this issue, briefly, coronary CTA is most suitable for use in patients with a low to intermediate pretest likelihood of ACS. Patients with definite ACS should be referred urgently to coronary angiography for intervention, and coronary CTA in this scenario is likely to delay therapy with no added benefit. Coronary CTA plays an uncertain role in the work-up of patients in whom there is a high but not definite likelihood of ACS with clinical acumen playing a heavy role in this situation.[12]

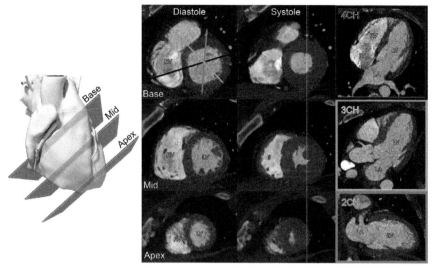

Fig. 1. Standard cardiac planes. CT images are reconstructed from a retrospectively gated cardiac CT, which enables viewing the heart at any stage (phase) of the cardiac cycle. The short axis plane is shown in diastole and systole. Note the normal, uniform thickening of the left ventricle in systole. The short axis reformations are made orthogonal to the long axis of the heart, as illustrated by the three-dimensional model on the left. The additional planes on the far right are planned from the short axis view in diastole and include the four-chamber (4CH), three-chamber (3CH), and two-chamber (2CH) views. LA, left atrium; LV, left ventricle; RA, right atrium; RV, right ventricle.

IMAGING TECHNIQUE
Conventional Cardiac Computed Tomography

Although several of the subsequently described manifestations of MI may be seen on routine, non-gated studies, most features are best identified on dedicated cardiac CT. This is typically performed with ECG-gating or triggering to minimize motion artifacts, which are inherent in nongated acquisitions. With retrospective ECG-gating, radiographic data are acquired throughout the cardiac cycle in a helical/spiral mode with simultaneous ECG acquisition. The data can then be reconstructed in any or all the cardiac phases. Images are typically reconstructed in mid-to-late diastole for coronary CT imaging. The radiation dose is high because of continuous acquisition throughout the cardiac cycle. Hence, an ECG-based tube current modulation is typically used, where the x-ray tube current is set at high value only for one preselected phase, and it is ramped down for the rest of the phases of the cardiac cycle. This technique is now reserved for indications that require all cardiac phases, such as evaluation of ventricular volumes/function or in patients with high or irregular heart rates. Prospective ECG-triggering is usually the current default mode of coronary CTA, where data are acquired in axial mode, and the tube is "on" only during a short time window in diastole (sequential or step-and-shoot mode). This technique results in significant radiation dose savings. Widening of the tube's "on" time is possible, which

means that data are acquired for a small additional window outside the chosen cardiac phase. A high-pitch helical mode is available in the latest generations of dual-source scanners, in which images are obtained with pitch as high as 3.4 ("flash" mode). This is performed with or without ECG-gating. This ECG-gating technique is called prospective-helical triggering, which allows acquisition of the entire data within a fraction of one cardiac cycle, minimizing motion and contrast doses.[13]

Advanced Imaging Techniques

The latest advances in scanner technique have opened exciting, new avenues for cardiac imaging with numerous opportunities for research and the advancement of clinical knowledge. These include delayed-enhancement CT imaging, CT perfusion imaging, CT strain imaging, myocardial extracellular volume analysis, and texture analysis.[14–16]

In dual-energy CT (DECT), also referred to as spectral CT or multienergy CT, radiographic data are acquired at more than one energy level. Materials and tissues show different attenuation properties at different energy levels depending on their atomic number and electron density. By obtaining data at multiple energy levels, these materials and tissues are delineated better than a conventional CT, in which most of these tissues yield similar attenuation. Generally, data are acquired only at two energy levels. Some scanners

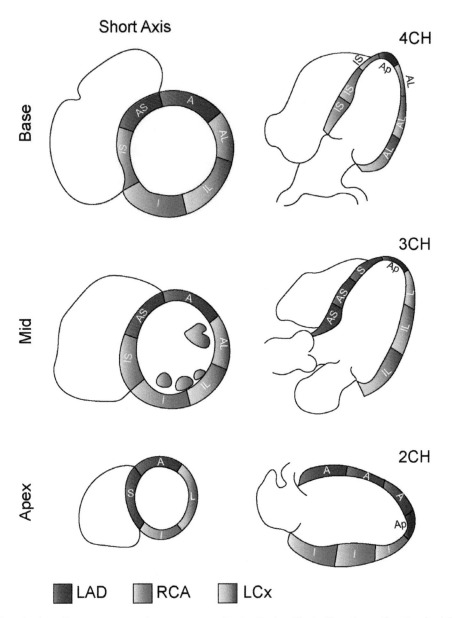

Fig. 2. Standard cardiac segments and coronary vascular territories. Illustration shows the standard 17-segment model of the heart in the short axis, four-chamber (4CH), three-chamber (3CH), and two-chamber (2CH) views. A, anterior; AL, anterolateral; Ap, apex; AS, anteroseptum; I, inferior; IL, inferolateral; IS, inferoseptum; L, lateral; LAD, left anterior descending; LCx, left circumflex artery; LV, left ventricle; RCA, right coronary artery; RV, right ventricle; S, septal. (Based on Cerqueira MD, Weissman NJ, Dilsizian V, et al. Standardized myocardial segmentation and nomenclature for tomographic imaging of the heart. A statement for healthcare professionals from the Cardiac Imaging Committee of the Council on Clinical Cardiology of the American Heart Association. Circulation 2002;105(4):539–42.)

accomplish this at the level of the x-ray source with varying technologies including the use of two x-ray tubes, rapid kilovolt (peak) switching, consecutive scans at different energy levels, or a split x-ray beam with high- and low-energy components. Alternatively, detector-based DECT scanners use one x-ray source and have two layers of detectors.

DECT allows the generation of multiple additional datasets beyond routine conventional CT images. For example, one can view iodine-only image sets, which highlight pixels containing iodine.

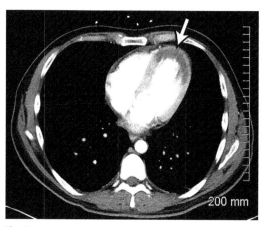

Fig. 3. Acute MI on routine CT. A 40-year-old man presented with chest pain and abdominal bloating to the emergency department. An axial CT image through the lower chest obtained as part of the routine abdominal and pelvic CT shows focal decreased attenuation of the true apex, apical lateral segment, and apical septal segments (*arrow*). As is seen with acute MI, myocardial wall thickness is preserved, although this can sometimes be difficult to judge on routine CT because of motion. Catheter angiography showed a 99% stenosis in the left anterior descending.

These may be used for qualitative and quantitative estimation of perfusion or for lesion characterization. Virtual noncontrast images, which remove iodine from pixels, are used to replace true noncontrast image and may help distinguish calcium from contrast enhancement. Virtual monoenergetic images mimic images obtained using a true monoenergetic x-ray beam and can help reduce artifacts caused by the polyenergetic nature of the conventional x-ray beam (eg, beam hardening). Virtual monoenergetic images, especially

at high energies (>70 keV), can result in fewer artifacts. Similarly, virtual monoenergetic images at lower energy levels are used to improve the contrast signal from iodine-enhanced structures. Numerous other data sets can be generated and may have a future role in cardiac imaging.[17]

NORMAL ANATOMY

Although many of the manifestations of MI are apparent on conventional planes orthogonal to the body axis, multiplanar reformats (MPR) with planes orthogonal to the axis of the heart may aid in identifying features of MI on CT (**Fig. 1**). MPRs are typically made in the two-chamber view (vertical long axis or paraseptal ling axis), four-chamber view (horizontal long axis), and short axis view (orthogonal to both long axes). A description should abide by the standard 17 myocardial segment model with an assignment of the affected territory to either the left anterior descending artery, right coronary artery, or left circumflex artery (**Fig. 2**).[18]

IMAGING FINDINGS IN THE ACUTE SETTING
Nongated Computed Tomography

Although findings related to acute MI are readily detected on cardiac-gated CT, they may also be incidentally detected on nongated CT.[19] On contrast-enhanced nongated chest CT, acute MI manifests as a focal area of diminished myocardial enhancement (**Fig. 3**) in a coronary artery vascular territory (see **Fig. 2**).[19] Wall thickness, which may help distinguish acute from chronic infarction, may be difficult to estimate because of motion. Nevertheless, normal-thickness myocardium is usually seen in acute MI, whereas thinned myocardium is typically seen in chronic MI.[20]

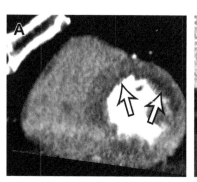
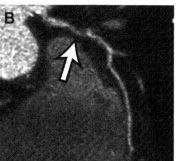
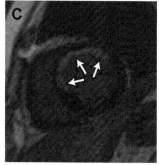

Fig. 4. Acute MI on ECG-gated cardiac CT and MR imaging. (*A*) Mid short axis view of the left ventricle derived from an ECG-gated cardiac CT shows focal hypoattenuation of the anteroseptal, anterior, and anterolateral myocardial segments with preserved myocardial thickness (*arrows*) indicative of acute MI. (*B*) Curved MPR shows stenosis (*arrow*) within the proximal left anterior descending artery. (*C*) Delayed-enhancement MR imaging performed in the short axis shows an area of a corresponding region of subendocardial late gadolinium enhancement compatible with MI (*arrows*). Note the preserved wall-thickness, a hallmark of acute MI and a distinguishing feature from chronic MI.

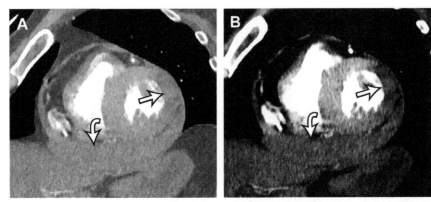

Fig. 5. The importance of appropriate window width and level. Mid short axis images of the left ventricle derived from an ECG-gated cardiac CT show the importance of appropriate window width and window level in the detection of myocardial infarction. Although the image with standard soft tissue window width and level (*A*) shows clearly the patient's hemopericardium (*curved arrow*), the decreased perfusion in the anterolateral and inferolateral segments (*straight arrow*) is more conspicuous with a window width of 100 HU and a window level centered at 50 HU (*B*).

Electrocardiogram-Gated Cardiac Computed Tomography

ECG-gated cardiac CT, which is commonly tailored for evaluation of the coronary arteries (coronary CTA), is well suited for demonstrating the noncoronary ancillary findings of acute MI, which is useful for prognostic and therapeutic guidance.[21] In the setting of suspected ACS, cardiac CT is not routinely obtained for the sole purpose of direct myocardial evaluation, which is usually reported as an adjunct to coronary CTA. Because coronary CTA is tailored to capture maximal arterial enhancement of the coronary arteries, it is well-timed for assessment of myocardial enhancement and, in a crude sense, is effectively an arterial phase myocardial perfusion CT at rest (nondynamic, single time point). If the examination was obtained with retrospective gating, functional information can be obtained revealing wall motion abnormalities and depressed ventricular function that not only increase specificity and sensitivity of coronary findings but also can be significant predictors of major adverse cardiac events.[21]

Findings of acute MI on CTA include a decrease in early myocardial enhancement in infarcted myocardium relative to normal myocardium (**Fig. 4**).[22,23] Typically, normally enhanced myocardium attenuation should be near 100 HU, whereas infarcted tissue approximates 50 HU. Individual differences in kilovolt (peak) and patient characteristics may cause variation in myocardial attenuation, and a practical approach is to consider myocardium less than 50% of the attenuation of normal myocardium to be infarcted.[24] Viewing these abnormalities requires a narrow window width and level to maximize the contrast between

normal and abnormal myocardium (eg, window 200, level 100) with manual adjustment necessary for individual patients.[25] To maximize contrast to noise, 5-mm-thick MPR or 5-mm minimum intensity projections are recommended (**Fig. 5**).[26] The myocardial abnormality should correspond to a vascular territory, and always begin from the endocardial surface and extend toward the subepicardial surface with the most extensive infarcts being transmural. Other patterns, such as subepicardial defects, midmyocardial defects, or nonvascular territory defects, should raise suspicion for artifact or other pathologies. It should be noted that in the acute setting, decreased myocardial perfusion can occasionally reflect regions of at-risk ischemic myocardium, but in most clinical scenarios, this would be more accurately assessed with other modalities, such as delayed-enhancement imaging (either CT or MR imaging).[27] On MR imaging, reporting the extent of transmural involvement in quartiles (1%–25%, 26%–50%, 51%–75%, and 76%–100%) is recommended because it has been well shown that patients with greater than 50% transmural extent of infarct are unlikely to see improved ventricular contractility after revascularization, and nearly no patients with greater than 50% transmural extent will see improvement.[28] Although not commonly used, this method can be extended to cardiac CT with delayed enhancement (10 minutes after contrast administration) (**Fig. 6**).[29,30] This description should use the standard American Heart Association 17-segment model to ensure consistency across modalities (see **Fig. 2**).[18]

Cardiac gating allows evaluation of myocardial thickness that is preserved in acute MI (as opposed to chronic MI, where myocardial thinning

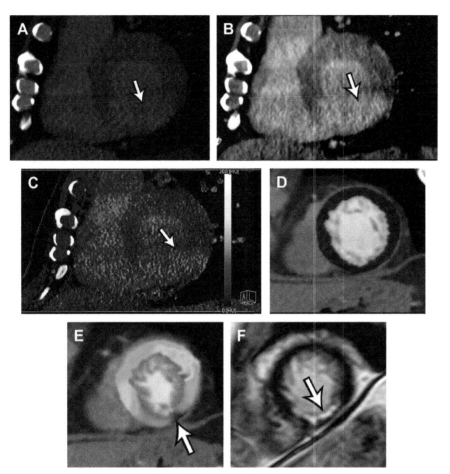

Fig. 6. Advanced imaging techniques in MI. (A–C) Short axis (SA) images of the left ventricle obtained from DECT 10 minutes following the administration of contrast show retained enhancement in the basal inferoseptal, inferior, and inferolateral myocardial segments (arrows). In this patient with acute coronary syndrome, this is compatible with infarcted myocardium. Conventional CT images (A) may not show the enhancement as well as monoenergetic CT images (B), which are extracted from the DECT data set. An iodine map (C) may render the abnormal iodine enhancement more conspicuous. (D–F) Strain imaging of the left ventricle in a different patient allows quantitative assessment of regional myocardial function. SA images of the left ventricle in diastole (D) and systole (E) with a color overlay of CT strain values shows decreased values in the hypokinetic inferior segment, colored blue during systole (arrow). SA MR imaging image (F) shows subendocardial late gadolinium enhancement indicative of infarct (arrow).

is evident).[20] Moreover, in retrospective acquisitions, functional data are extracted that can relay valuable information regarding regional wall motion abnormalities (Fig. 7). Regional wall motion is graded qualitatively as normal, hypokinetic, akinetic, or dyskinetic. Acute MI usually shows akinetic normal thickness myocardium confined to a coronary territory. The combination of a regional wall motion abnormality with coronary stenosis is associated with a particularly high rate of adverse cardiac events.[21]

Complications of Acute Myocardial Infarction

There are several potential complications of acute MI, and because many of them carry a significantly high associated mortality, it is important for the practicing radiologist to be familiar with their imaging manifestations, particularly the mechanical complications.

Mitral regurgitation

Mitral regurgitation following MI is common with an incidence of up to 50%, and it results from changes in left ventricle morphology or papillary muscle ischemia. The indirect sequelae of this manifests on imaging with findings of acute pulmonary edema (Fig. 8). Rare, but classically described in radiographs, unilateral pulmonary edema, usually in the right upper lobe is seen because of asymmetric increase in hydrostatic pressure of the right upper lobe caused by

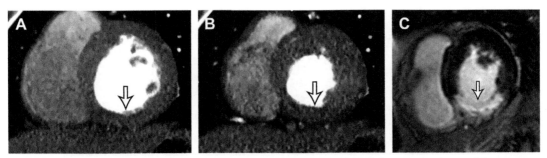

Fig. 7. Focal wall motion abnormality in MI. (*A, B*) Short axis images of the left ventricle obtained from a retrospectively ECG-gated cardiac CT obtained during diastole (*A*) and systole (*B*) show akinesis of the basal inferior segment (*arrow*) in a patient with acute MI. (*C*) Delayed-enhancement MR imaging in the same patient shows transmural late gadolinium enhancement in the basal inferoseptal, inferior, and inferolateral segments compatible with MI (*arrow*).

asymmetric blood flow from left atrium as a result of severe mitral regurgitation. This is a poor prognostic factor.[31] Papillary muscle rupture is a rare complication of papillary muscle ischemia, occurring in around 0.25% of cases of acute MI. It is catastrophic, as are all mechanical complications of acute MI, and direct visualization by imaging is uncommon but may include a flail mitral

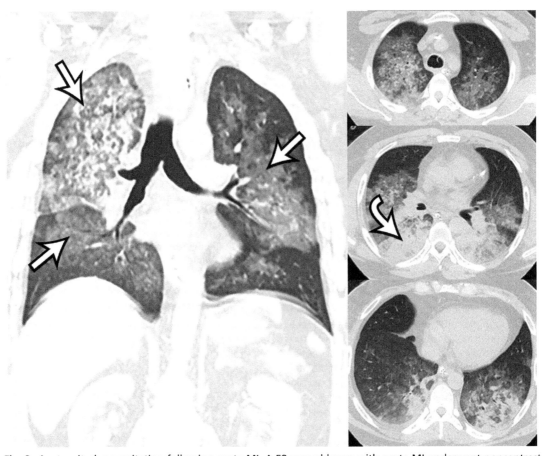

Fig. 8. Acute mitral regurgitation following acute MI. A 58-year-old man with acute MI underwent noncontrast CT for respiratory failure immediately following coronary angiography that had showed a significant lesion in the left anterior descending coronary artery. Compatible with pulmonary edema, CT images show confluent areas of ground glass opacity throughout the perihilar and central portions of the lungs (*straight arrows*) with dependent areas of consolidation (*curved arrow*). Acute mitral regurgitation is a complication of acute MI and may present with acute hydrostatic pulmonary edema.

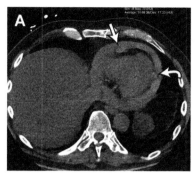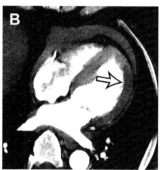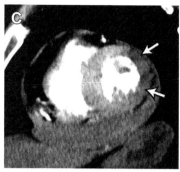

Fig. 9. Left ventricular free wall rupture and hemopericardium. A 67-year-old man with acute myocardial infarction presenting with hypotension and concern for cardiac tamponade on echocardiography. (*A*) Noncontrast axial CT shows a hyperdense circumferential pericardial effusion (average attenuation 36 HU) compatible with hemopericardium (*straight arrow*). A hyperdense defect traversing the epicardial fat (*curved arrow*) is suspicious for a site of myocardial rupture. (*B*) Contrast-enhanced axial CT shows a relative decrease in perfusion of the lateral myocardium with preserved wall thickness (*arrow*), compatible with acutely infarcted myocardium. (*C*) A reconstruction in the short axis plane aids in detection of the infarct (*arrows*) and facilitates identification of the affected myocardial segment and its corresponding vascular territory (the mid anterolateral and inferolateral myocardial segments corresponding to the left circumflex artery territory).

leaflet. The posteromedial muscle, which has a single blood supply, is more vulnerable to ischemia and consequently rupture.[32–34]

Free wall rupture

Left ventricular free wall rupture, although rare and occurring in only 2% to 4% of acute MI presentations, is an important entity to recognize because the associated potential pericardial tamponade carries a considerably high mortality. It is the second most common cause of in-hospital death for patients with STEMI.[35] Risk factors include female sex, age greater than 55, hypertension, and transmural infarction. Rupture may occur early (within 48 hours) or late (after 48 hours). The presentation is also categorized as acute or subacute with the acute form being associated with severe hypotension, acute pericardial tamponade, and sudden death. The tears may be caused by shear stress on a mural hematoma at the junction between an infarcted region and the adjacent compensatory hypercontractile myocardium. Subacute rupture takes a more insidious course, typically occurring within 3 to 5 days, and presents with a pericardial effusion with or without tamponade. It is caused by necrosis and neutrophil infiltration that results in thinned and weakened myocardium. In most cases of acute rupture, the patient dies before he or she is treated in a hospital.[36,37] If a patient is stable enough to undergo imaging, which is often performed to rule out other nefarious pathology, CT may show a pericardial effusion with an

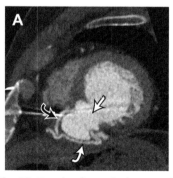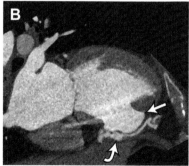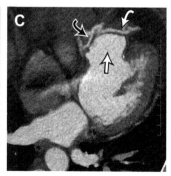

Fig. 10. Repair of ventricular septal rupture (VSR) and pseudoaneurysm. A 57-year-old man with a history of acute myocardial infarction complicated by VSR and pseudoaneurysm formation. Short axis (*A*), two-chamber (*B*), and four-chamber (*C*) reformations from a contrast-enhanced cardiac CT show hyperdense patch material from VSR repair (*curved black arrow*) and left ventricular free wall rupture repair (*curved white arrow*), the sequelae of prior myocardial infarction of the inferoseptal and inferior myocardial segments in the right coronary artery territory. There is a wide-mouthed aneurysm extending into the patch repair (*straight arrow*), an unanticipated complication of the repair.

attenuation greater than water, indicative of hemo-pericardium (Fig. 9). An associated infarct may also be apparent. With the administration of contrast, a thread-like defect in the myocardium that fills with left ventricular luminal density contrast may be seen in some cases; however, contrast in the pericardial effusion itself is rarely seen, possibly because of blockage of flow by the pericardial hematoma.[38] In the setting of cardiac tamponade, CT shows compression of the cardiac chambers, an enlarged superior vena cava, an enlarged inferior vena cava, periportal edema, reflux of contrast into the inferior vena cava or azygous vein, and enlarged hepatic and renal veins.[39]

Ventricular septal rupture

Ventricular septal rupture occurs in less than 1% of patients presenting with acute MI. The pathophysiology is similar to that of free wall rupture, and it occurs after a transmural infarction of the interventricular septum. It may be seen in left anterior descending, dominant right coronary artery, or dominant left circumflex artery infarcts because all of these coronary arteries may have septal branches. The resultant defect causes left-to-right shunting of blood and may lead to right ventricle complications, such as stunning or ischemia secondary to sudden systemic pressures in the right ventricle.[37] Imaging manifestations include a direct communication between the left ventricle and right ventricle, visualized by continuity of contrast between the chambers. If there is a differential of contrast opacification between the chambers, a jet of lesser or greater attenuation may be seen originating from one chamber and entering the next. Although the defect can occur anywhere in the septum, it is classically seen between the inferior basal septum and the hyperdynamic mid septum. Treatment of free wall rupture and ventricular septal rupture includes surgical repair, typically with a patch (Fig. 10). If a ventricular rupture is contained by local pericardial adhesions, it results in pseudoaneurysm (false aneurysm) formation.

SUMMARY

The manifestations of acute MI are readily identified on noncontrast and contrast-enhanced routine and cardiac-tailored CT. Knowledge of normal cardiac anatomy and vascular territories and the imaging findings of acute MI can aid in the day-to-day detection of this increasing common entity. The primary purpose of coronary CTA remains evaluation of the coronary arteries themselves, but when present, the manifestations

of MI and its associated abnormalities should be reported because they have important prognostic and clinical implications. Mechanical complications of acute MI can have catastrophic consequences, and it is important to be mindful of their imaging appearances. Awareness of potential mimickers and pitfalls, clinical and imaging, can help prevent unnecessary interventions and investigations.

REFERENCES

1. Amsterdam EA, Wenger NK, Brindis RG, et al. 2014 AHA/ACC guideline for the management of patients with non-ST-elevation acute coronary syndromes: a report of the American College of Cardiology/American Heart Association Task Force on practice guidelines. Circulation 2014;130(25):e344–426.

2. Anderson JL, Morrow DA. Acute myocardial infarction. N Engl J Med 2017;376(21):2053–64.

3. Thygesen K, Alpert JS, Jaffe AS, et al. Third universal definition of myocardial infarction. Circulation 2012;126(16):2020–35.

4. Kloner RA, Przyklenk K. Hibernation and stunning of the myocardium. N Engl J Med 1991;325(26):1877–9.

5. Conti CR. The stunned and hibernating myocardium: a brief review. Clin Cardiol 1991;14(9):708–12.

6. Fishbein GA, Fishbein MC, Buja LM. Myocardial ischemia and its complications. In: Buja LM, Butany J, editors. Cardiovascular pathology. Boston: Elsevier; 2016. p. 239–70.

7. Reimer KA, Lowe JE, Rasmussen MM, et al. The wavefront phenomenon of ischemic cell death. 1. Myocardial infarct size vs duration of coronary occlusion in dogs. Circulation 1977;56(5):786–94.

8. Fieno DS, Hillenbrand HB, Rehwald WG, et al. Infarct resorption, compensatory hypertrophy, and differing patterns of ventricular remodeling following myocardial infarctions of varying size. J Am Coll Cardiol 2004;43(11):2124–31.

9. Su L, Siegel JE, Fishbein MC. Adipose tissue in myocardial infarction. Cardiovasc Pathol 2004;13(2):98–102.

10. Baroldi G, Silver MD, De Maria R, et al. Lipomatous metaplasia in left ventricular scar. Can J Cardiol 1997;13(1):65–71.

11. Shriki JE, Shinbane J, Lee C, et al. Incidental myocardial infarct on conventional nongated CT: a review of the spectrum of findings with gated CT and cardiac MRI correlation. AJR Am J Roentgenol 2012;198(3):496–504.

12. Raff GL, Chinnaiyan KM, Cury RC, et al. SCCT guidelines on the use of coronary computed tomographic angiography for patients presenting with acute chest pain to the emergency department: a report of the Society of Cardiovascular Computed

Tomography Guidelines Committee. J Cardiovasc Comput Tomogr 2014;8(4):254–71.

13. Kalisz K, Buethe J, Saboo SS, et al. Artifacts at cardiac CT: physics and solutions. Radiographics 2016; 36(7):2064–83.

14. Jablonowski R, Wilson MW, Do L, et al. Multidetector CT measurement of myocardial extracellular volume in acute patchy and contiguous infarction: validation with microscopic measurement. Radiology 2015; 274(2):370–8.

15. Hinzpeter R, Wagner MW, Wurnig MC, et al. Texture analysis of acute myocardial infarction with CT: first experience study. PLoS One 2017;12(11):e0186876.

16. Nakauchi Y, Iwanaga Y, Ikuta S, et al. Quantitative myocardial perfusion analysis using multi-row detector CT in acute myocardial infarction. Heart 2012;98(7):566–72.

17. Kalisz K, Halliburton S, Abbara S, et al. Update on cardiovascular applications of multienergy CT. Radiographics 2017;37(7):1955–74.

18. Cerqueira MD, Weissman NJ, Dilsizian V, et al. Standardized myocardial segmentation and nomenclature for tomographic imaging of the heart. A statement for healthcare professionals from the cardiac imaging committee of the council on clinical cardiology of the American Heart Association. Circulation 2002;105(4):539–42.

19. Gosalia A, Haramati LB, Sheth MP, et al. CT detection of acute myocardial infarction. AJR Am J Roentgenol 2004;182(6):1563–6.

20. Nieman K, Cury RC, Ferencik M, et al. Differentiation of recent and chronic myocardial infarction by cardiac computed tomography. Am J Cardiol 2006; 98(3):303–8.

21. Schlett CL, Banerji D, Siegel E, et al. Prognostic value of CT angiography for major adverse cardiac events in patients with acute chest pain from the emergency department: 2-year outcomes of the ROMICAT trial. JACC Cardiovasc Imaging 2011;4(5): 481–91.

22. Mahnken AH, Bruners P, Katoh M, et al. Dynamic multi-section CT imaging in acute myocardial infarction: preliminary animal experience. Eur Radiol 2006;16(3):746–52.

23. Hoffmann U, Millea R, Enzweiler C, et al. Acute myocardial infarction: contrast-enhanced multi-detector row CT in a porcine model. Radiology 2004; 231(3):697–701.

24. Nance JW, Schoepf UJ. Myocardial ischemic disease: computed tomography. In: Abbara S, Kalva SP, editors. Problem solving in cardiovascular imaging. Philadelphia: Elsevier, Saunders; 2013. p. 490–504.

25. Blankstein R, Rogers IS, Cury RC. Practical tips and tricks in cardiovascular computed tomography: diagnosis of myocardial infarction. J Cardiovasc Comput Tomogr 2009;3(2):104–11.

26. Rogers IS, Cury RC, Blankstein R, et al. Comparison of postprocessing techniques for the detection of perfusion defects by cardiac computed tomography in patients presenting with acute ST-segment elevation myocardial infarction. J Cardiovasc Comput Tomogr 2010;4(4):258–66.

27. Nikolaou K, Sanz J, Poon M, et al. Assessment of myocardial perfusion and viability from routine contrast-enhanced 16-detector-row computed tomography of the heart: preliminary results. Eur Radiol 2005;15(5):864–71.

28. Kim RJ, Wu E, Rafael A, et al. The use of contrast-enhanced magnetic resonance imaging to identify reversible myocardial dysfunction. N Engl J Med 2000;343(20):1445–53.

29. Rodriguez-Granillo GA, Rosales MA, Baum S, et al. Early assessment of myocardial viability by the use of delayed enhancement computed tomography after primary percutaneous coronary intervention. JACC Cardiovasc Imaging 2009;2(9):1072–81.

30. Rodriguez-Granillo GA, Campisi R, Deviggiano A, et al. Detection of myocardial infarction using delayed enhancement dual-energy CT in stable patients. AJR Am J Roentgenol 2017;209(5):1023–32.

31. Attias D, Mansencal N, Auvert B, et al. Prevalence, characteristics, and outcomes of patients presenting with cardiogenic unilateral pulmonary edema. Circulation 2010;122(11):1109–15.

32. Kalra PR, Ohri SK, Morgan JM. Mitral regurgitation secondary to ruptured papillary muscle. Heart 2000;84(1):13.

33. Güvenç RÇ, Güvenç TS. Clinical presentation, diagnosis and management of acute mitral regurgitation following acute myocardial infarction. Journal of Acute Disease 2016;5(2):96–101.

34. Morris MF, Maleszewski JJ, Suri RM, et al. CT and MR imaging of the mitral valve: radiologic-pathologic correlation. Radiographics 2010;30(6):1603–20.

35. Figueras J, Alcalde O, Barrabes JA, et al. Changes in hospital mortality rates in 425 patients with acute ST-elevation myocardial infarction and cardiac rupture over a 30-year period. Circulation 2008; 118(25):2783–9.

36. Figueras J, Cortadellas J, Soler-Soler J. Left ventricular free wall rupture: clinical presentation and management. Heart 2000;83(5):499–504.

37. Jones BM, Kapadia SR, Smedira NG, et al. Ventricular septal rupture complicating acute myocardial infarction: a contemporary review. Eur Heart J 2014;35(31):2060–8.

38. Onoda N, Nonami A, Yabe T, et al. Postinfarct cardiac free wall rupture detected by multidetector computed tomography. J Cardiol Cases 2012;5(3): e147–9.

39. Restrepo CS, Lemos DF, Lemos JA, et al. Imaging findings in cardiac tamponade with emphasis on CT. Radiographics 2007;27(6):1595–610.

Chronic Infarcts and Mimickers of Infarcts

Alastair Moore, MD[a],*, Harold Goerne, MD[b,c], Prabhakar Rajiah, MBBS, MD[a],
Yuki Tanabe, MD[a], Sachin Saboo, MD[a], Suhny Abbara, MD[a]

KEYWORDS

- Chronic MI • Complications of chronic MI • Cardiac CT • Dual-energy CT
- Chronic MI on cardiac CT • Chronic MI on routine CT • Pitfalls of cardiac CT • Mimickers of MI

KEY POINTS

- Radiologists should be familiar with and confident in diagnosing the sequelae of chronic myocardial infarct (MI) on routine computed tomography (CT) of the chest, even in the face of clinical doubt, because the prognosis of silent MI, a common entity, carries a similar prognosis to clinically detected MI.
- Manifestations of chronic MI on CT, including subendocardial fatty metaplasia in a vascular distribution, focal wall thinning, and mural calcifications, can be detected on both cardiac tailored CT and routine chest CT.
- Complications of chronic MI include ventricular aneurysm, pseudoaneurysm, thrombus, and post-myocardial infarction syndrome (Dressler syndrome).
- Imaging mimickers of MI and its sequelae include physiologic fatty metaplasia, aneurysm formation from other causes, ventricular diverticula, artifact, and the normal structures of the heart, including the apical thin point and the membranous interventricular septum.

INTRODUCTION

Chronic myocardial infarction (MI) is a common entity. Indeed, more than a million cases of new MI occur annually in the United States,[1] and the prevalence of undiagnosed prior MI in nondiabetic patients ranges from 0.3% up to 6.4% in the elderly (diabetic patients have an even higher incidence, nearly 30% if there is known coronary artery atherosclerosis).[2]

Familiarity with the imaging manifestations of chronic MI and the potential complications is important for the practicing radiologist as findings are increasingly becoming apparent not just in cardiac computed tomography (CT) but also in routine CT of the chest. The clinical prognosis of silent MI is close to that of clinically detected MI, making its diagnosis important. Conversely, there are clinical situations mimicking MI, and an understanding of certain mimickers on CT may prevent further testing and unnecessary intervention. Last, there are imaging mimickers of MR imaging on CT.

In this article, the authors discuss the imaging manifestations of chronic MI in addition to the clinical and imaging mimickers of MI.

IMAGING MANIFESTATION OF CHRONIC MYOCARDIAL INFARCTION

Many sequelae of chronic MI can be readily identified on noncontrast and contrast-enhanced routine and cardiac-gated CT (**Fig. 1**). Subendocardial fatty metaplasia is a common feature of chronic MI and is identified as myocardium exhibiting attenuation less than −10 HU. Focal wall thinning, mural calcifications, and akinesis

[a] Department of Radiology, Cardiothoracic Imaging, UT Southwestern Medical Center, 5323 Harry Hines Boulevard, Dallas, TX 75390-8896, USA; [b] Department of Radiology, Cardiovascular Imaging Service, IMSS Western National Medical Center, Belisario Dominguez 1000, Guadalajara, Jalisco 44340, Mexico; [c] Cardiovascular Imaging Service, Imaging and Diagnosis Center (CID), Av. Americas 2016, Guadalajara, Jalisco 44610, Mexico
* Corresponding author. Department of Radiology Cardiothoracic Imaging, UT Southwestern Medical Center, E6.120 B, 5323 Harry Hines Boulevard, Dallas, TX 75390-8896.
E-mail address: alastair.j.e.moore@gmail.com

Radiol Clin N Am 57 (2019) 57–65
https://doi.org/10.1016/j.rcl.2018.08.007
0033-8389/19/© 2018 Elsevier Inc. All rights reserved.

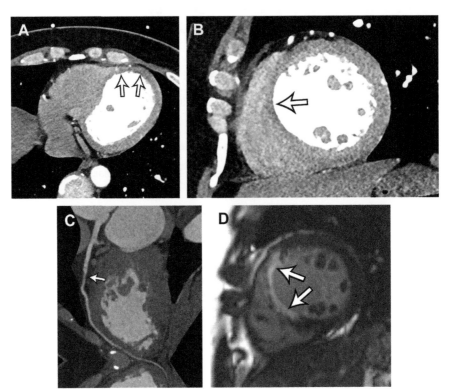

Fig. 1. Chronic MI axial (*A*) and short-axis (SA) (*B*) reconstructions from a contrast-enhanced coronary CTA demonstrate thinning of the anteroseptal wall with low attenuation (less than −10 HU) in the subendocardium (*arrows*) compatible with fatty metaplasia as a result of prior MI. (*C*) A curved multiplanar reformat image shows an area of moderate stenosis in the mid left anterior descending (LAD) artery (*arrow*). (*D*) An SA image from an MR imaging in the same patient shows transmural late gadolinium enhancement of the mid septal segments (*arrows*), confirming infarcted myocardium.

or dyskinesis (on retrospectively gated CT) are additional hallmarks of chronic MI (**Fig. 2**).[1,3,4]

Delayed enhancement imaging cardiac MR imaging has been well shown to demonstrate regions of scarring with the degree of transmural involvement reliably shown to predict return of normal function following revascularization.[5] This technique is an uncommon technique in CT, usually reserved for research or very specific clinical scenarios (**Fig. 3**). If CT imaging is obtained after contrast at 10 minutes delay, similar findings of retained contrast may be seen and correlate well with MR imaging.[6]

CHRONIC COMPLICATIONS OF MYOCARDIAL INFARCTION
Aneurysm

A common complication of MI is ventricular aneurysm (**Fig. 4**). A ventricular aneurysm is thinned, scarred myocardium that often moves dyskinetically with contraction. In contrast to pseudoaneurysm, all 3 layers of the myocardium remain intact, and aneurysms have a relatively low propensity for rupture. Imaging features include an outpouching from the left ventricle with a broad

base that increases in size with systole (dyskinesis).[7] Aneurysms may also be complicated by thrombus formation. Left untreated, left ventricular aneurysms may lead to heart failure, arrhythmias, and a high risk of thromboembolization. Endoventricular circular patch plasty (also known as the Dor procedure) is a surgical treatment with favorable long-term survival. It entails enclosing contractile and dysfunctional myocardium with a circular stitch and subsequent patch placement (see **Fig. 4**D).[8]

Pseudoaneurysm

If a ventricular rupture is contained by local pericardial adhesions, it results in pseudoaneurysm (false aneurysm) formation. A pseudoaneurysm contains no myocardium, which distinguishes it from an aneurysm. Pseudoaneurysms require prompt surgical correction because they tend to rupture, and therefore, distinguishing these from aneurysms, which have a more benign course, is important.[7,9] The CT feature of pseudoaneurysm includes a focal outpouching that communicates with the ventricular lumen. Classically, this has a

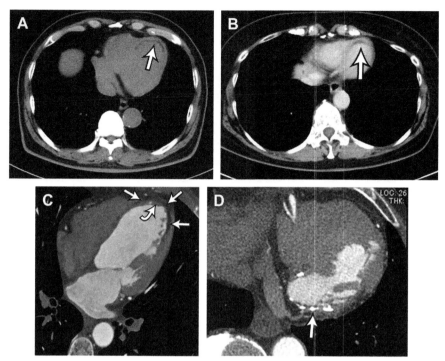

Fig. 2. Fatty metaplasia, myocardial thinning, and calcification. Axial noncontrast (*A*) and contrast-enhanced (*B*) routine CT images from the same patient demonstrate curvilinear fat attenuation (*arrow*) within the subendocardium in the LAD distribution consistent with prior LAD infarction. (*C*) A 4-chamber reconstruction from a cardiac CT in another patient shows apical thinning with subendocardial fat attenuation (*straight arrows*). There is probable thrombus in the apex (*curved arrow*), a complication of regional wall motion abnormality. (*D*) An axial image from a routine contrast-enhanced chest CT shows aneurysm formation in the basal inferior myocardium with calcifications (*arrow*). Aneurysm and myocardial calcifications are hallmarks of chronic MI.

narrow neck (<50% of the maximum diameter of the sac) and is more commonly associated with basal inferior and inferolateral ventricular segments. These features are often used to distinguish pseudoaneurysm from aneurysm (false aneurysms are rarely apical), although in practice features may overlap.[7,10]

Thrombus

Ventricular thrombus is a potential complication of focal wall motion abnormalities because of MI (**Fig. 5**). Thrombus is manifested as a low-attenuation intraluminal mass, either round or curvilinear, that is adherent to a dysfunctional

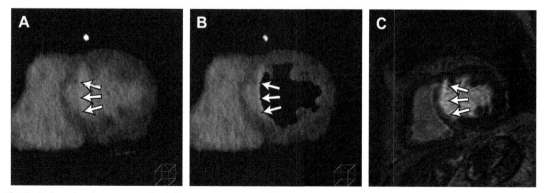

Fig. 3. Delayed-enhancement CT. (*A*) SA reconstruction from CT acquired 10 minutes following the administration of contrast shows a subtle region of retained contrast within the interventricular septum (*arrows*) indicative of myocardial scar from infarction. (*B*) Subtraction technique in the same slice renders the abnormality more conspicuous (*arrows*). (*C*) An SA image from an MR imaging in the same patient demonstrates subendocardial late gadolinium enhancement (*arrows*) within the septal segments, compatible with prior infarct.

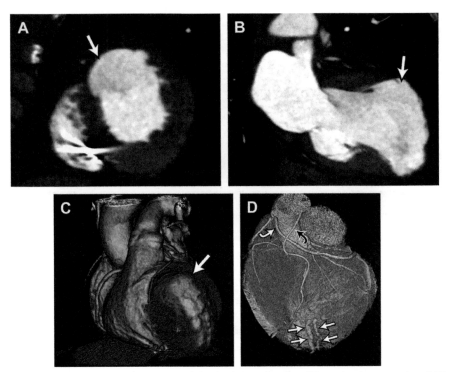

Fig. 4. Left ventricular aneurysm and Dor procedure. SA (*A*), 2-chamber (*B*), and volume-rendered 3D (*C*) reformations from a contrast-enhanced cardiac CT demonstrate an aneurysm (*arrow*) extending from the mid to anterior apical segments at the site of prior MI in the LAD territory. (*D*) A volume-rendered 3D reconstruction from a contrast-enhanced cardiac CT shows a left internal mammary artery to LAD artery bypass graft (*curved black arrow*), a saphenous vein graft (SVG) to oblique marginal artery bypass (*curved white arrow*), and a partly included SVG to right coronary artery bypass. There has been prior surgical repair of a left ventricle aneurysm (also known as the Dor procedure) (*straight white arrows*).

segment of myocardium. It typically yields attenuation between 25 and 80 HU, and a threshold of less than 65 HU may serve as a threshold for distinguishing it from normal myocardium, which typically exhibits an average attenuation near 100 HU.[11]

Dressler Syndrome

Postmyocardial infarction syndrome, also referred to as Dressler syndrome, is a combination of fever, chest pain, pleurisy, and pericarditis that occurs 2 to 3 weeks following MI and tends to recur. The cause is unclear but is probably an immune-mediated response. Historically, it was thought to be relatively common following MI, but the entity is quickly vanishing, likely due to the use of medicines such as angiotensin-converting enzyme inhibitors, statins, and beta-blockers.[12] Normal pericardium is usually less than 2 mm in thickness, and a thickness greater than 4 mm is suggestive of pericarditis. Pericardial effusion may be seen. In the appropriate setting, this can represent Dressler syndrome (**Fig. 6**). Calcifications and evidence of interventricular dependence on cine imaging

(such as septal bounce) are especially suggestive of constrictive pericarditis.[13]

CLINICAL AND IMAGING MIMICKERS

MI has clinical manifestations and imaging findings that are usually characteristic and definitive; however, some conditions may resemble or simulate MI. This section is divided into clinical and imaging mimickers. Clinical mimickers are conditions with signs and symptoms similar to MI that may be differential diagnostic considerations. Imaging mimickers include imaging findings that can simulate an MI.

Clinical Mimickers

Some clinical conditions may be accompanied by acute chest pain, elevated troponins, and electrocardiographic (ECG) changes simulating acute MI. The importance of early intervention in patients with acute MI leads to prompt invasive coronary angiography, and in these patients, no culprit lesion will be found. This clinical scenario is not an uncommon one as the false positive rate of

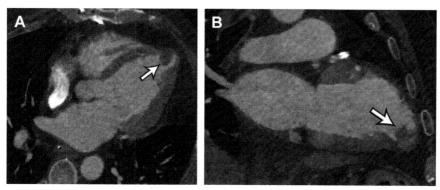

Fig. 5. Ventricular thrombus. Three-chamber (*A*) and 2-chamber (*B*) views from a contrast-enhanced cardiac CT show low-attenuation masslike density within the left ventricular apex (*arrow*) compatible with thrombus, a complication of focally decreased ventricular function as a result of chronic MI.

ST-segment elevation MI as reported in the literature is as high as 36%.[14]

Table 1 summarizes some of the most common causes of acute chest pain (cardiac or noncardiac origin).

Myocarditis

Patients with myocarditis may present with oppressive acute chest pain. Although typically seen in fewer than half of presenting patients, ECG changes similar to those seen with infarction

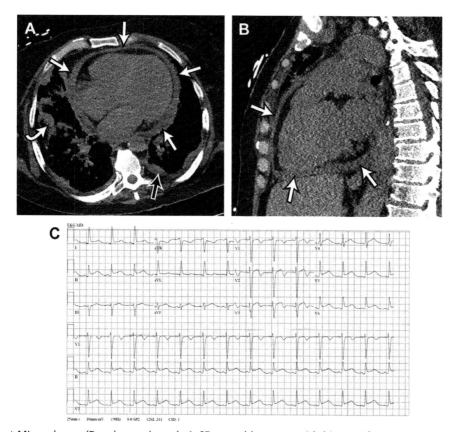

Fig. 6. Post-MI syndrome (Dressler syndrome). A 65-year-old woman with history of recent MI presented with chest pain and diffuse ST elevation on ECG. Axial (*A*) and sagittal (*B*) reconstructions from a noncontrast routine CT show a circumferential pericardial effusion (*white arrows*) that was new since the patient's discharge. Multifocal areas of consolidation were related to pulmonary edema (*curved arrow*), and a small left pleural effusion was present (*black arrow*). The patient's 12-lead ECG (*C*) shows ST segment elevation in most leads, compatible with pericarditis. The patient was diagnosed with Dressler syndrome on the basis of clinical and imaging findings.

Table 1	
Common causes of acute chest pain	
Cardiac	**Noncardiac**
Acute coronary syndrome	Aortic dissection
• ST elevation MI	Pulmonary embolism
• Non-ST elevation MI	Pneumothorax
• Unstable angina	Pneumonia
Myocarditis	Peptic ulcer disease
Pericarditis	Gastroesophageal
Stress-induced	reflux disease
cardiomyopathy	Esophageal perforation
Arrhythmia	Costochondritis
	Acute rib fracture

may be present and include ST-segment, T-wave, and Q-wave abnormalities. Bundle branch blocks or arrhythmias may also be seen.[15] Elevated troponin T can be seen in up to 35% of patients.[16] Coronary CT angiography (CTA) may be beneficial by ruling out coronary artery disease with a high negative predictive value close to 100%. Echocardiogram and nuclear medicine play a limited role in the diagnosis of myocarditis, and MR imaging is the imaging modality of choice for diagnosis.[17]

Stress-induced cardiomyopathy, also known as Takotsubo cardiomyopathy or broken heart syndrome, is characterized by transient apical systolic dysfunction. This myocardial stunning is hypothesized to be secondary to saturation of apical catecholamine receptors by adrenaline and noradrenaline released in response to a stressful situation. Similar to myocarditis, Takotsubo cardiomyopathy can simulate an infarction with the same clinical manifestations, but it occurs immediately after an event with great emotional stress. It typically presents in absence of obstructive coronary artery disease. Most patients have a full

recovery after a few weeks. On imaging, the typical appearance is dilation and akinesia of the myocardium affecting the apical and midregions with basal hyperkinesia.[18] The appearance has been described as apical ballooning, which resembles the shape of the Japanese octopus trap (takotsubo).

IMAGING MIMICKERS
Physiologic Fatty Infiltration

Fatty metaplasia is a common finding in chronic MI; however, myocardial fat be an incidental finding in normal hearts (Fig. 7). Deposits of fat can be seen with lipomatous hypertrophy of the interatrial septum, arrhythmogenic right ventricular dysplasia/cardiomyopathy, muscular dystrophy, and lipomas. Physiologic myocardial fat frequently occurs in the free wall of the right ventricle and is seen with increasing frequency and amount with increasing age. On autopsy, the reported prevalence in otherwise normal hearts approaches 85%.[19] By CT, the prevalence of right ventricular fat infiltration is 17% to 43%.[20,21] In contrast to fatty metaplasia secondary to MI, myocardium with physiologic fat shows no motion abnormality on retrospective CT, does not typically match a coronary artery territory, and is usually not linear and subendocardial in nature.

Ventricular Aneurysm

Chronic MI may lead to aneurysm formation, but there are several additional causes of ventricular aneurysm that may be encountered. Chagas disease, caused by the parasite *Trypanosoma cruzi*, may lead to irreversible myocardial damage and results in an apical aneurysm in half of the patients.[22] To distinguish it from sequelae of MI,

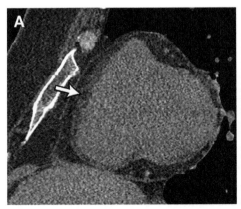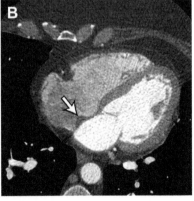

Fig. 7. (*A*) A short axis reformation from a noncontrast chest CT shows fat attenuation within the right ventricular free wall (*arrow*). Right ventricular myocardial fat is a common finding in normal patients. (*B*) An axial reconstruction from a contrast-enhanced CT shows fat attenuation within the interatrial septum consistent with lipomatous hyperplasia of the interatrial septum, a benign entity.

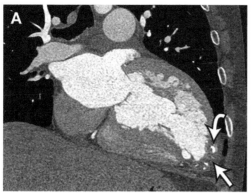
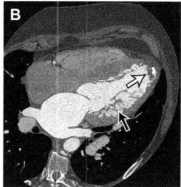

Fig. 8. Left ventricular noncompaction cardiomyopathy with thrombus. Two-chamber (*A*) and 4-chamber (*B*) views from a contrast-enhanced cardiac CT show prominent trabeculations within the entire ventricular lumen (*black arrow*) compatible with left ventricular noncompaction cardiomyopathy. In this scenario, the thrombus (*straight arrow*) with calcification (*curved arrow*) is associated with the cardiomyopathy and not underlying MI.

there is no obstructive coronary disease on imaging. Ventricular aneurysms can also occur under conditions in which the myocardium is disorganized and weak as in noncompaction cardiomyopathy (**Fig. 8**).[23] The aneurysm in noncompaction may also be congenital.[24] Midventricular hypertrophic cardiomyopathy can lead to apical aneurysms. The pathophysiology leading to aneurysm formation in these patients is unclear but may be related to midventricular systolic cavity obliteration.

Ventricular Diverticulum

Ventricular diverticula are usually observed at the apex. Similar to aneurysms, they contain all 3 layers of the ventricular wall. Distinguishing them from aneurysms, diverticula have a narrow neck, and differentiating them from pseudoaneurysms, they do contract synchronously with the left

ventricle (**Fig. 9**).[25] Pseudoaneurysms are also exceedingly rare at the apex, and in the rare cases where they are seen, they are usually associated with prior instrumentation or surgery.

Beam Hardening Artifact

If a very dense element, such as concentrated intraluminal contrast, is encountered by the polyenergetic x-ray beam in CT, lower-energy photons are selectively attenuated resulting in a beam composed of only higher-energy photons (beam hardening). These higher-energy photons will be less attenuated by remaining tissues, and when they reach the CT detector, they hence result in a higher signal than would have otherwise been expected. Erroneously, lower attenuation values are assigned to voxels along the x-ray path, contributing to the formation of dark bands. These dark bands may project into the myocardium,

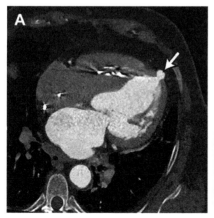
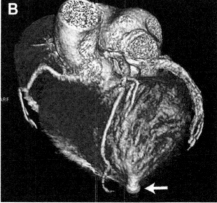

Fig. 9. Apical diverticulum. Four-chamber (*A*) and volume-rendered 3D (*B*) reformations from a contrast-enhanced cardiac CT show a small, focal outpouching extending from the apex of the left ventricle (*arrow*). True apical diverticulum is uncommon and is a normal variant. It shows contraction on functional imaging, distinguishing them from aneurysms and pseudoaneurysms.

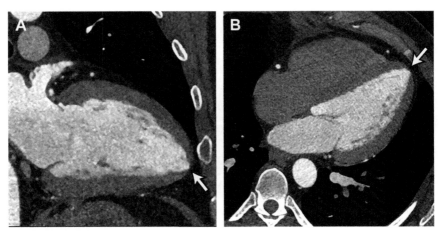

Fig. 10. Apical thin point. Two-chamber (*A*) and 4-chamber (*B*) reformations from a contrast-enhanced cardiac CT show the apical thin point (*arrow*), a normal structure that can be identified in nearly all normal patients and should not be confused with thinned, infarcted myocardium.

especially the subendocardial myocardium adjacent to the dense left ventricular lumen, simulating an area of myocardial hypoperfusion.[26]

NORMAL STRUCTURES

Myocardial thinning is a common feature of chronic MI, and the radiologist should be aware of 2 normal features of cardiac anatomy that may mimic this. The first feature is that the left ventricle is the apical thin point (**Fig. 10**). It is particularly

conspicuous on cardiac CT because of the ability to perform multiplanar reconstructions and is a normal feature in nearly all hearts. The thin point measures 2 mm or less in 97% and 1 mm or less in 67% of normal patients.[27,28] Another normal structure that may mimic sequelae of MI is the membranous septum, located in the basal region of the interventricular septum (**Fig. 11**). The membranous septum is a thin structure; it exhibits lower attenuation than the myocardium, and it does not show contractility.

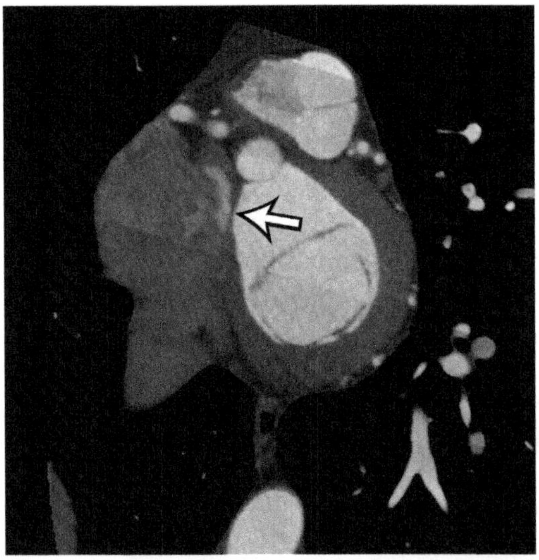

SUMMARY

Although the manifestations of chronic MI are easily identified on cardiac-CT, they can also be detected on both noncontrast and contrast-enhanced routine CT of the chest. An understanding of its imaging manifestations and potential complications is important, and this information should be included on routine radiology reports because it has important prognostic and therapeutic implications. Awareness of potential mimickers and pitfalls of MI, both clinical and imaging, can help prevent unnecessary interventions and investigations.

Fig. 11. The membranous septum. An SA reformation from a contrast-enhanced cardiac CT demonstrates the normal, thin membranous portion of the interventricular septum (*arrow*) near the base. This is a normal structure and does not represent abnormally thin infarcted myocardium.

REFERENCES

1. Shriki JE, Shinbane J, Lee C, et al. Incidental myocardial infarct on conventional nongated CT: a review of the spectrum of findings with gated CT and cardiac MRI correlation. AJR Am J Roentgenol 2012;198(3):496–504.
2. Valensi P, Lorgis L, Cottin Y. Prevalence, incidence, predictive factors and prognosis of silent myocardial infarction: a review of the literature. Arch Cardiovasc Dis 2011;104(3):178–88.

3. Gupta M, Kadakia J, Hacioglu Y, et al. Non-contrast cardiac computed tomography can accurately detect chronic myocardial infarction: validation study. J Nucl Cardiol 2011;18(1):96–103.

4. Nieman K, Cury RC, Ferencik M, et al. Differentiation of recent and chronic myocardial infarction by cardiac computed tomography. Am J Cardiol 2006; 98(3):303–8.

5. Kim RJ, Wu E, Rafael A, et al. The use of contrast-enhanced magnetic resonance imaging to identify reversible myocardial dysfunction. N Engl J Med 2000;343(20):1445–53.

6. Rodriguez-Granillo GA, Rosales MA, Baum S, et al. Early assessment of myocardial viability by the use of delayed enhancement computed tomography after primary percutaneous coronary intervention. JACC Cardiovasc Imaging 2009;2(9):1072–81.

7. Brown SL, Gropler RJ, Harris KM. Distinguishing left ventricular aneurysm from pseudoaneurysm. A review of the literature. Chest 1997;111(5):1403–9.

8. Sartipy U, Albåge A, Lindblom D. The Dor procedure for left ventricular reconstruction. Ten-year clinical experience. Eur J Cardiothorac Surg 2005; 27(6):1005–10.

9. Bisoyi S, Dash AK, Nayak D, et al. Left ventricular pseudoaneurysm versus aneurysm a diagnosis dilemma. Ann Card Anaesth 2016;19(1):169–72.

10. Hulten EA, Blankstein R. Pseudoaneurysms of the heart. Circulation 2012;125(15):1920–5.

11. Bittencourt MS, Achenbach S, Marwan M, et al. Left ventricular thrombus attenuation characterization in cardiac computed tomography angiography. J Cardiovasc Comput Tomogr 2012;6(2):121–6.

12. Bendjelid K, Pugin J. Is dressler syndrome dead? Chest 2004;126(5):1680–2.

13. Wang ZJ, Reddy GP, Gotway MB, et al. CT and MR imaging of pericardial disease. Radiographics 2003; 23(Spec No):S167–80.

14. McCabe JM, Armstrong EJ, Kulkarni A, et al. Prevalence and factors associated with false-positive ST-segment elevation myocardial infarction diagnoses at primary percutaneous coronary intervention-capable centers: a report from the Activate-SF registry. Arch Intern Med 2012;172(11):864–71.

15. Morgera T, Di Lenarda A, Dreas L, et al. Electrocardiography of myocarditis revisited: clinical and prognostic significance of electrocardiographic changes. Am Heart J 1992;124(2):455–67.

16. Lauer B, Niederau C, Kuhl U, et al. Cardiac troponin T in patients with clinically suspected myocarditis. J Am Coll Cardiol 1997;30(5):1354–9.

17. Friedrich MG, Sechtem U, Schulz-Menger J, et al. Cardiovascular magnetic resonance in myocarditis: a JACC white paper. J Am Coll Cardiol 2009; 53(17):1475–87.

18. Fernandez-Perez GC, Aguilar-Arjona JA, de la Fuente GT, et al. Takotsubo cardiomyopathy: assessment with cardiac MRI. AJR Am J Roentgenol 2010; 195(2):W139–45.

19. Tansey DK, Aly Z, Sheppard MN. Fat in the right ventricle of the normal heart. Histopathology 2005; 46(1):98–104.

20. Kirsch J, Williamson EE, Glockner JF. Focal macroscopic fat deposition within the right ventricular wall in asymptomatic patients undergoing screening EBCT coronary calcium scoring examinations. Int J Cardiovasc Imaging 2008;24(2):223–7.

21. Imada M, Funabashi N, Asano M, et al. Epidemiology of fat replacement of the right ventricular myocardium determined by multislice computed tomography using a logistic regression model. Int J Cardiol 2007;119(3):410–3.

22. Oliveira JS, Mello De Oliveira JA, Frederigue U Jr, et al. Apical aneurysm of Chagas's heart disease. Br Heart J 1981;46(4):432–7.

23. Sato Y, Matsumoto N, Yoda S, et al. Left ventricular aneurysm associated with isolated noncompaction of the ventricular myocardium. Heart Vessels 2006; 21(3):192–4.

24. Ootani K, Shimada J, Kitagawa Y, et al. Congenital left ventricular aneurysm coexisting with left ventricular non-compaction in a newborn. Pediatr Int 2014; 56(5):e72–4.

25. Rajiah P, Thomas J, Smedira N, et al. Double-chambered left ventricle due to fibroelastotic membrane: an unusual case. J Thorac Imaging 2012;27(1):W5–7.

26. Kalisz K, Buethe J, Saboo SS, et al. Artifacts at Cardiac CT: Physics and Solutions. Radiographics 2016;36(7):2064–83.

27. Bradfield JW, Beck G, Vecht RJ. Left ventricular apical thin point. Br Heart J 1977;39(7):806–9.

28. Johnson KM, Johnson HE, Dowe DA. Left ventricular apical thinning as normal anatomy. J Comput Assist Tomogr 2009;33(3):334–7.

Nonischemic Cardiomyopathies

Eric R. Flagg, MD, Ana Paula Santos Lima, MD, Kimberly G. Kallianos, MD,
Karen G. Ordovas, MD, MS*

KEYWORDS

• Cardiac CT • Cardiomyopathy • Nonischemic cardiomyopathy • Computed tomography

KEY POINTS

- Cardiac computed tomography scanning is a valuable modality for the assessment of nonischemic cardiomyopathies.
- New methods and technology are making myocardial tissue characterization with computed tomography scanning possible in ways previously only achieved by cardiac MR imaging.
- Cardiac computed tomography can offer a one-stop examination for the evaluation of cardiac function, wall motion, chamber volumes, myocardial characterization, and anatomic delineation, as well as being combined with evaluation of the coronary arteries.

INTRODUCTION

Computed tomography (CT) scanning can be used to assess the myocardium for both primary and secondary diseases. Although echocardiography is often the first-line modality, cardiac CT scanning can precisely depict the anatomy of the heart and offers certain advantages to echocardiography. Although the most common cardiac application of CT scanning is coronary imaging in the setting of ischemic heart disease, modern CT technology provides both excellent spatial and temporal resolution and can, therefore, identify both structural and functional abnormalities associated with nonischemic cardiomyopathies. Cardiac CT scanning can also aid in myocardial tissue characterization by quantification of the myocardial density and enhancement after contrast media, which are additional means to delineate myocardial injury and scar.

IMAGING TECHNIQUE
Basic Imaging Technique

Clinically important cardiac findings can be delineated at chest CT without electrocardiogram (ECG) gating,[1,2] but optimal evaluation of the cardiac anatomy and the myocardium requires high temporal resolution to minimize artifacts created by cardiac motion. Therefore, techniques are typically used in which the patient's ECG tracing is used to either selectively acquire images at specific points in the cardiac cycle or to retrospectively reconstruct images of the heart in certain segments of the cardiac cycle, techniques termed prospective triggering and retrospective gating, respectively. Both of these techniques are useful in the evaluation of nonischemic cardiomyopathies. With prospective triggering, the ECG tracing is used to selectively image during the desired cardiac phase segment. Diastolic triggering is most common, which occurs at approximately 70% to 75% of the R-R interval, because this is when cardiac motion is minimized. Although a general advantage of prospective triggering is a lower radiation dose compared with retrospective gating, in patients with cardiac arrhythmias, image quality may be poor and radiation doses may be much higher.[3] Retrospective gating involves image acquisition throughout the entire cardiac cycle with simultaneous recording of the ECG tracing.

Disclosure Statement: None of the authors have relevant disclosures.
Department of Radiology and Biomedical Imaging, University of California, San Francisco, 505 Parnassus Avenue, M-391, Box 0628, San Francisco, CA 9414, USA
* Corresponding author.
E-mail address: karen.ordovas@ucsf.edu

Radiol Clin N Am 57 (2019) 67–73
https://doi.org/10.1016/j.rcl.2018.08.003

The data can then be reconstructed into images of the heart at any phase of the cardiac cycle. This technique is useful for patients with variable heart rates and cardiac arrhythmias and additionally allows for qualitative and quantitative functional analysis through postprocessing.

Delayed Enhancement

Evaluation for myocardial delayed contrast enhancement (DCE) is a well-established technique that is based on the delayed accumulation of a contrast agent in areas of the myocardium that have an expanded extracellular space, either owing to injury to the myocytes or the accumulation of extracellular material.[4,5] It is useful for assessing for myocardial fibrosis in the setting of ischemic heart disease, and has increasingly shown value in the evaluation of nonischemic cardiomyopathy, both in terms of narrowing the differential diagnosis and contributing to prognosis of the disease.[5,6] Although DCE imaging has primarily been performed with gadolinium-enhanced cardiac MR (CMR) imaging, numerous studies have shown the feasibility and good correlation of myocardial DCE on iodinated-enhanced multidetector CT with that of DCE-CMR in the evaluation of ischemic and nonischemic cardiomyopathy.[7–9] Therefore, as CT radiation doses continue to decrease with modern CT technology, DCE-CT is an increasingly attractive alternative to DCE-CMR in patients who cannot undergo MR imaging.

Intravenous iodinated and gadolinium contrast materials have similar kinetics and, thus, imaging protocols are similar for DCE-CT and DCE-CMR. Image acquisition can be performed 5 to 15 minutes after contrast administration, although the precise acquisition timing is not well-established.[10] A limitation of DCE-CT is its inferior contrast resolution compared with DCE-CMR. However, multienergy CT has recently been shown to improve the performance of DCE-CT, specifically with the use of monoenergetic image reconstructions.[4,11]

Emerging Applications

Although the presence of myocardial delayed enhancement is an excellent indicator of focal areas of fibrosis, there are limitations to the quantification and reproducibility of measurements in diffuse myocardial diseases. Determination of extracellular volume (ECV) is a method of quantifying diffuse myocardial fibrosis or exogenous deposition in cardiomyopathies because it expands in both processes. This technique has been applied using contrast-enhanced CMR imaging and T1 mapping techniques.[12] However,

cardiac CT scanning has been preliminarily shown to be a comparable alternative in quantifying ECV. A prospective study by Lee and colleagues[13] involving 23 patients with nonischemic cardiomyopathy showed good agreement between equilibrium-enhanced CT and CMR imaging in the determination of ECV. Furthermore, estimation of ECV on the basis of material decomposition with multienergy noncontrast CT may even be feasible, as suggested by a recent animal phantom study.[14]

Another potential use of multienergy cardiac CT scanning is quantification of myocardial iron deposition. Commonly performed with T2* values in CMR imaging, several studies have also shown good correlation between CT scanning and CMR imaging in myocardial iron quantification with shorter examination times for CT scanning.[11] These expanding applications of CT scanning in the evaluation of nonischemic cardiomyopathies are only likely to increase with further advances in imaging technology and understanding of myocardial pathophysiology.

IMAGING FINDINGS AND PATHOLOGY
General

The most important features to evaluate the presence of cardiac disease on CT scans pertain to morphology and size of cardiac chambers and great vessels. When cardiac CT scanning is performed with a retrospective gating technique, evaluation of global and regional myocardial contractility can be performed. Finally, myocardial wall thickness, density, and enhancement pattern can aid in the characterization of nonischemic myocardial diseases.

Nonischemic Dilated Cardiomyopathy

Dilated cardiomyopathy can be readily diagnosed on cardiac CT scanning based on enlargement of the ventricles. In patients without an ischemic etiology, dilated cardiomyopathy is most commonly idiopathic, but can be seen as a sequela of myocarditis, drug toxicity, radiation, iron deposition, and systemic diseases, among other causes. The most common imaging presentation is a dilated left ventricle, with a maximum internal transverse diameter in the axial plane of greater than 5.6 cm,[15] with associated myocardial wall thinning (Fig. 1). On cine images, there is global hypokinesis, with no evidence of regional dysfunction. Ventricular volumes and ejection fraction can be quantified when multiple phases of the cardiac cycle are available for visualization of cine images. As seen with other modalities, normal ranges for indexed ventricular volumes and function are available for cardiac CT scanning.[16–18] The most

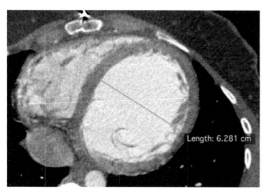

Fig. 1. Idiopathic dilated cardiomyopathy. Electrocardiographic-gated computed tomography image of the heart in the axial plane with intravenous contrast showing an enlarged left ventricle in a patient who had no evidence of coronary artery disease or other explanatory condition for dilated cardiomyopathy.

common imaging features that strengthen the diagnostic possibility of a nonischemic etiology for dilated cardiomyopathy are the absence of coronary calcifications and the absence of regional wall thinning or regional contractile abnormality. Delayed cardiac CT images can also rarely demonstrate myocardial enhancement in a nonischemic distribution, such as midwall or subepicardial.

Myocarditis

Myocarditis usually presents as chest pain, arrhythmias, and acute heart failure symptoms in young patients. It is usually caused by a viral infection and is commonly associated with pericarditis. On cardiac CT scans in the acute setting, the most common abnormality is seen on cine images, with global hypokinesis associated with normal ventricular size and normal myocardial wall thickness. Additionally, patchy delayed myocardial enhancement may occasionally be seen on cardiac CT in a transmural or subepicardial pattern.[19] Very frequently, patients have a pericardial effusion in conjunction with pericardial thickening and enhancement, consistent with associated pericarditis. If cardiac function is severely depressed, cardiac thrombi may be seen (**Fig. 2**). More commonly, cardiac CT scanning will show findings of sequela of myocarditis, such as myocardial calcification (**Fig. 3**) or fatty replacement in a nonischemic distribution, myocardial wall thinning, and ventricular dilatation.

Hypertrophic Cardiomyopathy

Hypertrophic cardiomyopathy (HCM) is characterized by left ventricular hypertrophy unexplained by another disease process, either cardiac or systemic, and is caused by a variety of cardiac sarcomere mutations. With an overall prevalence of 0.2% in the United States, it is clinically characterized by sudden cardiac death, heart failure, and arrhythmias. The penetrance of the HCM genotype is variable, and patients carrying HCM-related mutations may have morphologically normal myocardium and be asymptomatic, sometimes termed subclinical HCM.[20] There are several phenotypes of hypertrophy in HCM. The most common form is asymmetric septal hypertrophy, which is characterized on cardiac CT scanning by a septal thickness of greater than 15 mm or a ratio of septal thickness to inferior wall thickness of greater than 1.5 at the midventricular level (**Fig. 4**). The region of maximal hypertrophy often occurs in the mid and basal level anteroseptal wall, a phenotype that is strongly associated with left ventricular outflow

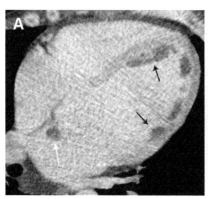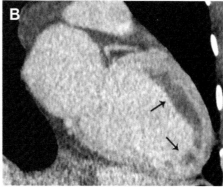

Fig. 2. Drug-induced myocarditis. Contrast-enhanced computed tomography image of the heart reformatted in the 4-chamber plane (*A*) and the vertical long axis plane (*B*) showing a multiple hypodense filling defects along the left ventricle wall (*black arrows*), consistent with ventricular thrombi. Thrombi may also form in the atria in patients with severely depressed cardiac function (*white arrow*).

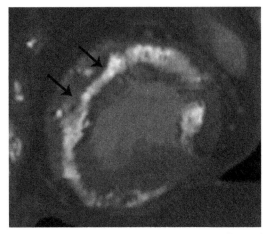

Fig. 3. Viral myocarditis. Contrast-enhanced computed tomography (CT) image of the heart in the short-axis plane showing extensive left ventricular mural calcification (*arrow*) in a patient with a history of viral myocarditis. This is the most commonly seen sequela of myocarditis on CT.

tract obstruction. In addition to septal hypertrophy causing subaortic stenosis, cine cardiac CT images reconstructed in the 3- or 4-chamber plane can demonstrate systolic anterior motion of the mitral valve leaflets, a phenomenon that further obstructs outflow and may cause mitral regurgitation. Other phenotypic forms of HCM include

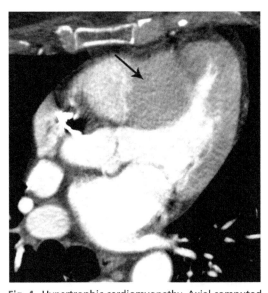

Fig. 4. Hypertrophic cardiomyopathy. Axial computed tomography image of the heart with intravenous contrast demonstrating marked asymmetric thickening of the interventricular septum (*black arrow*) with normal thickness of the lateral wall of the left ventricle, meeting criteria for the septal form of hypertrophic cardiomyopathy.

concentric (symmetric), apical (**Fig. 5**), midventricular, and masslike hypertrophy. Similar to CMR images, cardiac CT scans may show delayed enhancement, which often occurs in the right ventricle insertion points or the region of maximal hypertrophy and is an independent poor prognostic indicator.[7,21]

Cardiac Sarcoidosis

Sarcoidosis is a systemic disorder with a complex and poorly understood etiology that is characterized by granulomatous inflammation. It can affect virtually any organ system and is widely variable in its clinical presentation. Cardiac involvement is clinically established in 5% of those affected overall, but with an even higher prevalence at autopsy, and often presents with cardiac arrhythmias. However, the diagnosis can be clinically challenging and sometimes requires endomyocardial biopsy. Imaging plays an important role, and although CMR imaging and PET scans are the predominant modalities used, cardiac CT scans can also delineate abnormalities characteristic of cardiac sarcoidosis. In the acute phase of disease, cardiac CT scans can demonstrate myocardial wall thickening, either focal or diffuse. Chronic disease can manifest as wall thinning, reflective of fibrosis, and these regions may show delayed enhancement on cardiac CT scans. The pattern of delayed enhancement is characteristically epicardial or mesocardial, often involving the basal septum and sometimes the right ventricle. Per the JMWH revised guidelines for diagnosis of cardiac sarcoidosis, basal septal thinning, and a decreased left ventricular ejection fraction of less than 50% satisfy major criteria for diagnosis, both of which can be well-delineated by cardiac CT scans.[10,22]

Cardiac Amyloidosis

In a broad sense, amyloidosis is a protein deposition disease with a variety of causes that can have multisystem involvement and can be either primary or secondary. The clinical presentation depends on the underlying etiology, but cardiac amyloid deposition causes a restrictive cardiomyopathy that can lead to devastating heart failure. Diagnosis of the entity requires a high index of suspicion and multiple diagnostic tests are often used including ECG, echocardiography, CMR imaging, and sometimes myocardial biopsy. Cardiac CT scanning also has utility and often shows biventricular wall thickening and biatrial enlargement. Right atrial wall thickening can also occur and is considered a specific sign of cardiac amyloidosis. The early disease process is characterized by

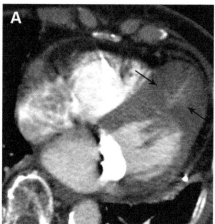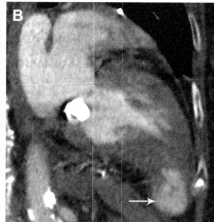

Fig. 5. Apical hypertrophic cardiomyopathy. (*A*) Contrast-enhanced computed tomography image of the heart showing marked circumferential wall thickening of the apical level left ventricle (*black arrows*) with cavity obliteration. (*B*) Image of the same patient reformatted in the vertical long-axis plane showing a focal, contrast-filled outpouching of the left ventricular apex (*white arrow*), consistent with an apical aneurysm, a known complication of the apical form of hypertrophic cardiomyopathy.

diastolic dysfunction, but cine images in more advanced disease will show global ventricular hypokinesis. A characteristically diffuse subendocardial pattern of delayed enhancement is often seen on DCE-CT, with peak delayed enhancement occurring earlier (5–7 minutes) than that seen in other cardiomyopathies.[23] As amyloid infiltration of the myocardium expands the extracellular space, it has been recently recognized that ECV is an additional powerful tool to assess for cardiac amyloidosis, and cardiac CT scans with delayed enhancement have been shown to perform well in calculating the ECV in patients with cardiac amyloidosis.[24,25]

Left Ventricular Noncompaction Cardiomyopathy

Left ventricular noncompaction is an entity in which there is an arrest of the normal myocardial compaction during embryogenesis, leading to a hypertrabeculated ventricle. It may be familial or sporadic, with several gene mutations having been associated with left ventricular noncompaction cardiomyopathy (LVNC) and the phenotype has a wide spectrum of clinical presentations. Patients may be completely asymptomatic and have normal cardiac function or they may present with heart failure, arrhythmias, or chest pain.[26] Diagnostic criteria exist for both echocardiography and CMR imaging and there is good correlation between cardiac CT scans and CMR images in the diagnosis of LVNC.[27] In patients with suspected LVNC on echocardiography, cardiac CT scans or CMR images are superior to

echocardiography for delineating the noncompacted segments and are also useful to assess for other cardiac defects that may suggest another diagnosis as the cause for hypertrabeculation. Characteristic imaging findings of LVNC at cardiac CT scans in adults include a ratio of noncompacted-to-compacted myocardium of greater than 2.3 measured in the left ventricular short axis plane at end diastole (**Fig. 6**). It commonly affects the mid and apical segments.

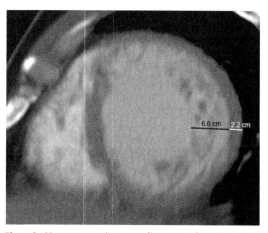

Fig. 6. Noncompaction cardiomyopathy. Contrast-enhanced cardiac computed tomography image in the short axis plane demonstrating hypertrabeculation (*black caliper*) of the nonseptal walls of the left ventricle with a thin compacted layer of myocardium (*white caliper*). The ratio of noncompacted-to-compacted myocardium in this patient is 3, meeting the criteria for noncompaction cardiomyopathy.

The compacted myocardium should appear as distinct from the endocardial noncompacted myocardium. Deep recesses within the hypertrabeculated regions are often seen and intertrabecular thrombi may be seen, because there is slow flow in these regions. Distinguishing LVNC from dilated cardiomyopathy can be challenging, because patients with LVNC often have increased left ventricular volumes and decreased systolic function.[19,26] The clinical significance, criteria for diagnosis, and treatment options of this entity are still evolving.

SUMMARY

Although not typically used as a primary modality for evaluation of nonischemic cardiomyopathies, cardiac CT scans can assess morphology, quantify function, delineate fibrosis, and likely in the near future provide tissue characterization with one examination. These attributes make cardiac CT scanning a comprehensive and powerful tool in the imaging armamentarium.

REFERENCES

1. Choy G, Kropil P, Scherer A, et al. Pertinent reportable incidental cardiac findings on chest CT without electrocardiography gating: review of 268 consecutive cases. Acta Radiol 2013;54(4):396–400.
2. Kanza RE, Allard C, Berube M. Cardiac findings on non-gated chest computed tomography: a clinical and pictorial review. Eur J Radiol 2016;85(2):435–51.
3. Desjardins B, Kazerooni EA. ECG-gated cardiac CT. AJR Am J Roentgenol 2004;182(4):993–1010.
4. Chang S, Han K, Youn JC, et al. Utility of dual-energy CT-based monochromatic imaging in the assessment of myocardial delayed enhancement in patients with cardiomyopathy. Radiology 2018;287(2):442–51.
5. Machii M, Satoh H, Shiraki K, et al. Distribution of late gadolinium enhancement in end-stage hypertrophic cardiomyopathy and dilated cardiomyopathy: differential diagnosis and prediction of cardiac outcome. Magn Reson Imaging 2014;32(2):118–24.
6. Assomull RG, Prasad SK, Lyne J, et al. Cardiovascular magnetic resonance, fibrosis, and prognosis in dilated cardiomyopathy. J Am Coll Cardiol 2006;48(10):1977–85.
7. Zhao L, Ma X, Feuchtner GM, et al. Quantification of myocardial delayed enhancement and wall thickness in hypertrophic cardiomyopathy: multidetector computed tomography versus magnetic resonance imaging. Eur J Radiol 2014;83(10):1778–85.
8. George RT, Silva C, Cordeiro MA, et al. Multidetector computed tomography myocardial perfusion imaging during adenosine stress. J Am Coll Cardiol 2006;48(1):153–60.
9. Gerber BL, Belge B, Legros GJ, et al. Characterization of acute and chronic myocardial infarcts by multidetector computed tomography: comparison with contrast-enhanced magnetic resonance. Circulation 2006;113(6):823–33.
10. Rodriguez-Granillo GA. Delayed enhancement cardiac computed tomography for the assessment of myocardial infarction: from bench to bedside. Cardiovasc Diagn Ther 2017;7(2):159–70.
11. Kalisz K, Halliburton S, Abbara S, et al. Update on cardiovascular applications of multienergy CT. Radiographics 2017;37(7):1955–74.
12. Haaf P, Garg P, Messroghli DR, et al. Cardiac T1 mapping and extracellular volume (ECV) in clinical practice: a comprehensive review. J Cardiovasc Magn Reson 2016;18(1):89.
13. Lee HJ, Im DJ, Youn JC, et al. Myocardial extracellular volume fraction with dual-energy equilibrium contrast-enhanced cardiac CT in nonischemic cardiomyopathy: a prospective comparison with cardiac MR imaging. Radiology 2016;280(1):49–57.
14. Kumar V, McElhanon KE, Min JK, et al. Non-contrast estimation of diffuse myocardial fibrosis with dual energy CT: a phantom study. J Cardiovasc Comput Tomogr 2018;12(1):74–80.
15. Kathiria NN, Devcic Z, Chen JS, et al. Assessment of left ventricular enlargement at multidetector computed tomography. J Comput Assist Tomogr 2015;39(5):794–6.
16. Stojanovska J, Prasitdumrong H, Patel S, et al. Reference absolute and indexed values for left and right ventricular volume, function and mass from cardiac computed tomography. J Med Imaging Radiat Oncol 2014;58(5):547–58.
17. Fuchs A, Mejdahl MR, Kuhl JT, et al. Normal values of left ventricular mass and cardiac chamber volumes assessed by 320-detector computed tomography angiography in the Copenhagen General Population Study. Eur Heart J Cardiovasc Imaging 2016;17(9):1009–17.
18. Lin FY, Devereux RB, Roman MJ, et al. Cardiac chamber volumes, function, and mass as determined by 64-multidetector row computed tomography: mean values among healthy adults free of hypertension and obesity. JACC Cardiovasc Imaging 2008;1(6):782–6.
19. Kalisz K, Rajiah P. Computed tomography of cardiomyopathies. Cardiovasc Diagn Ther 2017;7(5):539–56.
20. American College of Cardiology Foundation/American Heart Association Task Force on Practice; American Association for Thoracic Surgery; American Society of Echocardiography; American Society of Nuclear Cardiology; Heart Failure Society of America; Heart Rhythm Society; Society for Cardiovascular Angiography and Interventions; Society of

Thoracic Surgeons, Gersh BJ, Maron BJ, Bonow RO, et al. 2011 ACCF/AHA guideline for the diagnosis and treatment of hypertrophic cardiomyopathy: a report of the American College of Cardiology Foundation/American Heart Association Task Force on Practice Guidelines. J Thorac Cardiovasc Surg 2011;142(6):e153–203.

21. Chun EJ, Choi SI, Jin KN, et al. Hypertrophic cardiomyopathy: assessment with MR imaging and multidetector CT. Radiographics 2010;30(5):1309–28.

22. Jeudy J, Burke AP, White CS, et al. Cardiac sarcoidosis: the challenge of radiologic-pathologic correlation: from the radiologic pathology archives. Radiographics 2015;35(3):657–79.

23. Sparrow PJ, Merchant N, Provost YL, et al. CT and MR imaging findings in patients with acquired heart disease at risk for sudden cardiac death. Radiographics 2009;29(3):805–23.

24. Chevance V, Damy T, Tacher V, et al. Myocardial iodine concentration measurement using dual-energy computed tomography for the diagnosis of cardiac amyloidosis: a pilot study. Eur Radiol 2018; 28(2):816–23.

25. Treibel TA, Bandula S, Fontana M, et al. Extracellular volume quantification by dynamic equilibrium cardiac computed tomography in cardiac amyloidosis. J Cardiovasc Comput Tomogr 2015;9(6): 585–92.

26. Zuccarino F, Vollmer I, Sanchez G, et al. Left ventricular noncompaction: imaging findings and diagnostic criteria. AJR Am J Roentgenol 2015;204(5): W519–30.

27. Sidhu MS, Uthamalingam S, Ahmed W, et al. Defining left ventricular noncompaction using cardiac computed tomography. J Thorac Imaging 2014;29(1):60–6.

Computed Tomography Imaging of Cardiac Masses

Phillip M. Young, MD*, Thomas A. Foley, MD, Philip A. Araoz, MD, Eric E. Williamson, MD

KEYWORDS

- Cardiac masses • Cardiac CT • Cardiac imaging

KEY POINTS

- CT can add significant information relevant to the work-up and management of cardiac masses.
- CT is generally underused for evaluating masses, and the role will likely expand over time as the technology advances further.
- Many patients have an indication for thoracoabdominal or coronary evaluation anyway, and there is potential to add value by tailoring a single combined examination that optimizes evaluation of the cardiac mass in addition to answering other questions.

BACKGROUND

Cardiac masses are usually considered rare entities, but work-up for known, suspected, or artifactual intracardiac or juxtacardiac masses is fairly common in large medical facilities, and is challenging. First-line work-up for cardiac masses is usually echocardiography,[1] which often suffers from substantial limitations in acoustic windows, anatomic coverage, and tissue characterization ability. Although cardiac MR imaging is usually considered the most sophisticated modality for assessment and characterization of cardiac masses, in reality it suffers in many patients from relative limitations in anatomic resolution; artifacts (particularly on fast spin echo imaging used for tissue characterization); and the inherent two-dimensional planar acquisition technique, which requires a skilled operator, especially when the mass is not optimally visualized in the standard planes used for most cardiac MR examinations. In addition, many patients with malignant masses or comorbidities have trouble holding their breath for 20 or more seconds, which makes acquisition of the most helpful pulse sequence techniques difficult. MR imaging is also contraindicated in most patients with implanted cardiac devices, and for many patients an alternative advanced imaging modality is desirable.

Although not as commonly performed as echo or MR imaging, and not well supported by published guidelines,[2] cardiac computed tomography (CT) has some clear advantages and strong rationale for use as a preferred modality in evaluation of cardiac masses. Cardiac CT has fairly good capability for tissue characterization through assessment of density (distinguishing fat and calcium components from soft tissue) and perfusion. The latter is particularly helpful in establishing presence of thrombus versus enhancing tissue, and the pattern of enhancement in perfused masses may lead to insights that a mass is hypervascular, has a dominant fibrous component, or demonstrates features typical of a vascular malformation. Newer techniques, such as CT perfusion and dual-energy CT, may be useful in characterizing tissue and enhancement characteristics.

In addition, CT provides high-resolution volumetric coverage of lesions, which is unmatched by other modalities. It can be performed with dynamic assessment throughout the cardiac cycle, and allows assessment of relationship of a mass

Disclosures: Advisory Board, Arterys.
Department of Radiology, Mayo Clinic, 200 First Street Southwest, Rochester, MN 55905, USA
* Corresponding author.
E-mail address: young.phillip@mayo.edu

radiologic.theclinics.com

to myocardium, pericardium, coronary arteries, great vessels and pulmonary and systemic veins, cardiac valves, and adjacent tissues, such as lung and lymph nodes, in a way that no other imaging modality can match. All of this can aid assessment of potential for surgical resection and help inform the surgical approach. In fact, most patients with known or suspected malignant masses receive CT imaging of the chest, abdomen, and pelvis anyway to evaluate for metastatic disease. Too often, the opportunity is missed to perform a more sophisticated and comprehensive assessment of the heart during scanning that covers the anatomy anyway.

In most cases, masses are confidently characterized as benign or malignant based on morphologic features. Many benign lesions, such as thrombus, lipoma, fibroma, and myxoma, are confidently diagnosed. Malignant masses are often more challenging to specifically diagnose, but the differential diagnosis can often be narrowed, and more importantly the examination may document extent of the lesion and presence or absence of additional (extracardiac) metastatic lesions, perform preoperative coronary evaluation, and be used to help plan biopsy or resection.

TECHNICAL ISSUES

The scan protocol used can vary given the variety of clinical scenarios that may precede referral to CT.

If possible, clinical history and any available prior imaging (echocardiography, prior CT of the chest, or PET scan) should be reviewed before CT imaging. Our general practice for most examinations on patients sent without a known diagnosis is to obtain three-phase imaging (gated noncontrast, coronary CT angiography phase, and ~20-second delay phase) imaging for most examinations. For selected examinations where the presence of fibrotic tissue is suspected, a 5- or 6-minute delay low kilovolt scan is also obtained. We use retrospective gating with tube current modulation and iterative reconstruction almost universally for these examinations because multiphase evaluation can provide critical information about the extent and mobility of a mass and its effect on adjacent cardiac and noncardiac structures; ventricular and valvular function; and coronary artery anatomy, patency, and relationship of the coronary tree to the mass. If available, dual-energy or perfusion techniques are selectively used to gain additional information about the mass characteristics or usefully display that information to referring clinicians. If the scan is to be combined with imaging of the chest or abdomen

and pelvis, we generally scan the whole chest on the delay phase outlined previously, and can obtain abdominal and pelvic phase imaging with the same contrast bolus on the portal venous phase, 70 seconds after contrast injection.

SPECIFIC MASSES
Benign Masses

Thrombus
Thrombus is the most commonly encountered cardiac mass. Typically, thrombi appear as nonenhancing intracavitary filling defects that are often lobular, but may be linear or laminar, especially in the chronic state. They often occur in areas of low flow, such as in an atrial appendage, adjacent to a hypokinetic or akinetic segment, or in a ventricle with an aneurysm or reduced ejection fraction. They also may occur along valves especially in patients with hypercoagulable states (**Fig. 1**), or on catheters or device leads. In patients with implanted devices that have right atrial and ventricular leads, it is fairly common for thrombus to form along a site where the leads can rub together, and the insulating material around the leads can be damaged by the wear. Thrombi are almost always nonenhancing, and sometimes can calcify if chronic. Rarely, they may enhance in the chronic state because of neovascularity.[3]

Lipomatous hypertrophy of atrial septum
Lipomatous hypertrophy of the atrial septum is an entity that is characterized by mass-like accumulation of benign adipocytes in the atrial septum, generally in asymptomatic older patients (>75 years).[4] Metabolic activity in "brown" fat in these lesions may cause uptake on 18F-fluorodeoxyglucose PET/CT, and cause false-positive findings during cancer staging examinations, and the echogenic mass-like appearance may be concerning and difficult to characterize on echocardiography. However, these are easily characterized on CT, with classic fat attenuation, lobular appearance in the basal interatrial septum and posterior right atrium or SVC, and sometimes surrounding an undisturbed sinoatrial nodal artery (**Fig. 2**).

Myxoma
Myxomas are the second most common primary cardiac tumor in adults.[5] They are benign lesions characterized by myxoid tissue and spindle cells, often arising along the left side of the interatrial septum, sometimes with a stalk. They are more common in women than men, by a nearly 2:1 ratio.[6]

CT typically demonstrates a low-attenuation (usually water values for Hounsfield units), lobular

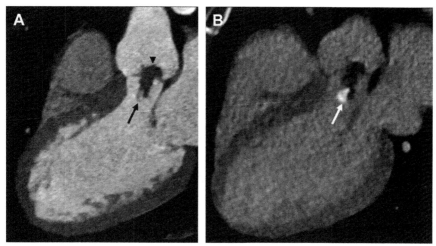

Fig. 1. CT in a 50-year-old woman who presented initially to neurology with worsening gait instability and slurred speech. MR imaging of the brain revealed multiple small supratentorial and infratentorial infarcts of varying ages in different vascular territories suspicious for embolic source. Transesophageal echocardiography demonstrated a large mobile mass on the noncoronary aortic valve cusp with varying echodensities. The interpretation was indeterminate, and the mass was given a differential diagnosis of atypical valvular myxoma, thrombus, atypical vegetation, or papillary fibroelastoma. CT was performed to further characterize the mass and perform preoperative coronary artery assessment to minimize the risk of embolization with instrumentation near the mass during invasive coronary angiography. (A) Three-chamber multiplanar reformatted image from the coronary CT angiography demonstrates a hypoattenuating mass (arrow) arising from the ventricular and aortic (arrowhead) surfaces of the noncoronary leaflet. (B) A 20-second delay phase image demonstrates nonenhancement of the mass and more clearly defines partial calcification of the mass (arrow). The findings are most suggestive of chronic thrombus, a diagnosis that was confirmed after resection.

mass with or without a stalk, usually attached to the left side of the atrial septum (**Fig. 3**). Enhancement is typically absent or minimal. Calcification may be present in some cases.

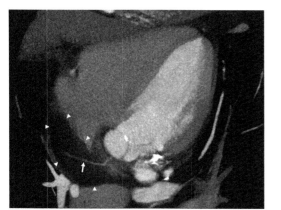

Fig. 2. A 70-year-old man developed paroxysmal atrial fibrillation and had an echocardiogram obtained that demonstrated a large, indeterminate echogenic mass. Cardiac CT was obtained to further evaluate this mass and evaluate patency of prior coronary bypass grafts. Oblique thin maximum intensity projection demonstrates a fat-attenuation right atrial mass attached to the posterior interatrial septum and right atrial wall (arrowheads) with the sinoatrial nodal artery running through it, undisturbed. This is classic mass-like lipomatous hypertrophy of the interatrial septum (arrow).

Papillary fibroelastoma

Papillary fibroelastomas frequently have a classic appearance on imaging, arising from a stalk attached to a valvular surface. Larger papillary fibroelastomas typically demonstrate a classic "frond-like" appearance that has been likened to

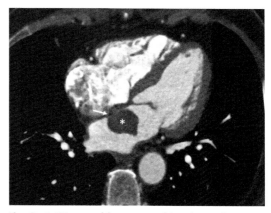

Fig. 3. A 67-year-old woman with a large, homogeneous, water-attenuation nonenhancing mass in the left atrium (asterisk), attached to the fossa ovalis (arrow). Cardiac CT clearly characterized the lesion as a benign myxoma, and was useful in preoperatively clearing the coronary arteries as part of a standard CT angiography for preoperative robotic surgery protocol.

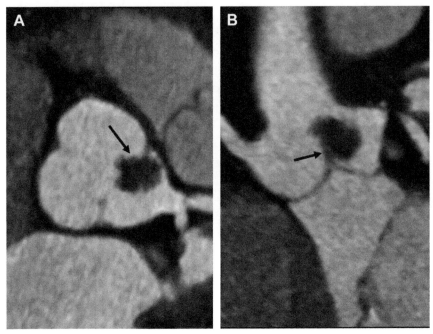

Fig. 4. Cardiac CT images in an 83-year-old man who had an aortic valve mass detected on transesophageal echocardiography performed during work-up for transient ischemic attacks. CT angiography was performed for additional evaluation of the mass and of the coronary arteries for preoperative clearance to avoid placing a catheter near the mass during conventional angiography. Oblique short (*A*) and long (*B*) images of the aortic valve demonstrate a lobular 1.5-cm mass with frond-like excrescences and a short stalk attaching it to the free edge of the left coronary cusp (*arrow*). The patient underwent successful resection.

a sea anemone or broccoli floret. However, smaller lesions may not demonstrate this as clearly on some imaging modalities, especially if the spatial resolution is not sufficient. CT can provide excellent characterization of many of these lesions owing to the high spatial resolution (**Fig. 4**).

Hematoma

Hematomas occasionally are confusing on alternative imaging modalities. They can appear mass-like and echogenic on echocardiography, and may be incompletely imaged. On CT or MR imaging performed covering the chest for noncardiac indications, they can appear as mixed density or rim enhancing, which can further cloud the picture. Imaging in multiple phases of enhancement may be helpful in some cases (**Fig. 5**). They demonstrate no internal enhancement with intravenous contrast, and can have calcific components when chronic.

Malignant Masses

Metastases

Cardiac metastases are more than an order of magnitude more common than primary cardiac malignancies[7] and imaging appearances vary substantially based on the primary tissue type and

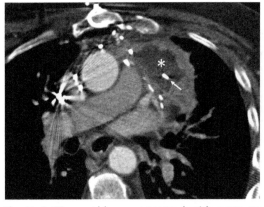

Fig. 5. A 68-year-old man presented with acute on chronic decompensated heart failure in the setting of ischemic cardiomyopathy. He had a prior history of four-vessel coronary artery bypass grafting 12 years previously. In addition to reduced left ventricular ejection fraction (30%) with regional wall motion abnormalities, echocardiography demonstrated an echogenic mass along the basal anterior wall of the left ventricle, lateral to the pulmonic valve. CT was ordered to assess the bypass grafts and the mass. Axial delayed postcontrast electrocardiogram gated image demonstrates a centrally nonenhancing, peripherally enhancing mass (*asterisk*) containing a surgical clip (*arrow*) along the course of an occluded bypass graft. The findings are indicative of a chronic hematoma.

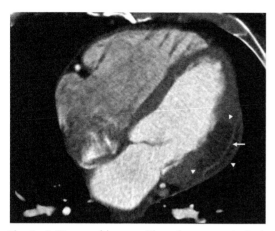

Fig. 6. A 55-year-old man with melanoma metastasis to the left ventricle. Because the patient needed follow-up of lung lesions, CT was used to image both areas of concern. Initial oblique multiplanar reformatted CT image demonstrates an infiltrative hypoenhancing mass in the lateral wall of the left ventricle (*arrowheads*), which surrounds an obtuse marginal branch of the circumflex coronary artery (*arrow*).

location. Often, the patient has a known primary tumor and additional metastatic lesions at the time of presentation, facilitating a correct diagnosis. CT is useful to confirm the presence of metastatic lesions incompletely characterized with other modalities (eg, whole-body PET or chest CT), distinguish whether an incidental lesion is malignant or benign; evaluate complications, such as ventricular or valvular dysfunction, inflow or outflow obstruction, pleural or pericardial involvement; or to evaluate response to therapy.

Although MR imaging is more commonly thought of as a gold standard noninvasive imaging modality for evaluating cardiac masses, with metastases the diagnosis is often known or suspected and the tissue characterization potential of MR imaging may not be as critical for evaluating metastases as in primary tumors. Rather, careful anatomic delineation of the mass may be sufficient. Advantages of CT include substantially higher spatial resolution, three-dimensional volumetric coverage, and better ability to visualize epicardial coronary arteries and mediastinal structures, which may help in potential surgical planning. There is also the ability to combine this examination with CT of the chest, which many patients with a known or suspected malignancy get anyway. CT can also provide useful information about response to therapy for a lesion by assessing changes in three-dimensional size, perfusion characteristics, and calcification (**Fig. 6**) that are arguably superior to any other imaging modality.

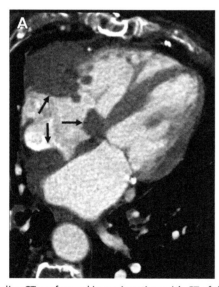
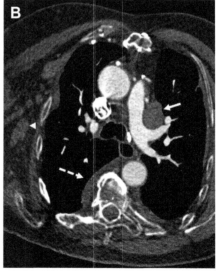

Fig. 7. Cardiac CT performed in conjunction with CT of the chest, abdomen, and pelvis in an 85-year-old man with a tricuspid valve mass seen on echocardiography and a history of non-Hodgkin lymphoma thought to be in remission. (*A*) Axial thick multiplanar reformat image demonstrates an infiltrative, enhancing mass involving the right atrioventricular groove, septal and anterior tricuspid leaflets, and posterior interatrial septum (*arrows*). (*B*) Full field of view chest reconstruction demonstrates additional enlarged left hilar (*arrow*) and right axillary (*arrowhead*) lymph nodes and an extrapleural mass in the right posterior hemithorax (*dashed arrow*). These findings are all typical features of lymphoma. The extent of the cardiac component was more clearly delineated with CT than with either transthoracic or transesophageal echocardiography, and the additional lesions seen in the chest add to the diagnostic confidence and are easier to biopsy than the cardiac lesions.

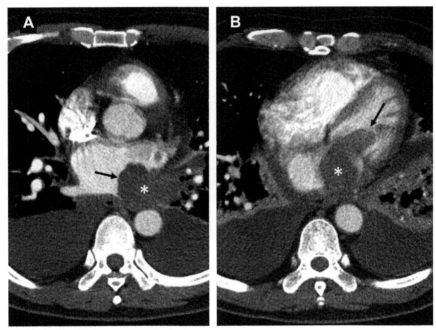

Fig. 8. CT images in a 50-year-old man with undifferentiated high-grade pleomorphic sarcoma. The patient presented with 2 months of progressive shortness of breath, coughing, and orthopnea. CT was performed to exclude pulmonary embolus, but demonstrated a large, lobular mass arising from the posterior left atrial wall (*asterisks*), occluding the left inferior pulmonary vein (*arrow* in A), and prolapsing through the mitral valve and partially obstructing mitral inflow (*arrow* in B). There are bilateral pleural effusions from pulmonary venous congestion.

Lymphoma

Although generally thought to be rare, the incidence of cardiac involvement in patients with lymphoma has probably been underestimated, and autopsy studies have reported 8% to 20% of lymphoma patients may have cardiac involvement.[8]

Primary cardiac lymphoma accounts for 1% to 2% of all cardiac neoplasms and represents an even lesser percentage of all extranodal lymphomas.[9,10] Primary cardiac lymphomas preferentially involve the right cardiac chambers and the pericardium, and often appear as homogeneous, infiltrative, enhancing masses that cross tissue borders. These masses may appear advanced at the time of presentation, and can present with a variety of symptoms related to involvement of valves, coronary arteries or myocardium, and pericardium. In any case, CT can provide exquisite delineation and characterization of cardiac lymphoma and potential complications, and can also be used for simultaneous assessment of noncardiac lymphoma staging (**Fig. 7**).

Undifferentiated pleomorphic sarcoma

Undifferentiated or pleomorphic sarcomas include lesions that have previously been classified with other, now outdated terms, such as malignant fibrous histiocytoma and undifferentiated sarcoma, and the group as now classified represents the largest group of primary cardiac malignancies.[11]

Like cardiac myxomas, they typically arise in the left atrium, but unlike myxomas they typically arise from the posterior wall rather than the atrial septum. Morphologically, these tumors are irregular, lobular,

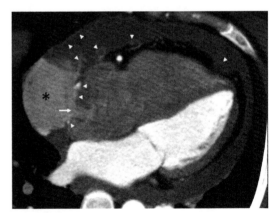

Fig. 9. Four-chamber thick multiplanar reformat CT image in a patient who presented with hemorrhagic pericardial effusion and findings suggestive of right atrial perforation on echocardiography subsequent to pericardiocentesis. CT demonstrates a ruptured (*arrow*) markedly enhancing right atrial mass with enhancing nodular tumor deposits scattered along the pericardium (*arrowheads*) and blood freely flowing into the pericardial space (*asterisk*). The findings are classic for ruptured right atrial angiosarcoma. Osseous metastatic lesions were also delineated on the scan.

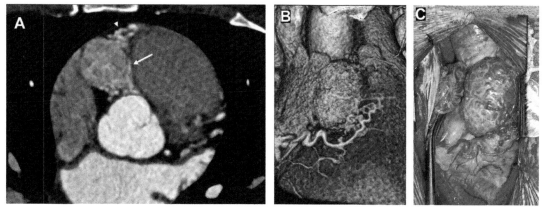

Fig. 10. A 45-year-old woman with an SDHB mutation and hypertension and suspicion for a paraganglioma. I-123 MIBG scan demonstrated mediastinal uptake and a cardiac CT was performed. Axial CT image (*A*) demonstrates a markedly hypervascular mass in the right atrioventricular groove (*arrow*) with enlarged coronary arteries and veins surrounding the lesion (*arrowhead*). The mass erodes the usual fat plane between the adjacent atrium and ventricle. Oblique reformatted CT image (*B*) showing the mass and its blood supply demonstrates high fidelity with the operative findings (*C*). This information can provide useful information to the surgeon planning to resect an infiltrative and extremely vascular mass, which can bleed extensively.

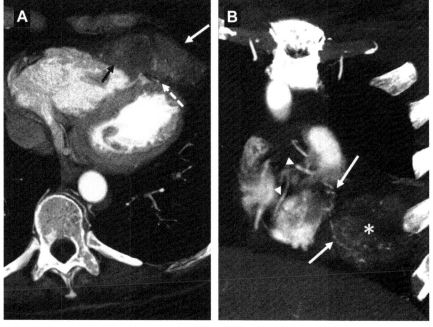

Fig. 11. A 69-year-old woman with a history of left breast cancer status post high-dose radiation therapy to the left breast 24 years previously who presented with a large mediastinal mass in the prior radiation port consistent with radiation-induced sarcoma (confirmed with biopsy). (*A*) Axial oblique multiplanar reformatted CT image demonstrates the mass (*white arrow*) invading the right ventricular apex (*black arrow*). Also notable is that the mass is separated from the left ventricular apex and left anterior descending coronary artery (*dashed arrow*) by a fat pane. (*B*) Oblique multiplanar reformatted CT image roughly equivalent to a right anterior oblique view demonstrates the relationship of the mass (*asterisk*) to its major blood supply from a conus artery branch (*arrows*) of the right coronary artery (*arrowheads*). This implies potential to resect the mass and reconstruct the right ventricular apex with little risk to the left ventricle or major epicardial coronary arteries. This was successfully accomplished and the patient was followed for several years with no evidence of local recurrence.

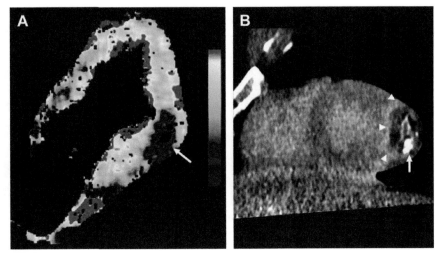

Fig. 12. CT perfusion and dual-energy imaging was performed during follow-up of patient illustrated in Fig. 6 after initiating pembrolizumab therapy. (*A*) Myocardial blood volume map demonstrates markedly low perfusion to this lesion. (*B*) Delayed postcontrast dual-energy imaging with 50-keV reconstruction in the short axis demonstrates central nonenhancement, marked peripheral enhancement (*arrowheads*), and central areas of calcification (*arrow*) have developed within this lesion. These findings in addition to complete metabolic response of this and other metastatic lesions seen on PET (not shown) indicates response to therapy.

and often invade and occlude adjacent structures, such as pulmonary veins and the left atrial appendage (**Fig. 8**). They tend to have an aggressive appearance and because of their location and degree of invasion of cardiac structures are frequently difficult or impossible to resect. Even obtaining tissue may be difficult because of their central location, but CT may be helpful in planning a potential biopsy route, such as transseptal core biopsy with intracardiac echo guidance.

Angiosarcoma

Angiosarcomas typically arise in the right atrium and right atrioventricular grove, and are the most common primary cardiac malignancy exhibiting tissue differentiation.[12–14] As their name would suggest, these tumors are extremely vascular and enhance avidly. Patients often present with chest pain or symptoms from hemorrhage of these vascular tumors, and CT is often the first imaging test in their work-up when they present emergently (eg, in the form of a CT for aortic dissection or pulmonary embolus). Echocardiography often does not evaluate the right ventricle well, and patients usually present on echo with nothing more than a complex or hemorrhagic pericardial effusion. MR imaging may be helpful, but if patients cannot hold their breath for at least 12 or 15 seconds, the images are limited. CT is useful in these cases to illustrate the presence and extent of hypervascular tumor (**Fig. 9**), and demonstrate metastatic lesions that would likely not be evident on the alternative modalities.

Paraganglioma

Paragangliomas arise from intrinsic cardiac paraganglia, which are commonly located in the atria (L > R), along atrioventricular grooves, and near the root of the aorta and pulmonary artery. They often arise in the setting of predisposing genetic mutations.[15]

On imaging they appear as well-defined, extremely vascular lesions that infiltrate adjacent tissues, and more commonly project into the pericardial space than intraluminally. They are rare in ventricular walls. Surgeons comment that these tumors are difficult to separate out from adjacent normal tissue and have to be "cut" out rather than shelled out. Because of this, and their highly vascular nature, CT imaging is helpful to define the anatomy and blood supply of these lesions (**Fig. 10**) to aid surgical planning.

FUTURE DIRECTIONS

It is difficult, perhaps impossible, to obtain enough data for a rare and heterogeneous group of tumors to prove that using CT to detect, characterize, stage, or otherwise evaluate cardiac masses improves outcome. However, it is easy to look at the impact CT has had in the rest of the body in assessing, characterizing, and staging tumors, helping plan surgery, and monitoring treatment response, and apply that knowledge to this set of diseases, especially because the latest generation of CT technologies allows virtually unparalleled potential to inform these things. In our

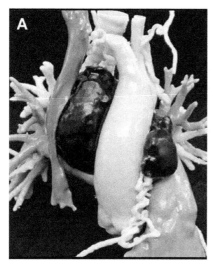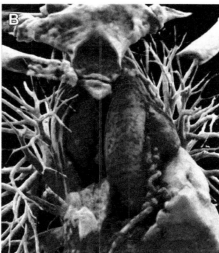

Fig. 13. A 43-year-old woman with a known SDHD mutation and history of prior paragangliomas who was found to have a large hypervascular mass centered between the great vessels. (*A*) In addition to showing typical characteristics of a cardiac paraganglioma, the CT data were used to create a three-dimensional printed model for the surgeon to review and plan what was eventually a successful surgery with modest blood loss. (*B*) In addition, the data can be used for cinematic three-dimensional rendering with a more realistic-appearing virtual model.

practice, CT has gained enough credibility to be considered essentially equivalent to a first-line test for many clinical scenarios involving work-up of a known or suspected mass. Already, volumetric multiphase imaging to assess relationship of a mass to coronary arteries, valves, pericardium, and the major structures of the heart is invaluable to helping plan a surgery (**Fig. 11**). Volume-rendered CT images, routine now in many practices, can convey potentially relevant surgical information in an intuitive fashion (see **Fig. 10**).

In addition, more recent technical advances in CT extend the ability to include advanced tissue characterization and perfusion. For example, dual-energy CT has been shown useful in distinguishing myxomas from thrombi based on iodine concentration, despite that native Hounsfield units between thrombus and myxoma were identical.[16] In our practice, we have found the ability to detect and quantify perfusion or iodine concentration extremely useful in characterizing and assessing tumors. These parameters may also be useful in assessing response of a lesion to a targeted chemotherapeutic agent, an increasing need in the age of molecular medicine (**Fig. 12**).

Three-dimensional printing using high-resolution CT data is extremely useful for presurgical planning, because it allows a surgeon to gain another level of insight by holding, turning, and manipulating a simulated model of the anatomy in question to help plan an operation before it begins. It is difficult to quantify the effect of techniques like this on outcomes, but surgical demand for these techniques has been strong in practices that have adopted

such services, especially for complex cases.[17] In these cases, many surgeons state that the ability to manipulate the anatomy in their hands and their minds can lead to a higher level of comfort entering surgery, shorter time in the operating room, and less blood loss. Advanced image processing algorithms also may help to provide some of this information with less effort and cost (**Fig. 13**).

SUMMARY

Although not generally considered a first-line imaging modality for work-up and follow-up of cardiac masses, CT is probably substantially underused for this purpose. The technology has substantial advantages over alternatives, such as echocardiography and MR imaging in some patients, and often provides additional or complementary information when used in addition to with these other modalities. In addition, many patients have an indication for a CT of the chest, abdomen, or coronary arteries anyway, and patients can benefit from a single examination tailored to multiple purposes. As CT and complementary technologies, such as three-dimensional printing and advanced modeling, continue to advance, CT will likely play an increasing role in imaging cardiac masses in many practices.

REFERENCES

1. Mankad R, Herrmann J. Cardiac tumors: echo assessment. Echo Res Pract 2016;3(4):R65–77.

2. Taylor AJ, Cerqueira M, Hodgson JM, et al. ACCF/
   SCCT/ACR/AHA/ASE/ASNC/NASCI/SCAI/SCMR 2010
   Appropriate use criteria for cardiac computed tomography. A report of the American College of Cardiology
   Foundation Appropriate Use Criteria Task Force, the
   Society of Cardiovascular Computed Tomography,
   the American College of Radiology, the American
   Heart Association, the American Society of Echocardiography, the American Society of Nuclear Cardiology,
   the North American Society for Cardiovascular Imaging, the Society for Cardiovascular Angiography and
   Interventions, and the Society for Cardiovascular Magnetic Resonance. J Cardiovasc Comput Tomogr 2010;
   4(6):407.e1-33.

3. Kim DH, Choi S, Choi JA, et al. Various findings of
   cardiac thrombi on MDCT and MRI. J Comput Assist
   Tomogr 2006;30:572–7.

4. Kuester LB, Fischman AJ, Fan CM, et al. Lipomatous
   hypertrophy of the interatrial septum: prevalence
   and features on fusion 18F fluorodeoxyglucose positron emission tomography/CT. Chest 2005;128:
   3888–93.

5. Tamin SS, Maleszewski JJ, Scott CG, et al. Prognostic and bioepidemiologic implications of papillary fibroelastomas. J Am Coll Cardiol 2015;65:
   2420–9.

6. Pinede L, Duhaut P, Loire R. Clinical presentation of
   left atrial cardiac myxoma. A series of 112 consecutive cases. Medicine 2001;80:159–72.

7. Burke A, Vermani R. Tumors of the heart and great
   vessels. Atlas of tumor pathology. 3rd Series,
   Fascicle 16. Washington (DC): Armed Forces Institute of Pathology; 1996.

8. Mahoney DO, Piekarz RL, Bandettini WP, et al. Cardiac involvement with lymphoma: a review of the
   literature. Clin Lymphoma Myeloma 2008;8(4):
   249–52.

9. Jonavicius K, Salcius K, Meskauskas R, et al. Primary cardiac lymphoma: two cases and a review
   of literature. J Cardiothorac Surg 2015;10:138.

10. Johri A, Baetz T, Isotalo PA, et al. Primary cardiac
    diffuse large B cell lymphoma presenting with supe-
    rior vena cava syndrome. Can J Cardiol 2009;25:
    e210–2.

11. Orlandi A, Ferlosio A, Roselli M, et al. Cardiac sar-
    comas: an update. J Thorac Oncol 2010;5:1483–9.

12. Leduc C, Jenkins SM, Sukov WR, et al. Cardiac an-
    giosarcoma: histopathologic, immunohistochemical,
    and cytogenetic analysis of 10 cases. Hum Pathol
    2017;60:199–207.

13. Hamidi M, Moody JS, Weigel TL, et al. Primary car-
    diac sarcoma. Ann Thorac Surg 2010;90:176–81.

14. Herrmann MA, Shankerman RA, Edwards WD, et al.
    Primary cardiac angiosarcoma: a clinicopathologic
    study of six cases. J Thorac Cardiovasc Surg
    1992;103:655–64.

15. Pasani B, Stratakis CA. SDH mutations in tumorigen-
    esis and inherited endocrine tumours: lesson from
    the phaeochromocytoma-paraganglioma syndromes.
    J Intern Med 2009;2669(1):19–42.

16. Hong YJ, Hur J, Kim YJ, et al. Dual-energy cardiac
    computed tomography for differentiating cardiac
    myxoma from thrombus. Int J Cardiovasc Imaging
    2014;30(Suppl 2):121–8.

17. Al Jabbari O, Abu Saleh WK, Patel AP, et al. Use of
    three-dimensional models to assist in the resection
    of malignant cardiac tumors. J Card Surg 2016;
    31(9):581–3.

Computed Tomography in Adult Congenital Heart Disease

Praveen Ranganath, MD[a], Satinder Singh, MD[b],
Suhny Abbara, MD[a], Prachi P. Agarwal, MD, MS[c],
Prabhakar Rajiah, MBBS, MD, FRCR[a],*

KEYWORDS

• CT • Congenital heart disease • Congenital • Heart

KEY POINTS

- The prevalence of adult congenital heart disease (ACHD) is increasing.
- Computed tomography (CT) plays an important role in the evaluation of ACHD, particularly when MR imaging is contraindicated or suboptimal or when evaluation of coronary arteries is required.
- CT protocols should be customized to answer the specific clinical question.
- The least possible radiation dose should be used without compromising on image quality.

INTRODUCTION

Although congenital heart diseases (CHD) are mostly diagnosed and treated in childhood, some remain untreated despite diagnosis in childhood and others present only in adulthood (**Table 1**).[1] Advances in cardiac surgical techniques, anesthesia, and perioperative care have significantly improved the life expectancy of patients with CHD.[2–5] Up to 95% of patients with complex CHD now survive into adulthood.[6–8] The average age of patients with CHD is continually increasing, and it is estimated that there are approximately 1 million patients with adult congenital disease (ACHD) in the United States.[8] Two-thirds of patients with CHD are now adults, and the number of these patients reaching an age older than 60 years is increasing rapidly.[9–11] Patients with ACHD need life-long care because residual or postoperative anatomic and hemodynamic abnormalities are common. Complications may develop secondary to the initial corrective surgical procedures that may require reoperation or interventions. In addition, with age, comorbidity due to acquired heart disease also comes into play. Periodic surveillance of ACHD with imaging is important to detect hemodynamic changes early, as symptoms may be late.[12] Proper imaging may be challenging due to complex anatomy and hemodynamics, requiring a thorough understanding of the CHD, common repair techniques, and common post-repair complications.

In this article, we review the role of computed tomography (CT) in the comprehensive evaluation of ACHD.

OVERVIEW OF IMAGING TECHNIQUES IN ADULT CONGENITAL HEART DISEASE

The goals of imaging in ACHD include reliable anatomic and functional assessment to guide

Disclosures: No financial disclosure or conflict of interest.
[a] Department of Radiology, Cardiothoracic Imaging, UT Southwestern Medical Center, 5323 Harry Hines Boulevard, Dallas, TX 75390-8896, USA; [b] Department of Radiology, University of Alabama Medical Center, 500 22nd Street South, Birmingham, AL 35233, USA; [c] Department of Radiology, University of Michigan, 1500 East Medical Center Drive, Ann Arbor, MI 48109, USA
* Corresponding author.
E-mail address: Prabhakar.Rajiah@utsouthwestern.edu

Radiol Clin N Am 57 (2019) 85–111
https://doi.org/10.1016/j.rcl.2018.08.013
0033-8389/19/© 2018 Elsevier Inc. All rights reserved.

Table 1 Types of adult congenital heart diseases	
Group	**Entities**
Usually diagnosed and treated in childhood	Tetralogy of Fallot (TOF) D- or L-transposition of great arteries Total anomalous pulmonary venous connection Coarctation of aorta Single ventricle
May be diagnosed in childhood, but not always treated	Atrial septal defect Ventricular septal defect Coarctation of aorta Small coronary fistulas
May be diagnosed in adults	Atrial septal defect Bicuspid aortic valve Partial anomalous pulmonary venous connection L-Transposition of great arteries Coronary artery anomalies Untreated TOF with mild right ventricular outflow tract obstruction

appropriate management. Radiography, echocardiography, CT, MR imaging, and invasive angiography are the imaging modalities commonly available for ACHD. The choice of the imaging modality is determined by the type of CHD, strengths and weaknesses of the imaging modality, availability, and institutional expertise. Often, a multimodality approach is required to glean all the necessary information.

Chest radiography provides basic information on cardiovascular anatomy and secondary changes in the lungs, pleurae, and pulmonary arteries, such as cardiac failure and pulmonary hypertension. *Transthoracic echocardiography (TTE)* is the first-line imaging technique used in ACHD due to its widespread availability, noninvasive nature, absence of radiation, and portability. Echocardiography is however limited in patients with poor acoustic windows, especially in chronic obstructive pulmonary disease, obesity, and chest wall deformities. Prior interventions and metallic devices also can make the examination challenging. Echocardiography is usually not suitable for assessment of the right ventricle (RV) due to its complex geometry, particularly with remodeling and regional dysfunction. Three-dimensional (3D) echocardiography can overcome geometric assumptions but often

underestimates volumes[13] and acoustic window restrictions remain. Moreover, systemic and pulmonary vasculature, baffles, conduits, and distal coronary arteries are often difficult to assess in an adult patient by TTE. Transesophageal echocardiography (TEE) has higher resolution than TTE and is used in specific cases, such as shunts and valvular abnormalities, but is more invasive and costlier. *MR imaging* is used when echocardiography is unable to address all the clinical questions. It can provide both anatomic and functional information without use of radiation. It is currently considered the reference standard for biventricular size and systolic function, especially for the RV,[14] although there are some disadvantages compared with CT. Additional advantages include myocardial tissue characterization, estimation of shunt and regurgitant fractions, and stress imaging, as well as evaluation of complex cardiovascular anatomy. Disadvantages of MR imaging include long examination time, claustrophobia,[15] and contraindications including metallic implants, particularly MR-incompatible pacemakers/implantable cardioverter defibrillators (ICDs).[16] Deposition of gadolinium in tissues including the brain[17] and nephrogenic systemic fibrosis in severe renal dysfunction also should be considered.[18] *Cardiac catheterization* is used to evaluate hemodynamics in ACHD and for interventional procedures. The drawbacks of cardiac catheterization are its invasiveness and associated complications as well as use of ionizing radiation.

COMPUTED TOMOGRAPHY

CT is an important imaging modality in the evaluation of ACHD with several advantages. CT is widely available and the examinations can be completed quickly, often reducing the need for anesthesia in uncooperative patients. Because of its high isovolumetric spatial resolution (on the order of 0.25 mm^3 voxel volume), CT has an advantage in imaging small structures (eg, coronary arteries). CT also offers good temporal resolution, which permits dynamic evaluation. Additional benefits include wide field of view without acoustic window restrictions and multiplanar reconstruction capabilities, which allows superior evaluation of extracardiac structures relative to echocardiography. Compared with most MR imaging sequences in which the optimal plane has to be premeditated and prescribed prospectively, CT allows for creation of any imaging plane retrospectively during the interpretation session. A disadvantage of CT, particularly in serial surveillance imaging, is the use of ionizing radiation, which may be associated with a theoretic risk of cancer, especially in younger patients and women.[19] Contrast-induced nephrotoxicity is a concern in patients with renal dysfunction, especially in patients with history of acute renal insufficiency and with repeated contrast injections; however, recent studies have shown that the incidence is low (0.85%).[20] Quantification of multivalvular regurgitation and shunts (if present at more than 1 level or if present in association with regurgitation) cannot be performed with CT. CT does not allow myocardial characterization, although some recent studies have shown the utility of delayed iodine enhancement[21] and even quantification of extracellular volume fraction.[22]

Common indications for the use of CT in ACHD are summarized in **Table 2**. CT is an attractive alternative in situations in which an MR image is either contraindicated (claustrophobia, metallic devices) or suboptimal due to patient-related factors (eg, poor compliance with breath holds, significant artifact from coils and stents). CT can provide comprehensive anatomic as well as dynamic functional information. Cardiac volumes and functions can be quantified with accuracy comparable to MR imaging.[23,24] CT is also ideal for the noninvasive evaluation of coronary arteries, including anomalies and acquired diseases. Additionally, CT offers evaluation of the entire coronary tree with a much shorter examination duration than MR imaging. CT can also evaluate extracardiac vascular and nonvascular structures, including the lungs and mediastinum. CT is an ideal imaging modality for presurgical/interventional planning, providing a roadmap of the anatomy and measurements. Presence of calcifications in aorta and conduits can be assessed. In addition, coronary CT angiography (CTA) can be used to evaluate coronary artery anatomy before redo sternotomies and major surgical interventions. Using the isotropic CT data, 3D models can be printed, which can be used by the surgeon/interventional expert for a hands-on understanding of complex anatomy. Three-dimensional printing has been shown to help in presurgical planning, reduce surgical/fluoroscopy time, and aid in medical and patient education.[25] CT is also an ideal imaging modality for evaluating complications of surgeries/interventions, including those related to prosthetic cardiac valve placement and ventricular assist devices.[26]

COMPUTED TOMOGRAPHY IMAGING TECHNIQUES

The CT scanning technique for ACHD varies depending on the anatomy and hemodynamic

Table 2
Utility of computed tomography in adult congenital heart disease

Utility	Comments
Cardiac anatomy and function	Mainly in situations when echocardiography is suboptimal and/or MR imaging is contraindicated or limited by artifacts
Coronary artery imaging	Ideal noninvasive imaging modality due to high spatial resolution
Extracardiac anatomy	Comprehensive evaluation including vasculature, mediastinum, lungs, and airways
Presurgical/ interventional	Provides roadmap and measurements Position of cardiovascular structures for redo sternotomy Position of coronary arteries Calcification in vessels or conduits
Three-dimensional printing	Assessment of anatomy Presurgical/interventional planning Education of patients and trainees Decreases operative/ fluoroscopy time
Postsurgical/ interventional	Evaluation of complications Evaluation of prosthetic valves/ventricular assist devices

features of the cardiac defect, type of surgical repair, suspected complications, patient's age, and level of cooperation. Therefore, the protocol should be tailored on a case-by-case basis to answer the specific clinical question.

Scan Technologies

Multidetector CT (MDCT) scanners (4–320 detector rows) with electrocardiogram (ECG) gating capabilities are required for obtaining good-quality images in ACHD. The recent wide-array detector scanners can image up to 16 cm of the patient with a stationary table in one gantry rotation (volumetric scanning), allowing a single heartbeat acquisition that minimizes motion artifact and contrast dose. Dual-source scanners have twice the temporal resolution of a single-source scanner, which also generates motion-free images. The latest generation of dual-source scanners also have a high-pitch helical mode (up to 3.4), which allows rapid acquisition with the expected gaps in data filled by data from the second x-ray tube. This technique allows single heartbeat scanning and use of low-dose contrast with a moving table (high-pitch helical "FLASH" acquisition).[27] Dual-energy images can be derived from different technologies and scanner configurations, namely dual-source, dual-layer, dual-spin, rapid kVp switching, split-beam, and photon-counting. Virtual monoenergetic images obtained from dual-energy scanners can be used to optimize the contrast at low energy levels and decrease artifacts at higher energy levels.[28]

Scan Modes

Cardiac CT is typically performed with ECG synchronization to minimize cardiac motion. An exception is the evaluation of large extracardiac structures (eg, great arteries and veins), for which a non-ECG gated scan at low pitch may suffice. High-pitch helical mode can achieve motion-free images even without ECG synchronization. This can be particularly helpful in individuals unable to hold their breath, although ECG synchronization is recommended for coronary or functional assessment. Prospectively triggered axial mode is often the default ECG mode for evaluation of cardiac anatomy, acquiring data from only a specific phase of the cardiac cycle rather than over the entire cardiac cycle. This mode has traditionally required a low and steady heart rate (<65 beats per minute), although newer scanners with high temporal resolution (particularly dual-source scanners) can image patients with higher heart rates. Single heartbeat scanning can be achieved through prospective triggering in a high-pitch helical mode with a dual-source scanner, although may require a slow heart rate. In contrast, retrospective ECG gating acquires data throughout the cardiac cycle as a helical scan with low pitch. Retrospective ECG gating is reserved for evaluation of ventricular function and for detailed coronary artery evaluation in patients with higher heart rates and arrhythmias.

Patient Preparation and Medications

Heart rate control is usually not required in ACHD unless coronary artery evaluation is needed. For these patients, beta-blockers, either oral (50–100 mg metoprolol 1 hour before) or intravenous (5–25 mg metoprolol before the procedure) are used to reduce the heart rate. Also, nitrates (0.4–0.8 mg sublingual nitroglycerin) are administered to dilate the coronary vasculature. Sedation is often not required but may be given to anxious and younger patients to avoid motion artifacts. Renal function should be checked before the scan; hydration or alternative imaging modalities should be considered if the renal function is too low. Patients with contrast allergies are premedicated with antihistaminics and steroids. Pregnancy tests are performed in female patients of childbearing age.

Contrast Injection

Contrast injection protocols are customized according to the cardiac anatomy and the clinical question (**Table 3**). Typically, a high concentration of iso-osmolar contrast media is injected through a large cannula placed in an antecubital vein using a power injector. Contrast flow rates are usually 3 to 6 mL/s. Contrast volume is calculated as the product of the injection rate and scan duration (plus 2 seconds and the time taken for the scanner to move from the site of bolus triggering to the actual acquisition). Both the contrast volume and flow rate are dependent on the body mass index. Image acquisition can be triggered either by bolus triggering, manual triggering, timing bolus, or an empirical delay. Contrast injection protocols can include biphasic, triphasic, split-bolus, long-injection, and delayed phase techniques (see **Table 3**).

Radiation Dose Reduction Strategies

With advances in scan technology and radiation dose reduction strategies, significant dose savings can be achieved, now routinely leading to sub milli-Sievert scans.[29,30] In accordance with the "As Low As Reasonably Achievable" (ALARA) principle, the lowest dose scan protocol that provides images of diagnostic quality to answer the clinical question should be selected. CT should be performed only if it is clinically appropriate and scanning should be limited to the anatomy of interest. Prospective ECG triggering is the default ECG gating mode, with retrospective ECG gating reserved for specific clinical situations. With retrospective gating, ECG-based tube current modulation is used to minimize the radiation dose by delivering peak radiation only to a single preselected phase of the cardiac cycle. Other radiation dose reduction methods include low tube voltage (kVp) settings, low tube current (mAs), anatomy-based tube current modulation, and iterative reconstruction algorithms (allowing for mA and kVp reduction while maintaining image noise). Use of high-pitch helical scanning on a dual-source scanner can also reduce radiation

Table 3
Types of computed tomography contrast injection protocols

Protocol Type	Brief Description	Typical Uses
Biphasic	1st phase: Contrast at high flow rate (80 mL at 5 mL/s) 2nd phase: Saline chaser at same flow rate (40 mL at 5 mL/s)	Coronary, systemic, pulmonary arterial angiography with acquisition timed to the vessel of interest
Triphasic	1st phase: Contrast at high flow rate (60 mL at 5 mL/s) 2nd phase: Contrast at slower flow rate (40 mL at 3 mL/s) or Contrast: saline mixture at same flow rate (50 mL of 50:50 mixture at 5 mL/s) 3rd phase: Saline chaser (40 mL at 5 mL/s)	Biventricular opacification for evaluation of cardiac morphology and quantification of volumes and function
Split-bolus	1st phase: Contrast at slow flow rate (60 mL at 3 mL/s) Pause: (30–60 s) 2nd phase: Contrast at high flow rate (70 mL at 5 mL/s) followed by saline chaser (50 mL at 4 mL/s)	Fontan physiology Evaluation of arterial and venous structures in the same study
Long injection	1st phase: High volume of contrast at slow rate (100 mL at 3–4 mL/s) 2nd phase: Saline chaser (40 mL at 4 mL/s)	For venous evaluation Fontan physiology
Delayed phase acquisition	1st phase: Contrast (100–150 mL at 3–5 mL/s) 2nd phase: Saline chaser (40 mL at 5 mL/s) 3rd phase: Late acquisition (30–60 s after arterial phase)	For venous occlusion

Sample injection protocols are given within parenthesis based on our experience.

exposure.[31] Thicker slices may compromise the spatial resolution, but this does not preclude the evaluation of large structures, such as aorta, and allows reduction of radiation dose.

A summary of the commonly used CT protocols in the evaluation of ACHD is provided in **Table 4**.

ADULT CONGENITAL HEART DISEASES

In the following sections, we provide a brief description of common pathologies in ACHD and discuss the role of CT in their evaluation.

Coronary Anomalies

Coronary artery anomalies can be generally categorized into 2 groups, namely primary coronary anomalies and at-risk coronaries in repaired CHD (eg, repaired conotruncal anomalies). Primary anomalies include those of origin, course, intrinsic anatomy, termination, and anastomotic vessels.[32–35] Echocardiography cannot image beyond the ostia, MR imaging is inadequate for distal branches, and catheter angiography is an invasive modality that does not provide 3D information. For these reasons, CT the ideal imaging modality for evaluation of coronary anomalies.

The coronary arteries develop from the peritruncal tissue and grow into the aortic root. Growth of the embryologic coronary artery into an abnormal location results in anomalous connection of a coronary artery.[36] Anomalous connection to the aorta can be asymptomatic or present with exercise-induced ischemia or sudden death.[32–34] Such anomalous connections are described in terms of ostial characteristics and coronary course. A single coronary artery may originate from either from a right-sided or left-sided sinus and is associated with other congenital defects in up to 40% of these cases (**Fig. 1**).[37] The coronary artery may have an anomalous origin from the opposite coronary sinus, that is, a left coronary artery originating from a right coronary sinus or a right coronary artery originating from a left coronary sinus. Such anomalous arteries have 1 of the 4 anomalous courses: Interarterial, retroaortic, transseptal/subpulmonic, and prepulmonic. An interarterial course is between the aorta and pulmonary artery (PA) (**Fig. 2A**). These arteries can also take a proximal intramural course in the aortic wall, which manifests as a slitlike or angulated ostia and abnormal change in caliber. The intramural course makes them vulnerable to myocardial ischemia and sudden cardiac death. In the retroaortic course, the coronary artery, usually a left circumflex artery (LCX), courses behind the aortic root (**Fig. 2B**). This entity is benign but it is important to recognize in patients who have

Table 4
Summary of common computed tomography imaging protocols in adult congenital heart disease

Type	Indication	Medication	Acquisition Mode	Contrast Injection	Scan Range	Resolution
Coronary artery	Anomalies Kawasaki disease Presurgical and postsurgical intervention	Beta-blockers Nitroglycerine	Prospective ECG: at slow heart rates Retrospective: at high heart rates	Biphasic: for isolated coronary anomalies from aorta Triphasic: for coronary fistulas, ALCAPA or in conjunction with other anomalies Triggered: from aorta (if known ALCAPA: from PA)	Carina to diaphragm Longer: if anomalies	High spatial and temporal
Volumes and function	Contraindications/ artifacts in MR imaging	Typically, none Beta-blocker if the HR is too high	Retrospective: with tube current modulation + thick slices Prospective: with 2 acquisition windows in end-diastole and systole	Triphasic protocol Trigger: from aorta	Carina to diaphragm	Good spatial and temporal resolution
Aorta	Aortic anomalies Size assessment	None	Prospective ECG triggered: for root Non-ECG gated: for arch	Biphasic: larger bolus than coronary Trigger: aorta	Apex of lung to diaphragm	Good spatial and temporal resolution
Pulmonary artery	Pulmonary arterial anomalies	None	Non-ECG gated (high/ regular pitch) Prospective ECG triggered: ventricular systolic phase acquisition for measurements	Biphasic Trigger: PA	Apex of lung to diaphragm	Good spatial resolution

	Indication		Acquisition	Contrast	Coverage	Resolution
Pulmonary vein	Pulmonary venous anomalies Before and after ablation	None	Non-ECG gated Prospective ECG triggered: ventricular systolic phase acquisition for measurements	Biphasic trigger: LA Late acquisition/ delayed phase: for venous obstruction	Apex of lung to diaphragm Scimitar: below diaphragm	Good spatial resolution
Systemic vein	Systemic venous anomalies Venous occlusicn	None	Non-ECG gated	Delayed phase Longer bolus, late acquisition Split bolus	Apex of lung to diaphragm	Good spatial and temporal resolution
Fontan	Cardiac anatomy/ function Fontan circuit evaluation	None	ECG gated Non-ECG gated	(Tailored for clinical indication) Triphasic: trigger from aorta (longer bolus-tracking time) Delayed phase: 60–150 s Split bolus Upper and lower extremity injection Dual energy with virtual monoenergetic images	Apex of lung to diaphragm	Good spatial and temporal resolution

Abbreviations: ALCAPA, anomalous left coronary artery from the pulmonary artery; ECG, electrocardiogram; HR, heart rate; LA, left atrium; PA, pulmonary artery.

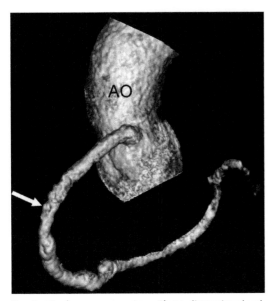

Fig. 1. Single coronary artery. Three-dimensional volume-rendered image shows a single coronary artery (*arrow*) originating from the right aortic sinus and supplying the entire ventricular myocardium. AO, aorta.

planned aortic root interventions or when a bypass graft to the LCX is considered to avoid inadvertent operative injury. In transseptal or subpulmonic course, the anomalous artery courses through the interventricular septum, below the level of RV outflow tract (RVOT) to reach the left side of the heart (**Fig. 2**C). In prepulmonic course, the anomalous coronary artery courses anterior to the RVOT (**Fig. 2**D), which is important in patients with tetralogy of Fallot (TOF) or those being considered for percutaneous pulmonic valve replacement. Of the described anomalies, surgical treatment may be needed for interarterial course, typically managed by ostial reimplantation or coronary artery bypass graft (usually combined with proximal ligation to avoid competitive flow) if there are 2 separate coronary ostia without an intramural course.[36] Intramural course can be managed by coronary unroofing or marsupialization (**Fig. 3**), fenestration, or coronary artery bypass graft (CABG). A separate entity known as myocardial bridging refers to an intramyocardial course of more distal coronary arteries instead of an epicardial course. This is generally considered to be benign due to the arterial compression occurring only in systole with normal coronary artery filling during diastole.[38]

Coronary arteries can originate from the pulmonary arteries, most commonly involving the left coronary artery (also known as ALCAPA; **Fig. 4**). In this anomaly, there is retrograde flow from the higher systemic pressure left coronary artery into the lower pressure PA with resultant collaterals from the right coronary arterial system, leading to myocardial steal. This abnormal flow pattern inevitably results in progressive left ventricular ischemia, fibrosis, dilation, and dysfunction. Associated mitral valve regurgitation resulting from papillary muscle ischemia and annular dilation is often present. If the left main coronary artery connects to the pulmonary trunk, symptoms often arise in infancy, necessitating early operative repair. If the left anterior descending, LCX, or the right coronary are involved, patients may present in early to mid-adulthood. The most important imaging feature to report in unrepaired patients is the position on the pulmonary trunk to which the left coronary artery connects.[34] Only connections to the right side of the pulmonary trunk are close enough to the empty aortic sinus to be amenable to direct ostial reimplantation. Connections to the left side of the trunk or other sites remote from the empty aortic sinus require more complicated repairs (ie, Takeuchi tunnel repair [**Fig. 5**], left subclavian artery graft, CABG). Anomalous origin of the right coronary artery, ARCAPA is less common.

Coronary fistulae represent abnormal connections between coronary arteries and other vascular structures, including the heart chambers (coronary-cameral fistula), aorta, PA, and venous structures.[35,39] Coronary fistulae can be clinically occult or may present with heart failure related to shunt physiology, and symptomatic heart failure is the principal operative indication. CT findings correlate with invasive angiography,[40–43] including the abnormal communication, dilated coronary arteries (**Fig. 6**), and secondary changes. The anatomy of the fistula, communication arising from the side versus end of coronary artery, and associated aneurysmal dilation are important parameters to delineate.[33,34,44] These characteristics can determine the need for specific additional operative techniques (eg, opening heart chambers, coronary arteriotomy) and have implications on perioperative mortality.[33,36]

Particular attention should be given to coronary anatomy imaging following repaired conotruncal anomalies. Following arterial switch and Ross procedures, the coronaries are either stretched or surgically reimplanted, which can lead to ostial stenosis and thrombosis.[45–48] When considering RVOT obstruction relief and pulmonic valve replacement in repaired TOF (discussed in the Conotruncal Anomalies section), delineation of coronary artery anatomy is critical to avoid possible extrinsic obstruction.[49] Any time sternal reentry is considered for reintervention, identification of anteriorly coursing coronaries or bypass

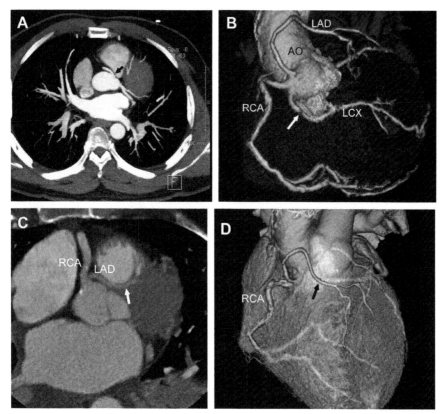

Fig. 2. Anomalous origin and course of coronary arteries. (*A*) Axial maximum intensity projection (MIP) image from a cardiac CT shows an anomalous origin of the right coronary artery (RCA) from the left coronary sinus with an interarterial course (*arrow*) between the aorta and pulmonary artery. (*B*) Three-dimensional volume-rendered reconstruction from another patient shows an anomalous origin of the left circumflex artery (LCX) from the right sinus, which then takes a retroaortic course (*arrow*) behind the aortic root. (*C*) Axial CT image shows anomalous origin of the left anterior descending artery (LAD) from the right coronary artery, which then takes a subpulmonic transseptal course through the ventricular myocardium (*arrow*) to reach the left. (*D*) Three-dimensional volume-rendered CT image shows anomalous origin of the LAD from the right sinus, taking a prepul-monic course (*arrow*) anterior to the right ventricular outflow tract. AO, aorta; RCA, right coronary artery. ([*B,D*] *Courtesy* Harold Goerne, MD, Guadalajara, Mexico.)

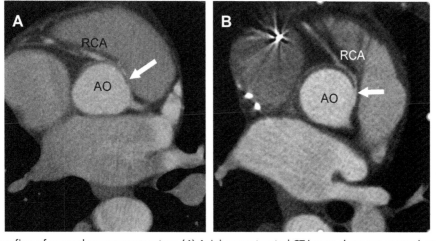

Fig. 3. Unroofing of anomalous coronary artery. (*A*) Axial reconstructed CT image shows an anomalous right cor-onary artery originating from the left sinus, with an intramural portion (*arrow*), which has a slitlike origin that is markedly narrowed. (*B*) Axial reconstructed CT image in the same patient following surgical unroofing shows improved patency of the ostium (*arrow*).

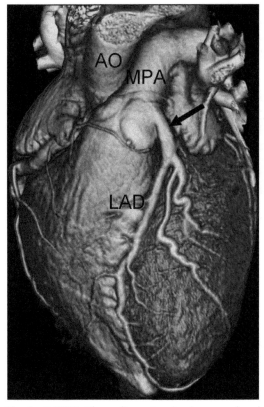

Fig. 4. ALCAPA. Three-dimensional volume-rendered reconstruction of a coronary CTA shows anomalous origin of the left main coronary artery (*arrow*) from the main pulmonary artery (MPA). (*Courtesy* Harold Goerne, MD, Guadalajara, Mexico.)

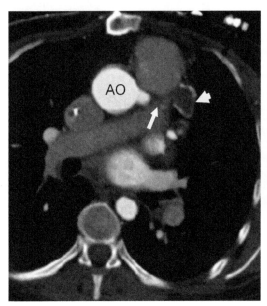

Fig. 5. Baffle thrombosis following Takeuchi repair: 33-year-old woman with history of ALCAPA status post Takeuchi repair at age 11 years followed by a CABG to the left anterior descending artery (LAD) at age 18 due to a positive stress test (inducible ischemia in the apical and septal wall) with sluggish flow through the baffle. Follow-up CT shows complete baffle thrombosis and occlusion (*arrow*) as well as aneurysmal dilation of the distal left main artery (*arrowhead*). The CABG to LAD was also found to be occluded (not shown) with markedly dilated left ventricle.

grafts is imperative to avoid injury during sternotomy. Current guidelines recommend coronary angiography by any advanced modality at least once in adulthood for surgically manipulated coronaries and at any time before RVOT intervention.[49]

Shunt Lesions

Congenital shunt lesions arise from abnormal or persistent communications between the right and left heart structures, which can lead to pathologic

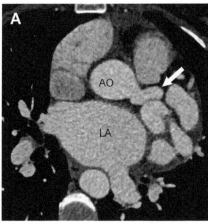
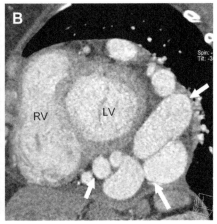

Fig. 6. Coronary artery fistula. (A) Axial cardiac CT shows large dilated coronary arterial branches originating from the left circumflex artery (*arrow*). (B) Short axis reconstruction of cardiac CT shows tortuous coronary arteries (*arrows*) in a different patient with coronary artery fistula that drains into the coronary sinus. Ao, aorta; LA, left atrium; LV, left ventricle; RV, right ventricle.

volume/pressure overload. This overload in turn may cause pulmonary arterial hypertension, Eisenmenger physiology, and right heart failure. Atrial arrhythmias, paradoxic emboli, and frequent respiratory infections are other complications of congenital shunt lesions. Many shunts present in childhood and are repaired. Unrepaired congenital shunt lesions first diagnosed in adulthood are usually small and cause progressive shunt-related symptoms.[50] CT is reserved for situations in which echocardiography fails or is suboptimal and cardiac MR imaging is not feasible or limited by artifacts.

Shunts can be broadly classified as left-to-right and right-to-left types, occurring at atrial, ventricular, arterial, or venous levels.[51] Atrial septal defects (ASD), ventricular septal defects (VSDs), atrioventricular septal or endocardial cushion defects (AVSDs), and patent ductus arteriosus (PDA) are some of the common types of shunts. Types of ASDs include the following: ostium secundum, which is seen in the midportion of the atrial septum (Fig. 7); ostium primum, seen near the atrioventricular junction (Fig. 8); sinus venosus defect, in the wall separating the left atrium from either the superior vena cava (SVC) (superior defect) (Fig. 9) or inferior vena cava (IVC) (inferior defect); and coronary sinus defect (unroofed coronary sinus defect) in the wall between the coronary sinus and left atrium (Fig. 10). Sinus venosus defects have a high association with partial anomalous pulmonary venous return, and coronary sinus defects have a high association with a persistent left SVC.[52]

VSD morphologies include the following: perimembranous (most common), in the membranous portion (Fig. 11A), which may be partially closed by septal leaflet of tricuspid valve with a residual aneurysm (Fig. 11B); muscular, in the muscular portion (Fig. 12); inlet type; and outlet type. Surgical repair involves either primary or patch closure; percutaneous repair involves implanted device closure.[50,53] In repaired VSDs, important complications to consider are residual septal defects and tricuspid valve injury.[54] Patch closures can calcify with age, and subtle defects can be well-characterized in CT that would otherwise be missed by echocardiography.

Atrioventricular canal or endocardial cushion defects are associated with Down syndrome and are frequently repaired in childhood. Associated defects include ostium primum ASDs, membranous VSDs, and cleft mitral valves with dysplastic valve leaflets. Surgical repair is more complicated than with ASD and VSD repair, often requiring multiple patches and reconstruction of each atrioventricular valve apparatus. Complications of AVSDs are valve stenosis, valve regurgitation, and ventricular outflow obstruction.[36]

PDA is patent connection between the aorta and left PA (Fig. 13) that is present in a small number of patients. In infants, symptomatic PDAs are often closed medically or ligated surgically without difficulty. In adults, percutaneous occluder device closure is preferred for small to moderate-sized symptomatic PDAs.[55] Associated aneurysms and calcification preclude percutaneous closure and portend an increased risk of intraoperative rupture, requiring adjustments to traditional operative approach (eg, need for cardiopulmonary bypass).[56] Aortopulmonary window or aortopulmonary septal defect is a rare lesion defined by the connection between the ascending aorta and main PA (but with intact aortic and pulmonic valves), resulting from failure of complete fusion

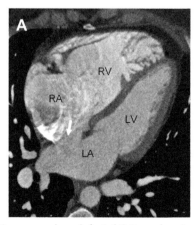
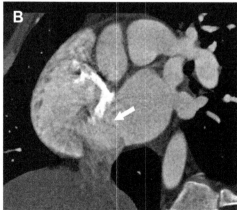

Fig. 7. Ostium secundum defect. (A) Four-chamber reconstructed cardiac CT image shows a large defect in the mid interatrial septum (arrow), consistent with a secundum type defect. (B) Sagittal reconstructed CT image from the same patient shows the large ostium secundum atrial septal defect (arrow).

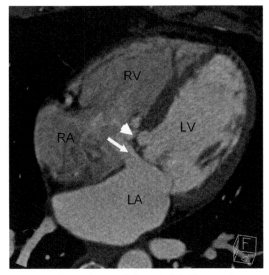

Fig. 8. Ostium primum defect. Axial CT scan shows a defect in the portion of atrial septum near the AV valve (*arrow*), consistent with an ostium primum defect. Note also a small defect in the membranous portion of the ventricular septum (*arrowhead*).

of the conotruncal ridges (**Fig. 14**). These defects have been classified based on the defect location along the aortopulmonary septum[57] and are often associated with other outflow tract, shunt, and aortic arch anomalies.

There are also numerous surgically created shunts and pathways in the cardiovascular system that are summarized in **Table 5** (**Fig. 15**).

Conotruncal Anomalies

Conotruncal anomalies are abnormalities of ventricular outflow tracts and include TOF,

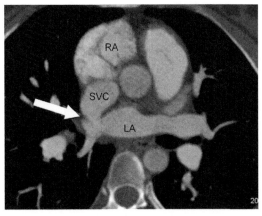

Fig. 9. Sinus venosus defect. Axial CT image shows communication (*arrow*) between the SVC and LA, consistent with a superior sinus venosus defect.

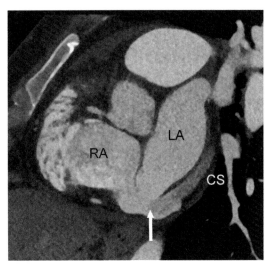

Fig. 10. Coronary sinus (CS) defect. Sagittal CT image shows a large communication (*arrow*) between the CS and the LA, consistent with a CS septal defect (unroofed CS).

transposition of the great arteries, truncus arteriosus, double-outlet right or left ventricle, interrupted aortic arch, and aortopulmonary septal defect. These conditions are typically repaired early in life, and imagers commonly encounter repaired conotruncal anomalies. CT is generally reserved for situations when MR imaging is not feasible or suboptimal. CT is particularly useful in patients with defibrillators placed due to increased risk of sudden death.

TOF refers to a specific combination of 4 defects: RVOT obstruction, RV hypertrophy, VSD, and an overriding aorta (**Fig. 16**). Major aortopulmonary collaterals (MAPCAs) are often seen as a result of the RVOT obstruction/severe pulmonary stenosis or atresia (**Fig. 17**). Numerous operative repairs have been described that are intended to offload the RV through elimination of intracardiac shunting (ie, closure of VSD) and relief of RVOT obstruction.[36] Following repair in infancy, most adult patients develop late post-repair complications related to progressive pulmonic regurgitation and right heart dysfunction. Branch PA stenosis, RVOT aneurysm (**Fig. 18**), recurrent VSDs, and development of MAPCAs are other commonly encountered post-repair complications. RV volumes and RVOT characteristics quantified by imaging play a key role in timing and planning reintervention, namely surgical or percutaneous transcatheter pulmonary valve replacement.[58,59] Patients with RVOT sizes 14 to 22 mm, relatively low distensibility, and straight or hourglass morphologies are best-suited for transcatheter valve replacement (**Fig. 19**).[60] CT allows delineation of

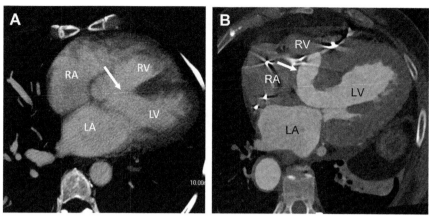

Fig. 11. Membranous VSD. (*A*) Four-chamber CT image shows a defect in the membranous portion of the ventricular septum (*arrow*). (*B*) Four-chamber image in another patient with a VSD shows a focal aneurysm (*arrow*) in the membranous portion of the ventricular septum.

coronary anatomy, which is critically important in identifying arteries at risk during repeat sternotomies and for compression during transcatheter pulmonary valve placement. CT also provides excellent characterization of the metallic endovascular stents and stent-mounted valves used in TOF repair that is often limited by susceptibility artifact with MR imaging. Occasionally, unrepaired TOF may be incidentally encountered in the adult population.

The defining lesion in transposition of the great arteries (TGA) is ventriculo-arterial discordance. The most common type of TGA, the D-TGA, is characterized by atrioventricular concordance and ventriculo-arterial discordance with the aorta usually located anterior and to the right of the PA (**Fig. 20**). There are 3 general types of D-TGA

surgical repairs (atrial switch, arterial switch, complex repair). The atrial switch procedure (Mustard or Senning procedure) uses atrial baffles, which divert the systemic and pulmonary venous flows to contralateral atria (**Fig. 21**). Baffle stenosis and leak, systemic right ventricular failure (**Fig. 22A**), tricuspid regurgitation, and bradyarrhythmia requiring pacemaker implantation are common complications of the atrial switch. CT is particularly useful for the evaluation of baffle anatomy and potential complications (**Fig. 22B, C, D**). Delineating the baffle, systemic venous, and pulmonary venous anatomy is important before placement of pacemaker. When baffle obstruction is suspected, lengthening the bolus-tracking sequence, delaying scan initiation, and adding delayed venous phase imaging are critical as blood return

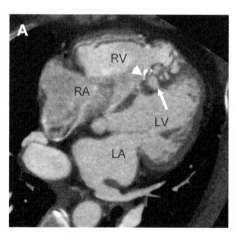
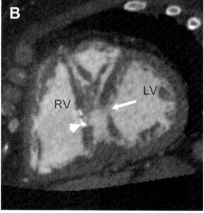

Fig. 12. Muscular VSD. (*A*) Axial CT image shows a large defect in the muscular portion of the ventricular septum (*arrow*). There is also evidence of prior patch repair (*arrowhead*). (*B*) Sagittal reconstructed CT image confirms the presence of a large defect in the muscular portion of the ventricular septum (*arrow*). There is also evidence of prior patch repair (*arrowhead*).

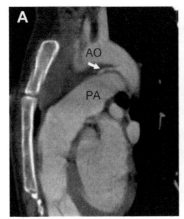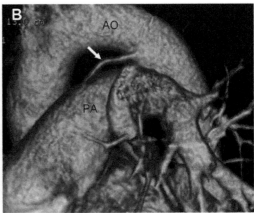

Fig. 13. Patent ductus arteriosus. (*A*) Sagittal reconstructed CT image in a 48-year-old patient shows patent ductus arteriosus (PDA) (*arrow*) between the proximal descending thoracic aorta and left PA near bifurcation. (*B*) Three-dimensional reconstruction in the same patient shows the presence of a small PDA (*arrow*).

to the heart often occurs slowly through collaterals.[44] Coronary sinus and marginal venous anatomy can also be evaluated with CT before placement of cardiac resynchronization therapy devices.

In contrast, the more commonly performed and preferred arterial switch procedure uses the Lecompte maneuver to restore ventriculo-arterial concordance. This procedure requires coronary reimplantation and significantly alters the stretch mechanics on the pulmonary trunk and aorta (**Fig. 23**A). For this reason, arterial switch-repaired D-TGA patients should be monitored for

coronary ostial stenosis, neopulmonary trunk and branch stenosis, and neo-aortic root dilation and aortic regurgitation. More complex surgical repairs (eg, Rastelli and Nikaidoh repairs) are selected when anatomy is not favorable for an arterial switch, such as with large VSDs, LVOT

Table 5
Common surgical shunts and pathways used in the treatment of congenital heart diseases

Type of Surgical Shunt	Description
Blalock-Taussig-Thomas- Classic	Subclavian artery to pulmonary artery: with transected subclavian artery
Blalock-Taussig-Thomas- Modified	Subclavian artery to pulmonary artery connection using a polytetrafluoroethylene (PTFE) graft
Potts	Descending thoracic aorta to left pulmonary artery
Waterson	Ascending aorta to right pulmonary artery
Glenn/hemi-Fontan	Superior vena cava to right pulmonary artery (uni/bidirectional)
Fontan	Inferior vena cava to pulmonary artery • Lateral tunnel: prosthetic intra-atrial baffle • Extracardiac conduit: prosthetic extracardiac tube graft

Fig. 14. Aortopulmonary window. Axial CT scan shows a large communication between the ascending aorta and the main PA (*asterisk*), consistent with an aortopulmonary window.

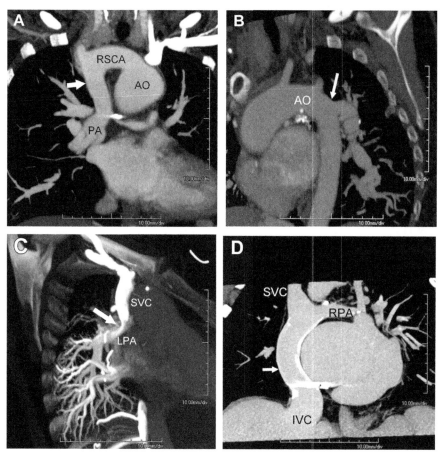

Fig. 15. Surgical shunts and procedures. (*A*) Coronal MIP image in a patient with pulmonary atresia shows a Blalock-Taussig-Thomas shunt (*arrow*) between the right subclavian artery (RSCA) and the right pulmonary artery (RPA). (*B*) Sagittal CT image shows Potts shunt (*arrow*) between the descending aorta and left pulmonary artery (LPA). A Potts shunt was a palliative procedure done to improve pulmonary circulation where a communication between descending aorta and left PA is created, now abandoned due to high rates of pulmonary hypertension. (*C*) Oblique reconstructed MIP image shows a Glenn shunt (*arrow*), which connects the SVC and the right PA. (*D*) Coronal reconstructed cardiac CT image shows appearance after Fontan procedure in which SVC and IVC (*arrow*) blood is rerouted to the pulmonary arteries bypassing the ventricle.

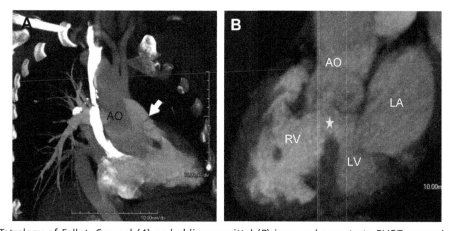

Fig. 16. Tetralogy of Fallot. Coronal (*A*) and oblique sagittal (*B*) images demonstrate RVOT narrowing (*arrow*) with large peri-membranous VSD (*star*) along with overriding aorta and hypertrophied right ventricle.

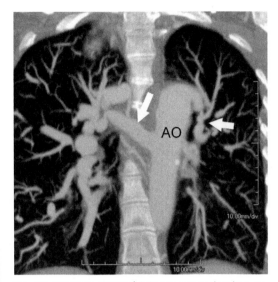

morphologic RV is characterized by absence of fibrous continuity between the atrioventricular and ventriculo-arterial valve, presence of moderator band, prominent trabeculations, and apical displacement of the atrioventricular (AV) valve. The aorta is usually located anterior and to the left of the PA.

Truncus arteriosus results from improper division of the aorta and pulmonary trunk by the aorticopulmonary septum, resulting in a common arterial trunk arising from a shared ventricular outflow tract. This defect is surgically repaired in the neonatal period through an RV-PA conduit and VSD patching. Evaluation of RV-PA conduit patency and integrity in repaired patients is critical in follow-up imaging. Aortopulmonary septal defect is another conotruncal abnormality described in the section on shunt lesions.

Fig. 17. MAPCAs. Coronal MIP reconstruction in a patient with severe pulmonary atresia shows development of extensive MAPCAs (*arrows*) originating from the descending thoracic aorta and supplying the lungs.

Single Ventricle and Other Complex Anomalies

obstruction, and certain double-outlet RVs (**Fig. 23**B, C). The Rastelli procedure can be complicated by outflow tract obstruction and conduit stenosis.[61–63] For post-Nikaidoh patients, the right coronary artery should be evaluated due to risk of injury related to the leftward movement of the aorta toward the VSD.

Congenitally corrected TGA (CC-TGA), also known as L-TGA can be incidentally discovered in the adult population. This anomaly may be confused with a normal heart because the hypertrophied systemic ventricle (ie, morphologic RV) is located on the left. L-TGA can be distinguished from normal anatomy by identifying the RV morphology and aortic position (**Fig. 24**). The

Single ventricle is a complex group of CHD, which is characterized by a morphologic or functional single ventricle. Common entities included in a single ventricle physiology are hypoplastic left heart syndrome, double-inlet left ventricle, tricuspid atresia, and pulmonic atresia (**Fig. 25**). These cases are surgically repaired in childhood through a multistage palliative approach (see **Table 5**). The first stage is performed in the neonatal period and the specific surgical strategy depends on the underlying disease. It typically involves a systemic artery–to-PA shunt or a complex surgery such as Norwood and Damus-Kaye Stansel procedures (**Fig. 26**). The second stage, performed at approximately 6 months of age, involves a Glenn or Hemi-Fontan procedure, which connects the superior venacaval flow to the PA (see **Fig. 15**C). The final stage, performed at 18 months to 3 years of age,

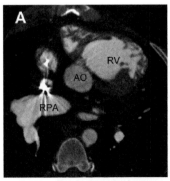
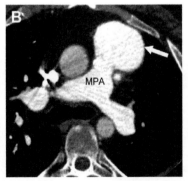
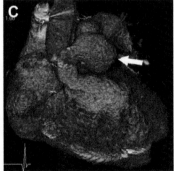

Fig. 18. Repaired TOF. (*A*) Axial CT image in a patient with repaired TOF shows a dilated and hypertrophied RV. (*B*) Axial CT scan in a separate patient with repaired TOF shows aneurysmal dilation of the RVOT (*arrow*). (*C*) Three-dimensional volume rendering of another patient treated with patch annuloplasty of the RVOT shows aneurysmal dilation of the RVOT patch (*arrow*).

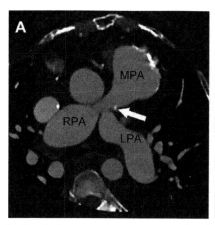
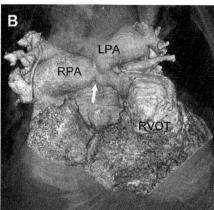

Fig. 19. Evaluation before percutaneous pulmonic valve placement. (*A*) Axial CT scan in a patient with repaired TOF who presented with pulmonic regurgitation and RV dysfunction shows severe narrowing of the main and left PAs (*arrow*). Note the aneurysmal dilation of the RVOT, which is calcified. (*B*) Three-dimensional volume-rendered image of the same patient shows the abnormal dilation of the RVOT and narrowing of the left and main PA (*arrow*).

is a Fontan procedure, which connects the IVC to the PAs, resulting in total cavopulmonary connection (see **Fig. 15**D). Following repair, there is higher risk of heart failure and poorer outcomes when the RV acts as the systemic ventricle. Ventricular dysfunction and shunt pathway thrombosis are other common post-repair complications. CT often is used in the evaluation of these patients when MR imaging is not feasible or expected to be suboptimal.

Awareness of the hemodynamics of Fontan circuit is essential to avoid pitfalls. In the Fontan pathway, there is the preferential blood flow of the SVC pathway to the right and IVC pathway to the left PA. This may cause different strengths of

contrast in the PAs and incomplete mixing in the Fontan, which may be incorrectly interpreted as filling defects, that is, pseudothrombus. Unexpected venous obstruction or unexpected anatomy variants such as persistent left SVC, and venovenous collaterals can further complicate adequate opacification of the Fontan pathway and PAs (**Fig. 27**A). Injection protocols must be tailored to avoid mixture of opacified and unopacified contrast that cause pseudothrombus. Common solutions to this problem involve a

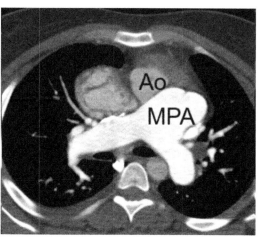

Fig. 20. D-TGA. Axial CT scan shows the aorta located anterior and to the right of PA, consistent with D-TGA. Ao, aorta.

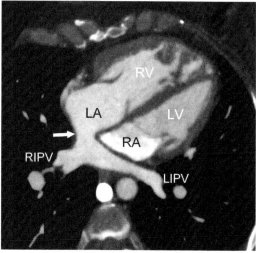

Fig. 21. Atrial switch procedure. Four-chamber CT scan in a patient with D-TGA and Mustard procedure shows the pulmonary venous flow baffled to the right side of the heart (*arrow*) and the systemic flow baffled to the left side of the heart (not shown). LIPV, left inferior pulmonary vein; RIPV, right inferior pulmonary vein.

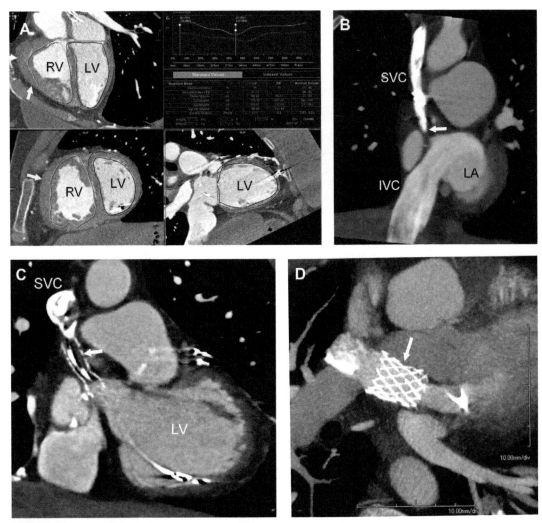

Fig. 22. Atrial switch procedure complications. (*A*) Multiplanar reconstructions show a dilated and hypertrophied systemic (morphologic right) ventricle (*arrow*) in a patient with D-TGA status post Senning-type atrial switch procedure. The ventricular volumes and function were quantified using CT since MRI was contraindicated due to the presence of a MR-incompatible pacemaker device. (*B*) Sagittal CT reconstruction in a patient with D-TGA status post Senning procedure, shows occlusion of the SVC baffle (*arrow*). (*C*) Coronal CT reconstruction in another patient with D-TGA status post Mustard procedure shows a thrombus in the SVC baffle (*arrow*). Note the pacemaker/ICD leads traversing the occluded SVC baffle. (*D*) Axial oblique reconstructed CT image in a patient with D-TGA status post Mustard procedure who underwent SVC stenting (*arrow*) for prior baffle occlusion.

delayed phase acquisition (**Fig. 27**B) and a split-bolus injection protocol with or without an additional delayed phase imaging (retrospective ECG gated scan at lower tube voltage, ~70 kVp, 60–150 s after injection). Simultaneous upper and lower extremity injections or simultaneous bilateral upper extremity injections are other options.[44,64–66] Creating virtual monoenergetic images from a dual-energy CT is another option to visualize the various structures in the same study.[66] Additionally, inexperienced technologists may mistake the neoaorta for the pulmonary trunk,

resulting in incorrect placement of the triggering region of interest, mistimed imaging acquisition, and inadequate opacification of the Fontan pathway and pulmonary circulation. Manual scan triggering and technologist education can help overcome this pitfall.

Cor triatriatum is characterized by division of the atrium into 2 chambers by a membrane. This anomaly is subcategorized as cor triatriatum sinister when the left atrium is involved (**Fig. 28**) and cor triatriatum dexter when the right atrium is involved. The membrane can be imperforate or

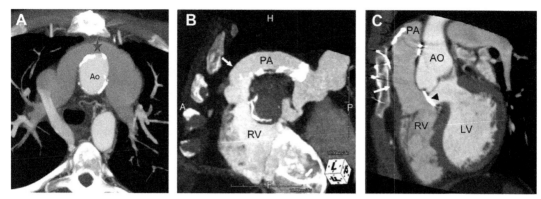

Fig. 23. Surgeries for D-TGA. (*A*) Axial CT of chest shows the typical appearance of the PA (*red star*) draped anterior to the ascending aorta in this patient status post arterial switch surgery with the Lecompte maneuver for D-TGA. (*B*) Rastelli procedure with a conduit from the RV to the PA (*arrow*). (*C*) Nikaidoh procedure, in which the aorta is translocated to the LVOT, VSD patched (*black arrowhead*), and RV-PA conduit placed (*white arrow*).

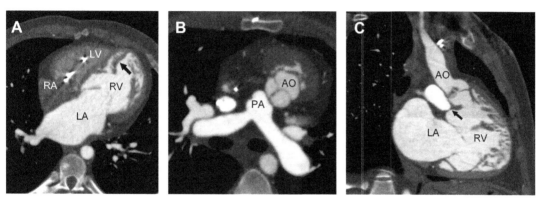

Fig. 24. L-TGA. (*A*) Axial CT scan shows a hypertrophied left-sided ventricle. However, note that a moderator band (*arrow*) is seen in this chamber, suggesting a morphologic RV. (*B*) Axial CT scan at a higher level shows that the aorta is located anterior and to the left of the PA, suggesting L-TGA. (*C*) Vertical long axis reconstruction of the CT shows that the aorta is connected to the left-sided ventricle, with muscular tissue (*arrow*) present between the atrioventricular and ventriculo-arterial valves confirming this to be a morphologic RV. Ao, Aorta; LA, left atrium; LV, morphologic left ventricle; RA, right atrium; RV, morphologic right ventricle.

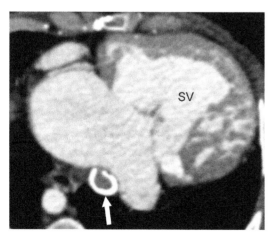

Fig. 25. Single ventricle. Axial CT scan in a patient with severe pulmonary atresia, shows a huge, dilated single ventricle (*arrow*). There is also an extracardiac Fontan (*arrow*) located posterior to the common atrium.

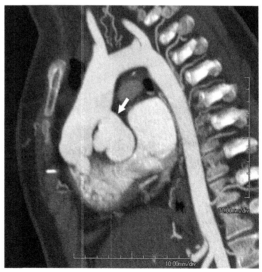

Fig. 26. Single ventricle surgery. Sagittal reconstruction CT in a patient with history of hypoplastic left heart syndrome shows Damus-Kaye-Stansel procedure with anastomosis of the aorta and main PA (*arrow*).

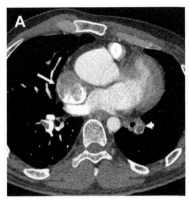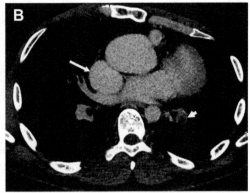

Fig. 27. Imaging Fontan. (*A*) Axial CT obtained in the arterial phase in a patient with Fontan procedure shows filling defects in the right and left PA branches (*small arrow*) and the Fontan pathway (*large arrow*). (*B*) Delayed phase CT image in the same patient shows persistence of the defect in the left PA (*small arrow*), consistent with pulmonary embolus (*small arrow*). The defect in the Fontan pathway has resolved, indicating that this was a mixing artifact/pseudothrombus (*large arrow*).

fenestrated. In cor triatriatum sinister, the left atrium is divided by a membrane into a posterosuperior chamber receiving pulmonary veins and anteroinferior chamber that connects to the left ventricle. Cor triatriatum is often identified incidentally on a chest CT performed for some other reason.

Valvular Anomalies

Severe valvular abnormalities can be seen as part of ACHD. Echocardiography and MR imaging are more commonly used in the evaluation of valvular anomalies. CT is used in situations in which these modalities are suboptimal, equivocal, or not feasible. Bicuspid aortic valve is the most common congenital heart valve disease, defined by 2 aortic valve leaflets instead of the normal 3 (**Fig. 29**). Mitral anomalies associated with AVSDs generally represent an absence of a portion of the valve apparatus, including a cleft mitral valve. Pulmonic stenosis or atresia can occur as part of a spectrum of

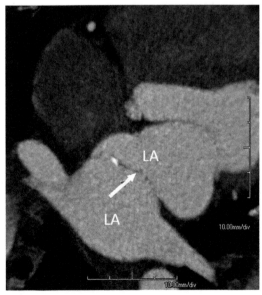

Fig. 28. Cor triatriatum. Axial reformatted CT image shows a membrane in the LA (*arrow*), located posterior to the left atrial appendage junction with LA, indicative of cor triatriatum.

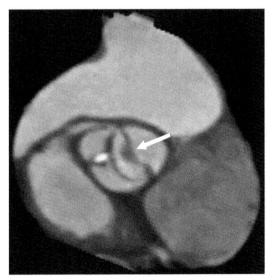

Fig. 29. Bicuspid aortic valve. Short-axis CT view through the aortic valve shows a bicuspid aortic valve (*arrow*) with two thickened leaflets and a calcified raphe between the right and left leaflets.

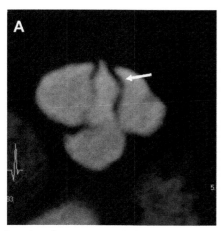 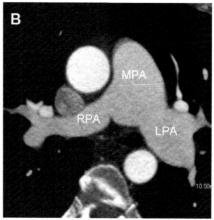

Fig. 30. Pulmonic valve stenosis. (*A*) Short-axis CT image through the pulmonic valve shows thickened leaflets (*arrow*), consistent with pulmonic stenosis. (*B*) Axial CT image in the same patient shows dilation of the main and left PA, which is characteristic of pulmonic valve stenosis.

other congenital disorders (eg, pulmonic valve anomalies in TOF) or rarely in isolation. The valve leaflets are thickened, the orifice area is small, and the main and left PAs are often dilated (**Fig. 30**). Such valve anomalies are managed in an approach similar to TOF or as a single ventricle physiology if extensive. Ebstein anomaly is characterized by apical displacement of the septal and/or posterior leaflets of the tricuspid valve (>8 mm/m^2), which results in atrialization of a portion of the RV (**Fig. 31**). This results in tricuspid

regurgitation and RV dysfunction. Associated ASDs are present in most cases. Although symptomatic neonates present with progressive heart failure, adults commonly present with supraventricular tachyarrhythmias (eg, Wolf-Parkinson-White syndrome).[36] Adults with repairs earlier in life may have tricuspid valve prostheses, sequelae of ASD repair, RV-PA conduits, and rarely a functional single ventricle physiology.

Thoracic Vascular Abnormalities

CT is commonly used for evaluation of thoracic vascular anomalies, involving the aorta, PA, systemic veins, and pulmonary veins.

Coarctation of the aorta is a discrete narrowing of the thoracic aorta seen distal to left subclavian artery origin, which may present incidentally in adulthood. CT allows characterization of the coarctation, concurrent collateral vessels, and any associated anomalies, such as bicuspid valve and postsurgical complications. Aortic hypoplasia is diffuse narrowing of the aortic arch/descending aorta, whereas interruption is atresia of a segment of aortic arch. Supravalvular aortic stenosis is seen in Williams syndrome. A left aortic arch with aberrant right subclavian artery is the most common aortic anomaly but does not form a vascular ring. Vascular rings encircle the trachea and esophagus and can potentially narrow these structures leading to respiratory or swallowing issues. Double aortic arch is the most common vascular ring followed by a right aortic arch with aberrant left subclavian artery. A right arch with mirror image branching

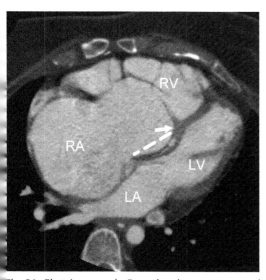

Fig. 31. Ebstein anomaly. Four-chamber reconstructed CT image in a patient with Ebstein anomaly shows apical displacement of the septal leaflet of tricuspid valve (*arrow*) with atrialized RV (*dashed line*).

pattern is usually not a ring, although has high association with cardiac anomalies. Circumflex aorta is a portion of arch extending behind the esophagus. Cervical arch is characterized by a high location in the lower neck. For all of these anomalies, CT can be used to accurately measure the thoracic aorta and evaluate for complications of prior aortic surgeries.

PA anomalies range from arterial agenesis that presents in infancy to vascular slings around the trachea that may be asymptomatic into adulthood. Pulmonary interruption is characterized by absence of the proximal PAs, that is, either the right or left PA, with intact distal intrapulmonary network, systemic collateral vessels, and a small ipsilateral lung (Fig. 32). In pulmonary agenesis, there is absence of ipsilateral lungs and bronchi along with pulmonary vasculature, whereas in aplasia, the lungs and pulmonary vasculature are absent, but there is a rudimentary bronchus. In pulmonary hypoplasia, the arteries, lung, and bronchus are all hypoplastic. Ductal origin of the PA is a rare anomaly in which the right or left PA does not communicate with the main PA, instead arising from the ductus arteriosus. A pulmonary sling is characterized by a left PA arising from the right PA, passing between the trachea and esophagus, and supplying the left lung (Fig. 33). When imaging these slings, attention should be paid to any concomitant tracheobronchomalacia and right main bronchial stenosis.

Anomalous pulmonary venous return can be partial (PAPVR; involving 1 to 3 veins) or total (TAPVR; involving all 4 veins). PAPVR is often an incidental diagnosis in asymptomatic adults, most commonly with abnormal left upper

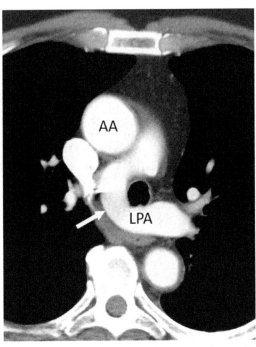

Fig. 33. Pulmonary sling. Axial CT scan shows the left PA coursing medially and then to the left behind the trachea (arrow) without significant airway compression. AA, ascending aorta.

pulmonary venous drainage into the left brachiocephalic vein followed by right superior pulmonary vein draining into the SVC (Fig. 34). Nearly half of all patients with PAPVR have concurrent sinus venosus type ASDs.[67] Scimitar

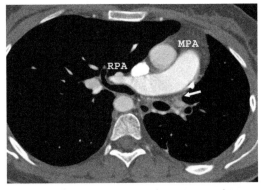

Fig. 32. PA interruption. Axial CT image shows a normal right PA, but absence of proximal left PA (arrow), which is consistent with PA interruption. Note the associated left lung hypoplasia.

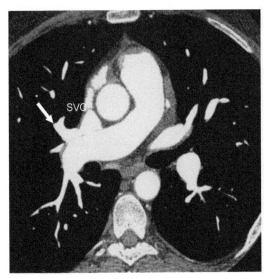

Fig. 34. PAPVR. Axial CT image shows an anomalous right upper lobe pulmonary vein (arrow) draining into the lower SVC.

syndrome is characterized by an anomalous PAPVR, typically on the right with an associated hypoplastic lung. The PAPVR in Scimitar syndrome typically extends inferiorly to drain infradiaphragmatically into the IVC, giving the appearance of a scimitar as it courses parallel to the right heart border (**Fig. 35**). PAPVR with significant shunts are treated surgically, depending on the location. Repair approaches can include creation of new pulmonary venous pathway using patches or the Warden procedure. The Warden procedure involves transverse division of the SVC, anastomosis of cephalic SVC to right atrial appendage, and use of the caudal SVC as a drainage conduit for the PAPVR into the left atrium (**Fig. 36**). TAPVR usually presents and is repaired in childhood. Depending on the drainage, it is classified as supracardiac (into the left brachiocephalic vein, most common), cardiac (into the right heart), and infracardiac (typically below the diaphragm). Operative correction of TAPVR requires reconnection of pulmonary venous drainage back to the left atrium. Pulmonary vein stenosis is a complication of the surgery.[68–70]

Systemic venous anomalies cover a wide range of abnormalities in the number and course of the SVC, IVC, and its tributaries. Persistent left SVC is the most common SVC anomaly, with most (80%–90%) of these draining into the coronary sinus (**Fig. 37**) and occurring with a concomitant right SVC. This can occasionally

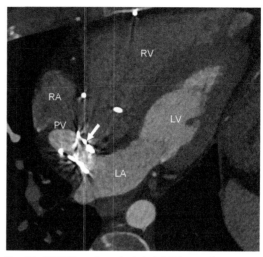

Fig. 36. PAPVR postsurgical. Axial CT scan after a Warden procedure shows a stent/baffle (*arrow*) connecting the right superior pulmonary vein to the LA. Also note the prior tricuspid valve annuloplasty. PV, pulmonary vein.

drain into the left atrium (between left atrial appendage and left pulmonary vein) due to an unroofed coronary sinus, which is called Raghib syndrome. This should be distinguished from a levoatriocardinal vein, an anomalous vein that connects the pulmonary vein (typically upper) or left atrium to a systemic vein (typically the left innominate vein). The pulmonary vein itself has normal communication with the left atrium. It is seen in left heart obstructive lesions as an alternative egress of pulmonary venous flow and hence there is a cephalad direction

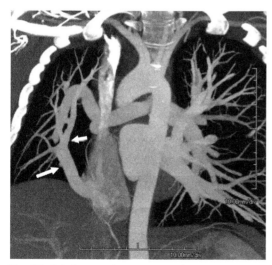

Fig. 35. Scimitar syndrome. Coronal CTA MIP image shows large anomalous pulmonary vein in the right lung that is draining inferiorly into the IVC (*arrows*). Note that the right lung is hypoplastic.

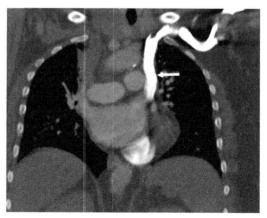

Fig. 37. Persistent left SVC. Coronal CT image shows a left-sided vena cava (*arrow*) that drained into the CS (not shown here).

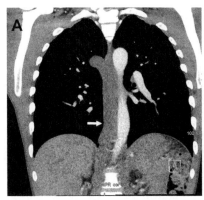
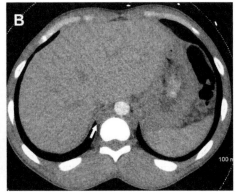

Fig. 38. Interrupted IVC with azygos continuation. (*A*) Coronal CT scan image shows a prominent right azygos vein (*arrow*). (*B*) Axial CT scan in the same patient at the level of the liver shows that the intrahepatic portion of the IVC is absent (*arrow*), consistent with interruption of IVC and azygos continuation.

of flow with a small left-to-right shunt.[71] Interrupted IVC is an absence of the intrahepatic IVC with concomitant lower body venous drainage into the dilated azygos and hemiazygos system (**Fig. 38**). This anomaly is associated with heterotaxy syndromes.[72] Retroaortic left brachiocephalic veins course behind the aorta to join the SVC (**Fig. 39**) and is associated with right-sided aortic arch, RVOT obstruction, and TAPVR.[73] Although systemic venous anomalies are rarely surgically repaired, knowledge of their presence and anatomy is critical in planning central venous access, cardiopulmonary bypass, and device implantation, including cardioverter defibrillators and pacemakers.

SUMMARY

CT plays an important role in the evaluation of ACHD, including for de novo presentation in adulthood and for follow-up cases from childhood. CT is particularly useful for the evaluation of cardiac/extracardiac anatomy and function in those patients with suboptimal echocardiography and infeasible or technically limited MR imaging. CT is the ideal noninvasive imaging modality for the evaluation of small structures, such as the coronary arteries. CT is critical in evaluating post-repair complications and in planning reinterventions.

REFERENCES

1. Bhatt AB, Foster E, Kuehl K, et al. Congenital heart disease in the older adult: a scientific statement from the American Heart Association. Circulation 2015;131:1884–931.
2. Dearani JA, Connolly HM, Martinez R, et al. Caring for adults with congenital cardiac disease: successes and challenges for 2007 and beyond. Cardiol Young 2007;17(Suppl 2):87–96.
3. Williams RG, Pearson GD, Barst RJ, et al. Report of the National Heart, Lung, and Blood Institute Working Group on research in adult congenital heart disease. J Am Coll Cardiol 2006;47:701–7.
4. Marelli AJ, Mackie AS, Ionescu-Ittu R, et al. Congenital heart disease in the general population: changing prevalence and age distribution. Circulation 2007;115:163–72.
5. Gatzoulis MAWG. Adults with congenital heart diseases: a growing population. Edinburgh (UK): Churchill Livingstone; 2003.
6. Moons P, Bovijn L, Budts W, et al. Temporal trends in survival to adulthood among patients born with

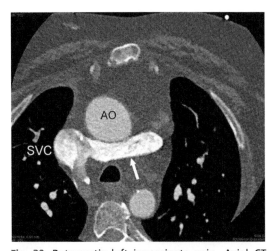

Fig. 39. Retroaortic left innominate vein. Axial CT scan in a patient with repaired TOF and right aortic arch shows a retroaortic left innominate vein (*arrow*).

congenital heart disease from 1970 to 1992 in Belgium. Circulation 2010;122:2264–72.

7. Warnes CA. The adult with congenital heart disease: born to be bad? J Am Coll Cardiol 2005;46:1–8.

8. Warnes CA, Williams RG, Bashore TM, et al. ACC/AHA 2008 guidelines for the management of adults with congenital heart disease: executive summary: a report of the American College of Cardiology/American Heart Association Task Force on practice guidelines (writing committee to develop guidelines for the management of adults with congenital heart disease). Circulation 2008;118:2395–451.

9. Tutarel O, Kempny A, Alonso-Gonzalez R, et al. Congenital heart disease beyond the age of 60: emergence of a new population with high resource utilization, high morbidity, and high mortality. Eur Heart J 2014;35:725–32.

10. Afilalo J, Therrien J, Pilote L, et al. Geriatric congenital heart disease: burden of disease and predictors of mortality. J Am Coll Cardiol 2011; 58:1509–15.

11. Stulak JM, Dearani JA, Burkhart HM, et al. Coronary artery disease in adult congenital heart disease: outcome after coronary artery bypass grafting. Ann Thorac Surg 2012;93:116–22 [discussion: 22–3].

12. Diller GP, Dimopoulos K, Okonko D, et al. Exercise intolerance in adult congenital heart disease: comparative severity, correlates, and prognostic implication. Circulation 2005;112:828–35.

13. Burchill LJ, Huang J, Tretter JT, et al. Noninvasive imaging in adult congenital heart disease. Circ Res 2017;120:995–1014.

14. Geva T. Is MRI the preferred method for evaluating right ventricular size and function in patients with congenital heart disease? MRI is the preferred method for evaluating right ventricular size and function in patients with congenital heart disease. Circ Cardiovasc Imaging 2014;7: 190–7.

15. Napp AE, Enders J, Roehle R, et al. Analysis and prediction of claustrophobia during MR Imaging with the claustrophobia questionnaire: an observational prospective 18-month single-center study of 6500 patients. Radiology 2017;283:148–57.

16. Stevens SM, Tung R, Rashid S, et al. Device artifact reduction for magnetic resonance imaging of patients with implantable cardioverter-defibrillators and ventricular tachycardia: late gadolinium enhancement correlation with electroanatomic mapping. Heart Rhythm 2014;11:289–98.

17. McDonald RJ, McDonald JS, Kallmes DF, et al. Gadolinium deposition in human brain tissues after contrast-enhanced MR Imaging in adult patients without intracranial abnormalities. Radiology 2017; 285:546–54.

18. Kodzwa R. Updates to the ACR manual on contrast media. Radiol Technol 2017;89:186–9.

19. Preston DL, Ron E, Tokuoka S, et al. Solid cancer incidence in atomic bomb survivors: 1958-1998. Radiat Res 2007;168:1–64.

20. Krause TM, Ukhanova M, Lee Revere F, et al. Risk predictors for postcontrast acute kidney injury. J Am Coll Radiol 2018. https://doi.org/10.1016/j.jacr.2018.04.015.

21. Chang S, Han K, Youn JC, et al. Utility of dual-energy CT-based monochromatic imaging in the assessment of myocardial delayed enhancement in patients with cardiomyopathy. Radiology 2018; 287:442–51.

22. Bandula S, White SK, Flett AS, et al. Measurement of myocardial extracellular volume fraction by using equilibrium contrast-enhanced CT: validation against histologic findings. Radiology 2013;269: 396–403.

23. Asferg C, Usinger L, Kristensen TS, et al. Accuracy of multi-slice computed tomography for measurement of left ventricular ejection fraction compared with cardiac magnetic resonance imaging and two-dimensional transthoracic echocardiography: a systematic review and meta-analysis. Eur J Radiol 2012;81:e757–62.

24. Maffei E, Messalli G, Martini C, et al. Left and right ventricle assessment with cardiac CT: validation study vs. cardiac MR. Eur Radiol 2012;22: 1041–9.

25. Kurup HK, Samuel BP, Vettukattil JJ. Hybrid 3D printing: a game-changer in personalized cardiac medicine? Expert Rev Cardiovasc Ther 2015;13: 1281–4.

26. Krishnan B, Yarmohammadi H, Eckman P, et al. Outflow thrombus in a left ventricular-assist device: visualization by CT angiography. J Cardiovasc Comput Tomogr 2014;8:473–4.

27. Achenbach S, Marwan M, Ropers D, et al. Coronary computed tomography angiography with a consistent dose below 1 mSv using prospectively electrocardiogram-triggered high-pitch spiral acquisition. Eur Heart J 2010;31:340–6.

28. Kalisz K, Halliburton S, Abbara S, et al. Update on cardiovascular applications of multienergy CT. Radiographics 2017;37:1955–74.

29. Ghoshhajra BB, Lee AM, Engel LC, et al. Radiation dose reduction in pediatric cardiac computed tomography: experience from a tertiary medical center. Pediatr Cardiol 2014;35:171–9.

30. Raff GL. Radiation dose from coronary CT angiography: five years of progress. J Cardiovasc Comput Tomogr 2010;4:365–74.

31. Li M, Sun G. Low-dose scan protocols in dual-source CT coronary angiography. Radiology 2012; 263:937–8 [author reply: 8].

32. Angelini P. Coronary artery anomalies: an entity in search of an identity. Circulation 2007;115: 1296–305.

33. Kayalar N, Burkhart HM, Dearani JA, et al. Congenital coronary anomalies and surgical treatment. Congenit Heart Dis 2009;4:239–51.

34. Perez-Pomares JM, de la Pompa JL, Franco D, et al. Congenital coronary artery anomalies: a bridge from embryology to anatomy and pathophysiology–a position statement of the development, anatomy, and pathology ESC Working Group. Cardiovasc Res 2016;109:204–16.

35. Yamanaka O, Hobbs RE. Coronary artery anomalies in 126,595 patients undergoing coronary arteriography. Cathet Cardiovasc Diagn 1990;21:28–40.

36. Kirklin JW, Kouchoukos NT. Kirklin/Barratt-Boyes cardiac surgery: morphology, diagnostic criteria, natural history, techniques, results, and indications. 3rd edition. Philadelphia: Churchill Livingstone; 2003.

37. Angelini PFV. Coronary artery anomalies: a comprehensive approach. Philadelphia: Lippincott Williams & Wilkins; 1999.

38. Nakanishi R, Rajani R, Ishikawa Y, et al. Myocardial bridging on coronary CTA: an innocent bystander or a culprit in myocardial infarction? J Cardiovasc Comput Tomogr 2012;6:3–13.

39. Ghandour A, Rajiah P. Unusual fistulas and connections in the cardiovascular system: a pictorial review. World J Radiol 2014;6:169–76.

40. Leschka S, Koepfli P, Husmann L, et al. Myocardial bridging: depiction rate and morphology at CT coronary angiography—comparison with conventional coronary angiography. Radiology 2008; 246:754–62.

41. Lim JJ, Jung JI, Lee BY, et al. Prevalence and types of coronary artery fistulas detected with coronary CT angiography. AJR Am J Roentgenol 2014;203: W237–43.

42. Tariq R, Kureshi SB, Siddiqui UT, et al. Congenital anomalies of coronary arteries: diagnosis with 64 slice multidetector CT. Eur J Radiol 2012;81: 1790–7.

43. Zhou K, Kong L, Wang Y, et al. Coronary artery fistula in adults: evaluation with dual-source CT coronary angiography. Br J Radiol 2015;88: 20140754.

44. Han BK, Rigsby CK, Leipsic J, et al. Computed tomography imaging in patients with congenital heart disease, part 2: technical recommendations. an expert consensus document of the society of cardiovascular computed tomography (SCCT): endorsed by the Society of Pediatric Radiology (SPR) and the North American Society of Cardiac Imaging (NASCI). J Cardiovasc Comput Tomogr 2015;9: 493–513.

45. Bonhoeffer P, Bonnet D, Piechaud JF, et al. Coronary artery obstruction after the arterial switch operation for transposition of the great arteries in newborns. J Am Coll Cardiol 1997;29:202–6.

46. Bonnet D, Bonhoeffer P, Piechaud JF, et al. Long-term fate of the coronary arteries after the arterial switch operation in newborns with transposition of the great arteries. Heart 1996;76: 274–9.

47. Legendre A, Losay J, Touchot-Kone A, et al. Coronary events after arterial switch operation for transposition of the great arteries. Circulation 2003; 108(Suppl 1):II186–90.

48. Pasquali SK, Hasselblad V, Li JS, et al. Coronary artery pattern and outcome of arterial switch operation for transposition of the great arteries: a meta-analysis. Circulation 2002;106:2575–80.

49. Warnes CA, Williams RG, Bashore TM, et al. ACC/AHA 2008 guidelines for the management of adults with congenital heart disease: a report of the American College of Cardiology/American Heart Association Task Force on practice guidelines (Writing Committee to Develop Guidelines on the Management of Adults With Congenital Heart Disease). Developed in collaboration with the American Society of Echocardiography, Heart Rhythm Society, International Society for Adult Congenital Heart Disease, Society for Cardiovascular Angiography and Interventions, and Society of Thoracic Surgeons. J Am Coll Cardiol 2008;52:e143–263.

50. Konstantinides S, Geibel A, Olschewski M, et al. A comparison of surgical and medical therapy for atrial septal defect in adults. N Engl J Med 1995; 333:469–73.

51. Rajiah P, Kanne JP. Cardiac MRI: part 1, cardiovascular shunts. AJR Am J Roentgenol 2011;197: W603–20.

52. Rajiah P, Kanne JP. Computed tomography of septal defects. J Cardiovasc Comput Tomogr 2010;4: 231–45.

53. Humenberger M, Rosenhek R, Gabriel H, et al. Benefit of atrial septal defect closure in adults: impact of age. Eur Heart J 2011;32:553–60.

54. Yilmaz AT, Ozal E, Arslan M, et al. Aneurysm of the membranous septum in adult patients with perimembranous ventricular septal defect. Eur J Cardiothorac Surg 1997;11:307–11.

55. Liddy S, Oslizlok P, Walsh KP. Comparison of the results of transcatheter closure of patent ductus arteriosus with newer Amplatzer devices. Catheter Cardiovasc Interv 2013;82:253–9.

56. O'Donovan TG, Beck W. Closure of the complicated patent ductus arteriosus. Ann Thorac Surg 1978;25: 463–5.

57. Doty DB, Richardson JV, Falkovsky GE, et al. Aortopulmonary septal defect: hemodynamics, angiography, and operation. Ann Thorac Surg 1981;32: 244–50.

58. Ammash NM, Dearani JA, Burkhart HM, et al. Pulmonary regurgitation after tetralogy of Fallot repair: clinical features, sequelae, and timing of pulmonary

valve replacement. Congenit Heart Dis 2007;2: 386–403.

59. Geva T. Repaired tetralogy of Fallot: the roles of cardiovascular magnetic resonance in evaluating pathophysiology and for pulmonary valve replacement decision support. J Cardiovasc Magn Reson 2011; 13:9.

60. Chung R, Taylor AM. Imaging for preintervention planning: transcatheter pulmonary valve therapy. Circ Cardiovasc Imaging 2014;7:182–9.

61. Hazekamp MG, Gomez AA, Koolbergen DR, et al. Surgery for transposition of the great arteries, ventricular septal defect and left ventricular outflow tract obstruction: European Congenital Heart Surgeons Association multicentre study. Eur J Cardiothorac Surg 2010;38:699–706.

62. Lee JR, Lim HG, Kim YJ, et al. Repair of transposition of the great arteries, ventricular septal defect and left ventricular outflow tract obstruction. Eur J Cardiothorac Surg 2004;25:735–41.

63. Williams WG, McCrindle BW, Ashburn DA, et al. Outcomes of 829 neonates with complete transposition of the great arteries 12-17 years after repair. Eur J Cardiothorac Surg 2003;24:1–9 [discussion: 10].

64. Han BK, Lesser JR. CT imaging in congenital heart disease: an approach to imaging and interpreting complex lesions after surgical intervention for tetralogy of Fallot, transposition of the great arteries, and single ventricle heart disease. J Cardiovasc Comput Tomogr 2013;7:338–53.

65. Han BK, Rigsby CK, Hlavacek A, et al. Computed tomography imaging in patients with congenital heart disease part i: rationale and utility. An expert consensus document of the Society of Cardiovascular Computed Tomography (SCCT): endorsed by the Society of Pediatric Radiology (SPR) and the North American Society of Cardiac Imaging (NASCI). J Cardiovasc Comput Tomogr 2015;9:475–92.

66. Ghadimi Mahani M, Agarwal PP, Rigsby CK, et al. CT for assessment of thrombosis and pulmonary embolism in multiple stages of single-ventricle palliation: challenges and suggested protocols. Radiographics 2016;36:1273–84.

67. Ho ML, Bhalla S, Bierhals A, et al. MDCT of partial anomalous pulmonary venous return (PAPVR) in adults. J Thorac Imaging 2009;24:89–95.

68. Hyde JA, Stumper O, Barth MJ, et al. Total anomalous pulmonary venous connection: outcome of surgical correction and management of recurrent venous obstruction. Eur J Cardiothorac Surg 1999; 15:735–40 [discussion: 40–1].

69. Lacour-Gayet F. Surgery for pulmonary venous obstruction after repair of total anomalous pulmonary venous return. Semin Thorac Cardiovasc Surg Pediatr Card Surg Annu 2006;9:45–50.

70. Ricci M, Elliott M, Cohen GA, et al. Management of pulmonary venous obstruction after correction of TAPVC: risk factors for adverse outcome. Eur J Cardiothorac Surg 2003;24:28–36 [discussion: 36].

71. Agarwal PP, Mahani MG, Lu JC, et al. Levoatriocardinal vein and mimics: spectrum of imaging findings. AJR Am J Roentgenol 2015;205:W162–71.

72. Bass JE, Redwine MD, Kramer LA, et al. Spectrum of congenital anomalies of the inferior vena cava: cross-sectional imaging findings. Radiographics 2000;20:639–52.

73. Kulkarni S, Jain S, Kasar P, et al. Retroaortic left innominate vein - Incidence, association with congenital heart defects, embryology, and clinical significance. Ann Pediatr Cardiol 2008;1:139–41.

Congenital Thoracic Aortic Disease

Luis A. Landeras, MD*, Jonathan H. Chung, MD

KEYWORDS

- Aortic arch anomalies • Vascular rings • Coarctation • Aortic arch interruption • Aortic hypoplasia
- CT angiography

KEY POINTS

- Computed tomography angiography should be a first-line imaging modality for evaluation of the thoracic aorta and should be performed with electrocardiographic gating to improve accurate aortic root and ascending aorta evaluation.
- The presence of a retroesophageal diverticulum (diverticulum of Kommerell) suggests the presence of a ligamentum arteriosum contralateral to the aortic arch and the presence of a vascular ring.
- Right aortic arch with mirror branching imaging is associated with congenital heart disease in more than 90% of cases.

INTRODUCTION

Congenital variants and anomalies of the thoracic aorta encompass a variety of disorders with variable clinical manifestations ranging from asymptomatic to life threatening. Despite the relative low prevalence of clinically significant congenital thoracic aortic disorders, it is important to be familiar with these conditions, as they may explain a patient's symptoms, may draw attention to associated anomalies, and will determine future therapeutic interventions.

We review the embryology of the thoracic aorta and its branches in light of congenital anomalies to highlight the pathophysiologic mechanisms of various anomalies. Likewise, we will examine the role of imaging with focus on the use of computed tomography angiography (CTA) in the evaluation of these pathologies and present suggested imaging protocols. Finally, we provide insights into the diagnosis of specific thoracic aortic anomalies with emphasis on the evaluation of vascular rings.

EMBRYOLOGY

The normal thoracic aorta and great vessel formation is a complex process that starts with vasculogenesis at 20 to 22 days from conception. Networks of endothelial channels form by aggregation and fusion of angioblasts, which result in paired ventral and dorsal aortae and aortic arches. The ventral aortae fuse to form a single ventral aorta, the aortic sac. The dorsal aortae also partially fuse into a single dorsal aorta that forms the midline descending aorta. This begins distally and proceeds in a retrograde fashion.[1] There is associated craniocaudal development of 6 aortic arches, the so-called branchial arch arteries, which communicate with the ventral aortic sac and paired dorsal aortae. These arches do not exist simultaneously but rather present sequentially with subsequent complete or partial regression. The aortic sac proximally communicates with the heart through the truncus arteriosus. The truncus subsequently divides into the ventral

Disclosure Statement: The authors have nothing to disclose.
Department of Radiology, The University of Chicago, 5841 South Maryland Avenue, MC 2026, Chicago, IL 60637, USA
* Corresponding author.
E-mail address: llanderas@radiology.bsd.uchicago.edu

Radiol Clin N Am 57 (2019) 113–125
https://doi.org/10.1016/j.rcl.2018.08.008
0033-8389/19/

aorta and pulmonary trunk by the spiral aortopulmonary septum.

As noted previously, the 6 aortic arches are not present at the same time, and the fifth arch is rarely seen in humans due to nonexistence or incomplete formation and very early regression (**Fig. 1**). These different embryologic components contribute to form the normal aorta and arch vessels in the following manner[2]: The first and second arches regress almost completely with the residual first arch modeling into the maxillary and external carotid arteries, and the second arch contributes to form the hyoid and stapedial arteries. The third arches form the common carotid and proximal internal carotid arteries. The distal internal carotid arteries are formed from the aorta dorsalis. The left fourth arch develops into the left aortic arch between the left common carotid and the left subclavian artery. The right fourth arch predominantly atrophies with a small portion forming the proximal right subclavian artery. The ventral portion of the sixth arches contribute to form the proximal right and left pulmonary arteries. The dorsal portion of the left sixth arch forms the ductus arteriosus connecting the left pulmonary artery to the aortic arch. The dorsal portion of the right sixth arch involutes. The seventh intersegmental branches arise from the dorsal aorta, with the left intersegmental branch forming the left subclavian artery. The right seventh intersegmental contributes to form the distal aspect of the right subclavian artery with the mid and proximal portions formed by a remnant of right dorsal aorta and right fourth arch, respectively. The ventral aortic sac develops right and left horns, with the right horn forming the brachiocephalic artery, and the left horn forming the proximal ascending portion of the arch. Deviations of this developmental pattern with persistent or regression of different segments can explain most of the thoracic aorta anomalies.

The theoretic model of Edwards'[3] double ring provides a simplified approach and helps to understand the development of the arch and branch vessel anomalies. In this model, bilateral aortic arches and ductus arteriosi encircle the trachea and esophagus (**Fig. 2**). Similarly, faulty regression of specific segments of the aortic arch help to understand the resultant arch anomalies. This model does not explain the lateral position of the descending aorta or the eventual size of vessels.[4]

IMAGING

Imaging strategies available for assessment of the thoracic aorta include radiography, echocardiography, vascular ultrasound, esophagography, CTA, magnetic resonance angiography, and catheter angiography.

Chest radiography is inexpensive, widely available, and may provide clues of direct or indirect congenital thoracic anomalies. In particular, arch laterality or bilaterality may be suggested by the pattern of indentation of the trachea air column and position with respect to the thoracic spine pedicles. It is also useful to exclude other potential etiologies of a patient's symptoms and help to guide subsequent imaging.

Transthoracic echocardiography also provides excellent cardiac and proximal aorta morphologic and functional assessment, particularly in small pediatric patients, without the use of radiation. Its main limitations relate to small fields of view, suboptimal acoustic windows, poor transmission through air/bone, and its operator dependency with commonly insufficient visualization peripheral vascular segments.

Esophagography may be obtained earlier in the diagnostic imaging workup, particularly in the setting of gastrointestinal symptoms. Indentation of the posterior esophagus should raise concern for a double aortic arch, right arch with aberrant left subclavian artery or left arch with an aberrant right subclavian artery. Given its direct lack of direct vascular visualization, other imaging modalities are required for complete assessment. A negative esophagogram excludes a vascular ring.

MR imaging offers large fields of view, excellent soft tissue contrast, great spatial resolution, and multiplanar capabilities, and requires no radiation, making it a good option for the evaluation of pediatric patients. However, MR scanners are not as widely available and these examinations are relatively long and commonly require deep sedation or anesthesia in young children with intubation, further limiting trachea evaluation. In addition, it provides limited evaluation of the airway and lung parenchyma. Lately, there is also concern regarding the unknown effects of gadolinium deposition in the brain.

Advantages of CT include large fields of view, superb spatial resolution, excellent temporal resolution, and rapid acquisition with no need for sedation or general anesthesia. The use of inspiratory and expiratory imaging can also provide additional information when evaluating central airways. In the setting of vascular ring evaluation, it allows simultaneous evaluation of vasculature, airways, and the esophagus. The main drawbacks relate to use of ionizing radiation and intravenous (IV) contrast material, with potential risk of allergic reactions and nephrotoxicity.

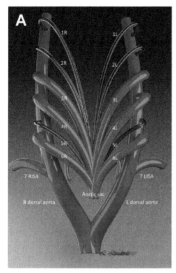 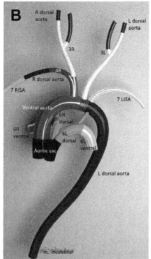 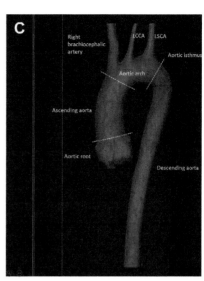

Fig. 1. Thoracic aorta development. (*A*) Schematic representation of the Rathke diagram demonstrates development of the aorta, pulmonary artery and arch branches from 6 pairs of aortic arches connecting the ventral aorta sac and the dorsal aortae. Transparent glass arches correspond to the segments that involute, either completely or near completely. (*B*) Schematic of the normal left aortic arch and branch vessels with colors indicating their different embryologic origins. The main contributors to the fully developed aorta include the ventral aorta (*orange*) (ascending aorta, proximal arch, and right brachiocephalic artery), the left fourth arch (*pink*) (distal aortic arch), and left dorsal aorta (*dark red*) (descending aorta). The aortic root and main pulmonary artery arise from the divided truncus arteriosus (aortic sac) (*blue*). The right and left main pulmonary arteries and the left ligamentum arteriosus derive from the sixth arches (*green*). The common carotids originate from the right and left third aches (*white*). The 7th intersegmental arteries (*yellow*) contribute to form the distal aspect of the right subclavian artery and the entire left subclavian artery. (*C*) Normal left aortic arch and branch arteries in volume-rendered image with conventional arch branching pattern. LCCA, left common carotid artery; LISA, left intersegmental artery; LSCA, left subclavian artery; RISA, right intersegmental artery.

COMPUTED TOMOGRAPHY PROTOCOL

Advances in CT technology continue to improve the evaluation of the thoracic aorta. Nowadays, it can be commonly performed without sedation during quiet breathing. Although the latest dual-source and wide-detector scanners allow high z axis coverage, 64 multidetector CT (MDCT) scanners still allow appropriate evaluation of these patients.

CTA imaging is limited to a single angiographic phase. Protocols need to be individualized to provide the minimal radiation dose, typically with 70 to 100 kVp imaging, automatic tube current modulation, prospective electrocardiogram triggering, iterative reconstruction, and high pitch, if available. The ability to image patients at 70 to 80 kVp is limited on older MDCT scanners due to the insufficient x-ray tube current output. In addition, when imaging at 70 to 80 kVp, it is important to move monitoring leads or other external objects out of the scanned region, as extensive artifacts could develop. A right upper extremity IV access is preferred, as dense contrast in the left innominate vein can preclude assessment of smaller structures, particularly in arch pathologies. Alternatively, a lower extremity could be used. Usually,

1 to 3 mL/kg of low-osmolar iodinated contrast material with 300 to 370 mg/mL concentration should be used up to a total volume of 100 to 120 mL. It is advisable to follow with an admixture of IV contrast and saline (50%–50% or 70%–30%) to allow proper evaluation of the right heart chambers. A saline flush allows a compact bolus with less recirculation and ensures all the intended contrast is indeed administered and not left in the IV tubing system. Power injection is preferred to obtain homogeneous opacification with rates of 1 to 5 mL/s depending on patient size and available venous access.

Bolus test timing and bolus tracking are both viable alternatives to initiate image acquisition. Bolus tracking requires identifying a target vessel, placing a region of interest over it and triggering after a specific threshold attenuation is reached (usually 100 HU). Test bolus offers the advantage of more closely monitoring the opacification of other cardiovascular structures, including assessment of superior vena cava (SVC) washout, which if excessively hyperattenuating could limit assessment of neighboring structures due to beam-hardening artifact. Alternatively, a fixed empirical

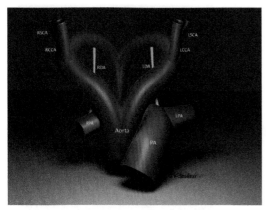

Fig. 2. Schematic 3D representation of Edward's Hypothetical Double Arch. Bilateral aortic arches and ductus arteriosi encircle the trachea and esophagus and each arch gives origin to common carotid arteries and subclavian arteries separately. The ventral portions of the sixth arches form the pulmonary artery and the dorsal portions of the sixth branchial arch become ductus arteriosus. LCCA, left common carotid artery; LDA, left ductus arteriosus; LPA, left pulmonary artery; LSCA, left subclavian artery; RCCA, right common carotid artery; RDA, right ductus arteriosus; RPA, right pulmonary artery; RSA, right subclavian artery.

delay of 12 to 15 seconds after contrast initiation for children weighing less than 10 kg or 20 to 25 seconds for larger children has been suggested.[5]

THORACIC CONGENITAL AORTIC ANOMALIES

A clear understanding of the definitions of the aorta and associated vascular structures is fundamental for clear communication, as terminology of this anatomy can be confusing. The aorta is commonly divided into 4 sections: the aortic root (which includes the aortic valve annulus, the sinuses of Valsalva, and sinotubular junction), the ascending aorta, the aortic arch, and the descending aorta. The aortic arch is the portion of the aorta, whether patent or atretic, that connects the ascending and descending aorta and gives rise to the arteries supplying the head, neck, and upper extremities. The aortic arch can be subdivided into the proximal arch (between the innominate artery and left common carotid artery), distal arch (between left common carotid and subclavian artery), and aortic isthmus (between the left subclavian artery and ligamentum arteriosum).[6]

Aortic arch laterality is determined by which bronchus is crossed by the arch. Uncommonly, arch laterality may be difficult to establish and arch branching pattern can be used as a surrogate for arch laterality with a few general rules: the first arch branch vessel that contains the common carotid artery is contralateral to the aortic arch, except in the presence of a retroesophageal brachiocephalic artery, which would be the last vessel from the arch, leaving then an ipsilateral right common carotid as the first arch branch from the arch. The aberrant or retroesophageal subclavian artery is always contralateral to the arch, but it should be carefully used when the entire aorta courses posterior to the esophagus.

Another important concept is the definition of a vascular ring, which is an abnormality of the aortic arch, its branches, or remnants that result in encircling of the trachea and the esophagus with variable degrees of compression.[7] When the vascular structures forming the ring are atretic or if caused by the ligamentum arteriosum, it may be difficult to identify a vascular ring. The "3 Ds" should suggest a vascular ring in the setting of an atretic nonvisible segment: Dimple contralateral to the arch (ductus); Diverticulum opposite to the side of the arch; Descending aorta on the opposite side to the arch (retroesophageal aorta/circumflex aorta).

NORMAL AORTIC ARCH

The normal pattern is a left arch with a left descending thoracic aorta and left ductus, either patent or ligamentous, extending from the proximal descending aorta, just distal to the origin of the left subclavian artery, to the left pulmonary artery. The arch branches are, in proximal to distal order, the right brachiocephalic artery, the left common carotid artery, and the left subclavian artery. This normal pattern results from proper regression of the hypothetical right arch (right dorsal aorta) between the right subclavian artery (seventh intersegmental artery) and the descending aorta, and involution of the right duct (right sixth arch dorsal portion).

The typical arch branching pattern occurs in 70% to 80% of the population.[4,8] The most common arch variant branching pattern results from a common origin of the left common carotid artery and right brachiocephalic artery, or, less commonly, with the left common carotid arising directly from the right brachiocephalic artery. This pattern prevalence is estimated at 13% and 9%, respectively. Although typically referred to as a bovine-type arch, the actual aortic arch pattern seen in cattle includes a single trunk off the aortic arch that provides a right subclavian artery, a bicarotid trunk, and left subclavian artery.[9] Another common variant arch anatomy includes the left vertebral artery arising directly from the aortic arch with a prevalence of 5% to 10%.

LEFT ARCH VARIANTS

Left Aortic Arch with Aberrant Right Subclavian Artery

This represents the most common congenital anomaly of the arch with a prevalence of 0.5% to 2.0%.[10] This implies abnormal regression of the right arch (right fourth arch proximal) between the right common carotid and right subclavian arteries, including the right ductus arteriosus. The distal right dorsal aorta becomes the proximal right subclavian artery. The aberrant right subclavian artery becomes the last arch branch and courses retroesophageal (Fig. 3). This is commonly an isolated anomaly, but can be associated with other congenital anomalies. Patients with Trisomy 21 have a higher prevalence reported to be 35%. Most cases are asymptomatic, but in approximately 10% of adult patients may have dysphagia symptoms resulting from dilation, calcification, and hardening of the aberrant subclavian artery against the esophagus and commonly referred to as dysphagia lusoria. In questionable cases, esophageal manometry may be useful to determine the clinical significance of the esophageal compression as the cause of symptomatology.

Left Aortic Arch with Diverticulum of Kommerell

A diverticulum of Kommerell, also referred to as a retroesophageal diverticulum, occurs when the aberrant right subclavian artery arises from a diverticular outpouching of the thoracic aorta. The diverticulum is thought to represent a remnant of the right dorsal aorta related to persistence of the right sixth arch dorsal portion (right ductus), which normally involutes. A vascular ring is completed by the right-sided ductus or ligamentum arteriosum. The presence of a retroesophageal diverticulum should suggest a ductus or ligamentum arteriosum on the contralateral side of the aortic arch and therefore completes a vascular ring that is commonly loose. If no retroesophageal diverticulum is present, the ductus or ligamentum arteriosum is on the same side of the aortic arch.

Circumflex Left Aortic Arch

In this abnormality, the descending aorta is located on the right, and the left arch demonstrates an abrupt course through the midline posterior to the esophagus above the level of the carina to reach the descending aorta. A right ductus or ligamentum arteriosum is usually present and connects the right-sided descending aorta to the right pulmonary artery forming a vascular ring. The arch branching pattern is classically like a left arch with aberrant right subclavian artery. The arch itself is retropharyngeal and the aberrant right subclavian artery arises from the arch after it is right-sided. This anomaly is thought to be the result of regression of the right fourth arch between the right subclavian artery and right common carotid with persistent right sixth arch dorsal portion (ductus) in the presence of a right-sided descending aorta. Less commonly, it can also result from regression of the right aortic arch more distally between the right subclavian artery and the ductus arteriosus, with absence of an aberrant right subclavian artery and no vascular ring.[11]

RIGHT ARCH VARIANTS

A right aortic arch occurs in 0.1% of the population.[12] It is caused by persistence of the right fourth arch and variable regression of the left fourth arch and dorsal aorta. In right arch anomalies, the arch typically begins on the right and starts to descend ipsilaterally, and gradually transitions toward the left, so that at the level of the diaphragm, joins the descending aorta on the left. A vascular ring may occur depending on the level of the left fourth arch resorption, the laterality and course of the ligamentum arteriosum, and the descending aorta.

Right Aortic Arch with Aberrant Left Subclavian Artery

This anomaly results from persistence of the right fourth arch with regression of the left fourth arch between the left common and subclavian arteries when using the hypothetical model of Edward's.[3] The branching sequence consist of the left common carotid, right common carotid, right subclavian artery and anomalous retroesophageal left subclavian artery as the last vessel to arise from the proximal descending aorta and demonstrates a retroesophageal course. Typically, a right-sided ductus or ligament arteriosum courses between the right-sided descending aorta and right pulmonary artery. This variant is not a vascular ring and it mirrors a left aortic arch with aberrant right subclavian. The typical pattern with right ductus or ligamentum is not associated with major congenital heart disease (CHD).[7,13] In the setting of a left ductus or absence ductus, the arch anomaly is associated with major intracardiac anomalies.

Right Aortic Arch with Aberrant Left Subclavian Artery with Retroesophageal Diverticulum

This results from regression of the left fourth arch between the left common carotid and left subclavian arteries with persistence of the left sixth

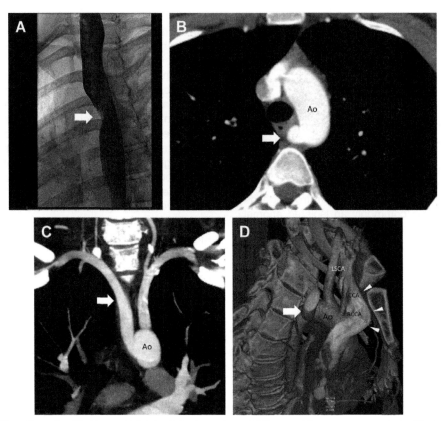

Fig. 3. Left aortic arch with aberrant right subclavian artery. A 28-year-old woman presented with dysphagia to solids. (*A*) Spot fluoroscopic image demonstrates discrete retroesophageal oblique impression (*arrow*). (*B*) Axial CT image, (*C*) coronal CT MIP, and (*D*) 3D volume-rendered reconstruction demonstrate a left aortic arch with anomalous left subclavian artery (*arrow*) coursing obliquely posterior to the esophagus as the last arch branch. Arrowheads, left innominate vein; Ao, aorta; LCCA, left common carotid artery; LSCA, left subclavian artery; RCCA, right common carotid artery.

arch. The branching pattern is the left common carotid, right common carotid, and right subclavian arteries followed by the anomalous retroesophageal left subclavian artery, but in this case arising from a diverticulum (**Fig. 4**). The larger caliber of the vessel and abrupt transition is best demonstrated on coronal imaging. The remnant of the left dorsal arch accounts of the retroesophageal diverticulum and the typical persistence of the left sixth arch commonly results in a left ductus or ligamentum arteriosum, which connects the retroesophageal diverticulum and the left pulmonary artery completing a vascular ring. This is the second most common cause of a vascular ring (30% of these cases) after a double aortic arch, although it is often relatively loose. This arch variant is infrequently associated with CHD. An atretic left arch should be raised as a differential in this situation.

Right Aortic Arch with Mirror Image Branching

This is the second most common form of right arch anomaly after the right arch with aberrant left subclavian artery.[4] It results from partial regression of the left fourth arch after the origin of the left subclavian artery (seventh intersegmental branch). The arch branching is typically the left brachiocephalic artery, followed by right common carotid and, last, the right subclavian artery (**Fig. 5**). The descending aorta is on the right and the ductus is present on the left (75% of these cases). In almost all cases, the involution occurs between the left ductus and the dorsal descending aorta[14] and characteristically, the left sixth arch persists as a ductus or ligamentum arteriosum between the left brachiocephalic artery anteriorly and the left pulmonary artery posteriorly. There is no vascular ring formation but is strongly associated with CHD in up to 98% of the cases, including tetralogy of Fallot, truncus arteriosus, tricuspid atresia, and transposition of great artery with pulmonary valve stenosis. The differential includes a double aortic arch with atretic left arch, although in this situation the descending aorta is usually left-sided.

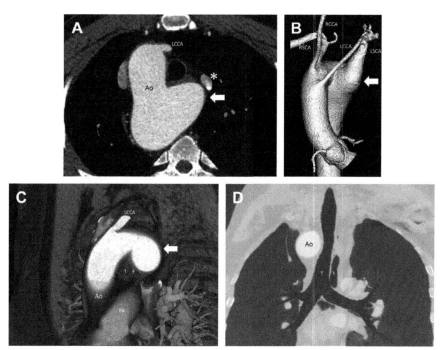

Fig. 4. Right aortic arch with aberrant left subclavian artery arising from a retroesophageal diverticulum. A 72-year-old asymptomatic man: (A) Axial CT image demonstrates a right aortic arch with diverticular structure (arrow) arising from the posterior arch with mild mass effect over the trachea and esophagus. Incidentally, there is duplicated left SVC (asterisk). (B) A 3D volume-rendered reconstruction demonstrates better the large Kommerell diverticulum (arrow) giving origin to the anomalous left subclavian artery. The dimple in the diverticulum corresponds to the ligamentum arteriosum. (C) A 3D volume-rendered reconstruction in grayscale demonstrates again the large retroesophageal diverticulum (arrow) and the nonopacified ligamentum arteriosum (red asterisk) that completes the vascular ring. (D) Coronal minimal intensity projection slab depicts only mild impression of the right aortic arch despite the vascular ring. Ao, aorta; E, esophagus; LCCA, left common carotid artery; LSCA, left subclavian artery; PA, pulmonary artery; RCCA, right common carotid artery; RSCA, right subclavian artery; T, trachea.

In very rare cases and typically not associated with congenital heart disease, the involution occurs between the left subclavian artery and the left ductus, resulting in a right aortic arch with mirror image branching but with a left ductus connecting a retroesophageal diverticulum and the pulmonary artery and completing a vascular ring.[14,15] In approximately 25% the ductus is located on the right, the result of left sixth arch regression with persistence of the right sixth arch with actual mirror image of the normal left arch anatomy. This is not associated with a vascular ring or intracardiac defect. Occasionally, the ductus is bilateral and may or may not be associated with cardiac anomaly. An absent ductus is associated with major intracardiac anomaly.

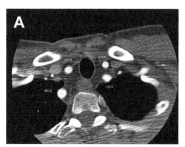
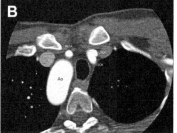
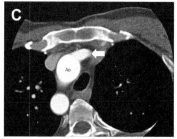

Fig. 5. Right aortic arch with mirror branching image. (A) Axial CT image at the thoracic inlet level demonstrates asymmetric distribution of the arch vessels. (B) Axial CT image at a lower level shows a right aortic arch and the bifurcation of the left brachiocephalic artery. (C) Axial CT image at a lower level demonstrates the takeoff of the left brachiocephalic artery (arrow) and a right descending aorta. Ao, aorta; LCCA, left common carotid artery; LSCA, left subclavian artery; RCCA, right common carotid; RSCA, right subclavian artery.

Right Aortic Arch with Aberrant Brachiocephalic Artery

This is a very rare anomaly due to the regression of the left fourth arch between the ascending aorta and left common carotid with persistent left dorsal and left ductus arteriosus.[16] The first arch branch is the right common carotid, followed by the left common carotid and the left brachiocephalic artery. A left ductus or ligamentum arteriosum persists on the left connecting the brachiocephalic artery to the left pulmonary artery and forming a vascular ring.

Right Arch with Isolation of the Left Subclavian Artery

Isolation refers to an arch vessel arising typically from the pulmonary artery through a ductus arteriosus and without communication to the aorta.[17] The most common form is a right aortic arch with isolation of the left subclavian artery and is associated with CHD in 50% of cases. It results from involution of the left arch at 2 separate segments, between the left common carotid and left subclavian arteries, and between the left ductus arteriosus and left subclavian artery. If the ductus arteriosus closes, this anomaly may result in subclavian steal phenomenon with subsequent vertebrobasilar insufficiency.

Circumflex Right Aortic Arch

This is a rare anomaly in which the descending thoracic aorta is located on the left and closely resembles a right arch with aberrant left subclavian artery arising from a diverticulum. This anomaly is a mirror image of the circumflex left aortic arch. The right aortic arch crosses the midline posterior to the esophagus above the level of the carina (**Fig. 6**). After crossing the midline, it gives rise to a diverticulum and this gives a ductus or ligamentum arteriosum that connects to the left pulmonary artery, completing a vascular ring.[18] This is the third most common type of vascular ring. Arch branch pattern includes an aberrant left subclavian artery arising from a diverticulum after the aorta has crossed the midline or a mirror image branching pattern. The differential includes a double aortic arch with atretic left arch from which it is essentially indistinguishable. This anomaly may result from regression of the left fourth arch between the left subclavian artery and left common carotid with persistent left sixth arch dorsal portion (ductus) and in the presence of a left-sided descending aorta. This results in a circumflex aorta with aberrant left subclavian artery. Alternatively, it may also result from regression of the left fourth arch between the left subclavian artery and the left ductus arteriosus or ligamentum arteriosum with mirror imaging branching.[18,19]

DOUBLE AORTIC ARCH

Double aortic arch is the most common cause of a symptomatic vascular ring and accounts for 50% to 60% of vascular rings.[20] When symptomatic during infancy or childhood, it characteristically presents with respiratory symptoms or feeding difficulties.[19] However, it is not uncommon to see asymptomatic adults. It results from lack of involution of the right and left fourth arches and the right and left dorsal aortae, each giving rise to a separate common carotid and subclavian arteries. Usually only 1 of the 2 sixth arches persist, giving rise to a ductus or ligamentum arteriosum. This anomaly is rarely associated with CHD, but when present typically is tetralogy of Fallot followed by the transposition of great arteries but incidence is not higher than the general population.

Typically, the proximal aorta bifurcation into right and left arches is higher than the level of distal confluence of the arches. The right arch is commonly larger and higher than the left arch (55%–70% of cases).[13,20] Less commonly, the left arch is dominant (20%–35%) (**Fig. 7**). In a minority, both arches are equal in size (5%–10%). The descending aorta is typically located on the left and classically opposite to the dominant arch, but may be seen on the right or midline. The ductus arteriosum is commonly located on the left, but may be present on the right or rarely be bilateral. The smaller arch may be focally or diffusely stenotic or atretic, more commonly the left arch (**Fig. 8**).

Two scenarios are possible with a partially atretic left arch. In one, the atretic segment is present between the left common carotid and left subclavian artery and mimics a right arch with aberrant left subclavian artery from a retroesophageal diverticulum. In another possibility, a more distal atretic segment beyond the left subclavian artery can be confused with a right arch with mirror image branching. It is important to differentiate these entities as double aortic arches even when atretic segments constitute actual vascular rings while right aortic arches with mirror branch imaging commonly do not. Findings that suggest an atretic arch include symmetric appearance of the bilateral common carotid and subclavian arteries originating from their respective ipsilateral arches on an axial image just above the level of the arches (the 4-vessel or 4 artery sign).[4] In contrast, a right arch with mirror image branching, the left subclavian artery arises from the left brachiocephalic

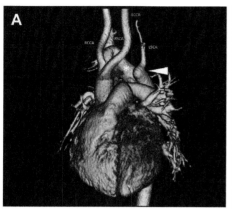
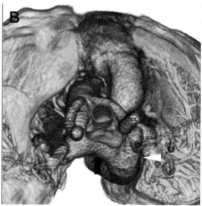

Fig. 6. Circumflex right aortic arch. (*A*) A 3D volume-rendered coronal oblique projection from contrast-enhanced CT demonstrates right-sided aortic arch (*asterisk*) with an aberrant left subclavian artery arising from a diverticulum (*arrowhead*) after the aorta has crossed the midline and a left descending aorta. (*B*) A 3D volume-rendered projection including also the air-filled structures shows the circumflex right aortic arch retroesophageal segment (*arrow*) and again a diverticulum (*arrowhead*) arising from the aorta after crossing the midline implying the presence of a left ductus ligament. DAo, descending aorta; LCCA, left common carotid artery; LSCA, left subclavian artery; RCCA, right common carotid; RSCA, right subclavian artery.

artery with significant asymmetry. In addition, it may be apparent tethering and distortion of the left common carotid or subclavian artery posteriorly from the patent aortic arch caused by traction from the atretic segment. Other clues include arch laterality, presence and orientation of a ductal diverticulum and dimple, and focal airway narrowing.[21]

Arch dominance determination has significant surgical consequences, as thoracotomy is usually performed in the nondominant side. Coronal multiplanar reformat (MPR) and 3-dimensional (3D) volume-rendered images are particularly useful. In apparently equal-sized aortic arches, one of the arches typically gets smaller in the posterior aspect near the descending aorta. It is also important to remind the surgeon that an apparent right aortic arch with retroesophageal diverticulum or right

aortic arch with left descending aorta could be an atretic left aortic arch in addition to a left ligament.[7]

CERVICAL AORTIC ARCH

Cervical aortic arch refers to an aortic arch extending superiorly in the neck above the clavicles. This may be on the left or right side and is usually an incidental finding. Patients usually present with a pulsatile neck mass. This may result from persistence of a third aortic arch (more commonly on the right) and abnormal regression of the fourth aortic arches. Another theory suggests failure of caudal migration of the fourth arch, or even that the third and fourth arches fuse, with lack of caudal migration.[22,23] Cervical arch branching pattern anomalies include right aortic arch with mirror image, aberrant subclavian artery with a Kommerell

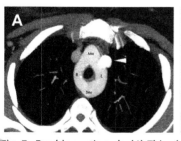
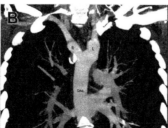
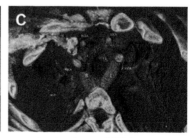

Fig. 7. Double aortic arch. (*A*) Thin-slab maximum-intensity projection from contrast-enhanced CT demonstrates 2 arches surrounding the trachea and esophagus with a slightly larger left arch. A duplicated left SVC is also present (*arrowhead*). (*B*) Thick-slab coronal maximum-intensity projection from contrast-enhanced CT demonstrates again a slightly larger left arch and a midline descending aorta. (*C*) A 3D volume-rendered image shows the 4-vessel sign with symmetric distribution of the bilateral common carotid and subclavian arteries. AAo, ascending aorta; DAo, descending aorta; L, left arch; LCCA, left common carotid artery; LSCA, left subclavian artery; R, right arch; RCCA, right common carotid; RSCA, right subclavian artery.

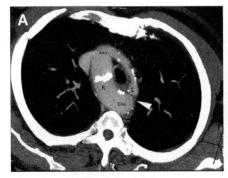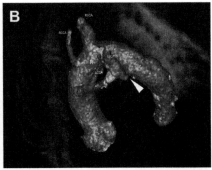

Fig. 8. Double aortic arch with focal left atretic segment. (*A*) Thick-slab maximum-intensity projection from contrast-enhanced CT demonstrates 2 arches surrounding the trachea and esophagus with a larger and higher right arch. Focal atretic segment with fibrous cord is present on the left posteriorly (*arrowhead*). (*B*) A 3D volume-rendered image shows a smaller left aortic arch in close relation to an ipsilateral descending aorta but without definite communication (*arrowhead*). The left arch extends posterior to the left subclavian artery with a diverticular outpouching compatible with atresia of the distal left arch with a fibrotic band tethering the left subclavian artery. AAo, ascending aorta; DAo, descending aorta; L, left arch; LCCA, left common carotid artery; LSCA, left subclavian artery; R, right arch; RCCA, right common carotid; RSCA, right subclavian artery.

diverticulum, and separate origins of the internal and external carotid arteries from the aortic arch.

AORTIC HYPOPLASIA

Hypoplasia of the aorta refers to an abnormally diffuse reduced caliber of the aorta that commonly results in obstruction to the antegrade flow. Narrowing may involve the entire aortic arch or a limited portion. It could be defined based on reference standards adjusted to body mass index (>−2 Z score).[6] In the presence of a normal ascending aorta, proximal arch, distal arch, and isthmus hypoplasia can be diagnosed if their diameters are less than 60%, 50%, or 40% compared with the ascending aorta, respectively.[24,25] Tubular hypoplasia requires a minimal length greater than 5 mm in infants. Aortic arch hypoplasia can be an isolated finding or be associated with other obstruction left-sided lesions, such as congenital

mitral stenosis, mitral atresia, hypoplastic left heart syndrome, aortic stenosis, aortic atresia, interrupted aortic arch, and coarctation of the aorta. Treatment is typically considered for a hemodynamically significant lesion with a gradient greater than 15 to 20 mm Hg.[26]

COARCTATION OF THE AORTA

Coarctation of the aorta characteristically refers to focal narrowing of the aorta usually near the ligamentum arteriosum distal to the left subclavian artery (**Fig. 9**). It accounts for 7% of all congenital heart disease with a prevalence of 4 per 10,000 live births. Histopathologically, there are cystic changes in the media with elastin fragmentation and increased collagen deposition that results in a thickened aortic wall.[27] Two proposed mechanisms try to explain its origin: (1) the ductal theory postulates the presence of ectopic ductal tissue

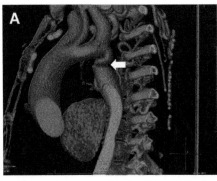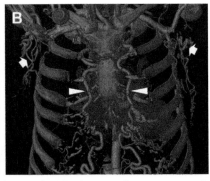

Fig. 9. Coarctation of the aorta. (*A*) A 3D volume-rendered sagittal projection reveals severe narrowing involving the isthmic portion of the aorta (*arrow*) with large posterior intercostal arteries. (*B*) A 3D volume-rendered frontal projection image shows multiple, large tortuous collaterals circulation, including internal mammary (*arrowheads*), thoracodorsal (*short arrows*) arteries.

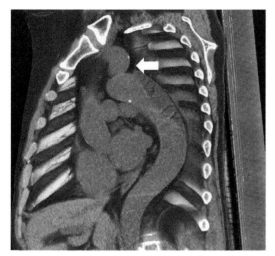

Fig. 10. Pseudocoarctation of the aorta. A 3D volume-rendered sagittal projection reveals focal buckling (*arrow*) with associated tortuosity and elongation of the descending thoracic aorta without a discrete focal stenosis. Notice the lack of collateral pathways.

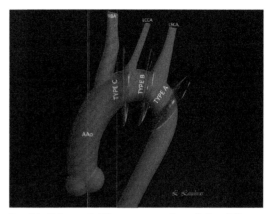

Fig. 11. Schematic 3D representation of the different interrupted aortic arches based on Celoria and Patton classification of IAA. Transparent discs represent the focal discontinuity of the different types of aortic arch interruption. Type A has an interruption distal to the left subclavian artery. In type B, the absent segment locates between the left common carotid artery and left subclavian artery. Type C gap is distal to the brachiocephalic artery. The descending thoracic aorta reconstitutes from the pulmonary artery through a ductus arteriosus. AAo, ascending aorta; LCCA, left common carotid; LSCA, left subclavian artery; RBA, right brachiocephalic artery.

extending into the aorta, and (2) the hemodynamic theory suggests the coarctation results from abnormally decreased preductal flow.[26] It may occur as an isolated lesion in approximately 80% of cases. It is commonly associated with Turner syndrome, bicuspid aortic valve, intracranial aneurysms, ventricular septal defect, atrial septal defect, and Shone complex (left ventricular outflow obstruction and parachute mitral valve).[6] Typically, patients present with arterial hypertension in the upper extremities and a systolic murmur.

Characteristic findings included focal eccentric narrowing of the juxtaductal thoracic aorta with multiple collateral vessels bypassing the stenotic segment. Coarctation of aorta can be treated surgically with tube grafts or aortoplasty, percutaneous balloon angioplasty, and stent placement.

PSEUDOCOARCTATION

Pseudocoarctation is a rare anomaly consisting of kinking and buckling of the arch and descending aorta at the level of the ligamentum arteriosum.[28] There is no actual pressure gradient across the stenosis and therefore the lesion is not hemodynamically significant with no collateral vessel formation (Fig. 10).

Patients are classically asymptomatic and it is considered a benign anomaly that generally requires no surgical intervention. Occasionally, symptomatic patients and those with aneurysmal formation may require treatment.[4] The pathogenesis of aneurysm beyond the kinked segment may relate to abnormal turbulent flow.

INTERRUPTED AORTIC ARCH

Interrupted aortic arch (IAA) refers to the focal discontinuity between the ascending and descending thoracic aorta with flow to the descending aorta dependent on a patent ductus arteriosus. The separation can be complete or fibrous tissue cord may be present. IAA prevalence is estimated in 2 per 100,000 live births.[3] There is a significant association with patients with DiGeorge syndrome who present an interrupted aortic arch in 5% to 20% of cases, whereas 40% to 50% with interrupted aortic arch will have DiGeorge syndrome.[29] The most commonly used classification system recognizes 3 groups: type A, distal to the left subclavian artery; type B, distal to the left common carotid artery takeoff; and type C, proximal to the origin of the left common carotid artery (Fig. 11). Type B accounts for 50% to 60% of cases, type A represent 30% to 40% of cases (Fig. 12), and type C is the least common (<5% of cases).[26] In any of these types, the right subclavian artery may demonstrate a normal origin (subtype 1) or anomalous origin (distal to the left subclavian artery, subtype 2; or from the right ductus arteriosus, subtype 3).[30] IAA is commonly associated with large ventricular septal defect (VSD) and left ventricular outflow obstruction. Less commonly, it may present with a large aortopulmonary window or truncus anomaly.

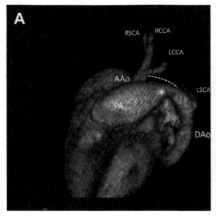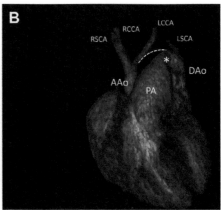

Fig. 12. Interrupted aortic arch type B. (*A*) A 3D volume rendering from a superolateral perspective reveals focal interruption of the aortic arch (*dotted line*) with pulmonary artery communicating with the descending aorta through a large ductus arteriosus (*asterisk*). (*B*) A 3D volume-rendered frontal projection demonstrates interruption of the aortic arch (*dotted line*) just beyond the left common carotid artery. Large ductus arteriosus again showed (*asterisk*). AAo, ascending aorta; DAo, descending aorta; LCCA, left common carotid artery; LSCA, left subclavian artery; PA, pulmonary artery; RCCA, right common carotid; RSCA, right subclavian artery.

Patients present in the first 2 weeks of life with shock or severe heart failure after spontaneous closure of the ductus arteriosum. On physical examination, a gray appearance of the lower body due to hypoperfusion is characteristic with difference in systolic blood pressure and oxygen saturation between the right upper extremity and lower extremities. IAA is usually treated with side-to-side anastomosis rather than conduit interposition. Postoperative complications include persistent subaortic and aortic stenosis, and residual VSD.

SUMMARY

Congenital aortic anomalies include a variety of pathologic disorders with clinical presentations ranging from asymptomatic to life threatening. CTA imaging provides a rapid and reliable way to accurately diagnose these variants and anomalies as well as evaluate associated lesions, which helps in management.

ACKNOWLEDGMENTS

The authors acknowledge Dr Carlos F. Ugas and Dr Aracelly Matos, Department of Pediatric Radiology, Instituto del Niño San Borja, Lima, Peru, for contributing **Figs. 6** and **12**.

REFERENCES

1. Waldo K, Kirby M. Development of the great arteries. In: de la Cruz MV, Markwald RR, editors. Living morphogenesis of the heart. Boston: Birkauser; 1998. p. 187–217.

2. Kau T, Sinzig M, Gasser J, et al. Aortic development and anomalies. Semin Intervent Radiol 2007;24: 141–52.

3. Edwards JE. Anomalies of the derivatives of the aortic arch system. Med Clin North Am 1948;32: 925–49.

4. Hanneman K, Newman B, Chan F. Congenital variants and anomalies of the aortic arch. Radiographics 2017;37(1):32–51.

5. Siegel MJ. Multiplanar and three-dimensional multidetector row CT of thoracic vessels and airways in the pediatric population. Radiology 2003;229(3): 641–50.

6. Restrepo CS, Melendez-Ramirez G, Kimura-Hayama E. Multidetector computed tomography of congenital anomalies of the thoracic aorta. Semin Ultrasound CT MR 2012;33(3):191–206.

7. Weinberg PM. Aortic arch anomalies. J Cardiovasc Magn Reson 2006;8(4):633–43.

8. Priya S, Thomas R, Nagpal P, et al. Congenital anomalies of the aortic arch. Cardiovasc Diagn Ther 2018;8(Suppl 1):S26–44.

9. Layton KF, Kallmes DF, Cloft HJ, et al. Bovine aortic arch variant in humans: clarification of a common misnomer. AJNR Am J Neuroradiol 2006;27(7):1541–2.

10. Türkvatan A, Büyükbayraktar FG, Olçer T, et al. Congenital anomalies of the aortic arch: evaluation with the use of multidetector computed tomography. Korean J Radiol 2009;10(2):176–84.

11. McLeary MS, Frye LL, Young LW. Magnetic resonance imaging of a left circumflex aortic arch and aberrant right subclavian artery: the other vascular ring. Pediatr Radiol 1998;28(4):263–5.

12. Maldonado JA, Henry T, Gutiérrez FR. Congenital thoracic vascular anomalies. Radiol Clin North Am 2010;48(1):85–115.

13. Etesami M, Ashwath R, Kanne J, et al. Computed tomography in the evaluation of vascular rings and slings. Insights Imaging 2014;5(4):507–21.

14. Schlesinger AE, Krishnamurthy R, Sena LM, et al. Incomplete double aortic arch with atresia of the distal left arch: distinctive imaging appearance. AJR Am J Roentgenol 2005;184(5):1634–9.

15. D'Souza VJ, Velasquez G, Glass TA, et al. Mirror-image right aortic arch: a proposed mechanism in symptomatic vascular ring. Cardiovasc Intervent Radiol 1985;8(3):134–6.

16. Moes CA, Mawson JB, MacDonald C, et al. Right aortic arch with retroesophageal left aberrant innominate artery. Pediatr Cardiol 1996;17(6):402–6.

17. Luetmer PH, Miller GM. Right aortic arch with isolation of the left subclavian artery: case report and review of the literature. Mayo Clin Proc 1990;65(3):407–13.

18. Knight L, Edwards JE. Right aortic arch. Types and associated cardiac anomalies. Circulation 1974;50(5):1047–51.

19. Kanne JP, Godwin JD. Right aortic arch and its variants. J Cardiovasc Comput Tomogr 2010;4(5):293–300.

20. Ekstrom G, Sandblom P. Double aortic arch. Acta Chir Scand 1951;102(3):183–202.

21. Gould SW, Rigsby CK, Donnelly LF, et al. Useful signs for the assessment of vascular rings on cross-sectional imaging. Pediatr Radiol 2015;45(13):2004–16 [quiz: 2002–3].

22. Kellenberger CJ. Aortic arch malformations. Pediatr Radiol 2010;40(6):876–84.

23. Stojanovska J, Cascade PN, Chong S, et al. Embryology and imaging review of aortic arch anomalies. J Thorac Imaging 2012;27(2):73–84.

24. Ho SY, Anderson RH. Coarctation, tubular hypoplasia, and the ductus arteriosus. Histological study of 35 specimens. Br Heart J 1979;41(3):268–74.

25. Singh S, Hakim FA, Sharma A, et al. Hypoplasia, pseudocoarctation and coarctation of the aorta—a systematic review. Heart Lung Circ 2015;24(2):110–8.

26. Hellinger JC, Daubert M, Lee EY, et al. Congenital thoracic vascular anomalies: evaluation with state-of-the-art MR imaging and MDCT. Radiol Clin North Am 2011;49(5):969–96.

27. Rao PS. Coarctation of the aorta. Curr Cardiol Rep 2005;7(6):425–34.

28. Kessler RM, Miller KB, Pett S, et al. Pseudocoarctation of the aorta presenting as a mediastinal mass with dysphagia. Ann Thorac Surg 1993;55(4):1003–5.

29. Pongiglione G. Aortic arch interruption: Orphanet encyclopedia 2004. Available at: http://www.orpha.net/data/patho/GB/uk-AAI.pdf. Accessed June 29, 2018.

30. Collins-Nakai RL, Dick M, Parisi-Buckley L, et al. Interrupted aortic arch in infancy. J Pediatr 1976;88(6):959–62.

Computed Tomography of Acquired Aortic Diseases

Xhorlina Marko, MD, Constantino S. Peña, MD*

KEYWORDS

• CTA • Aorta • Atherosclerosis • Aortic aneurysm • Aortitis

KEY POINTS

- Computed tomography angiography (CTA) has replaced catheter angiography in the evaluation of aortic disease.
- CTA is able to evaluate occlusive and aneurysmal disease of the aorta.
- Inflammatory conditions of the aorta can also be assessed with CTA.

INTRODUCTION

Computed tomography (CT) angiography (CTA) has become the standard of practice for imaging the aorta. By rapidly imaging the aorta during a contrast bolus, CTA provides an efficient technique to evaluate the vasculature in a large portion of the body. The ability to reliably perform CTA with high temporal and spatial resolution resulting in submillimeter isotropic images (equal spatial resolution in all 3 dimensions) has allowed for postprocessing techniques that further enrich the arterial assessment. Although there are risks involved in obtaining a CTA scan, such as contrast-induced nephropathy and radiation exposure, the benefits of CTA outweigh the risks in appropriate patients. When imaging the aorta, CTA has replaced catheter angiography in the diagnosis of acquired disease such as aortoiliac disease, aneurysm, and infectious and inflammatory disease of the aorta.

IMAGING OF AORTA

The aorta is the largest vessel in the body. Although there are several imaging modalities available to evaluate the aorta, CTA has the ability to evaluate the aortic wall and lumen easily, quickly, and reproducibly without the need for invasive technologies such as direct angiography or intravascular ultrasonography. CTA relies on a volumetric CT acquisition when the vessels are fully enhanced with iodinated contrast material. The images are of high spatial resolution and isotropic, allowing detailed three-dimensional (3D) reconstructions. In the thorax, electrocardiogram-based cardiac gating (prospective or retrospective) can be used to reduce cardiac motion, particularly with the evaluation of the aortic root.[1]

Magnetic resonance (MR) is a second modality that can be used to evaluate the morphology of the aorta. MR carries a significant advantage in that it does not require ionizing radiation. MR angiography (MRA) examinations usually require the use of gadolinium chelates as a contrast agent and this limits their use in patients with renal dysfunction. Noncontrast MRA examinations are becoming more useful in clinical practice; however, they may lack the spatial resolution of present gadolinium-enhanced scans. CTA examination is much more readily available and reproducible, making it the primary morphologic examination of the aorta in clinical practice.

COMPUTED TOMOGRAPHY PROTOCOL FOR EVALUATION OF AORTA

The general protocol for performing aortic CTA is shown in **Table 1**. A non–contrast-enhanced CT

Miami Cardiac and Vascular Institute, Baptist Health South Florida, 8900 North Kendall Drive, Miami, FL 33176, USA
* Corresponding author.
E-mail address: tinopena@msn.com

Radiol Clin N Am 57 (2019) 127–139
https://doi.org/10.1016/j.rcl.2018.08.012

Table 1 Computed tomography angiography of the aorta: general 3-phase protocol	
Noncontrast phase	Acquired helically and non–cardiac gated at 3–5 mm slice thickness If there is concern for the aortic root, prospectively cardiac gated scan obtained
Arterial phase	25 mL saline bolus at 3.5 mL/s to confirm intravenous patency 75–125 mL of contrast material at 3.5–5 mL/s with saline chaser Timing bolus or bolus tracking used to identify peak enhancement Biphasic injection can also be performed to increase the imaging window Contrast injection rate may vary with the patient's body mass index Cardiac gated acquisition reconstructed at 1-mm intervals between 2-mm thick images
Delayed phase	Acquired helically and non–cardiac gated at slice thickness 3–5 mm If there is concern for the aortic root, prospectively cardiac gated scan obtained

acquisition is used for the evaluation of acute or subacute hemorrhage, as may be seen in a contained aortic rupture or intramural hematoma. It may also be used to compare and ensure that increased density seen on a contrast-enhanced image is contrast material and not from a native area of increased density, such as wall calcifications.

The contrast-enhanced phase is acquired during arterial enhancement after a rapid injection (3–5 mL/s) of iodinated contrast material for a total volume of 75 to 125 mL. When determining an arterial imaging protocol, the amount of contrast enhancement (contrast injection: rate, amount, iodine concentration), length of the injection, length of the scan, and time to beginning the acquisition are critical in order to image the vessel during peak arterial enhancement for the length of the scan. In order to image during the arterial phase, 2 primary techniques are used to define the time to peak enhancement of the desired vessel: bolus triggering or timing bolus.

The final acquisition is usually a delayed phase. The amount of delay may depend on the indication for the examination and the structures that require delayed visualization. To evaluate the portal venous system, the delay may be between 40 and 70 seconds after the arterial injection, whereas, to evaluate for a possible endoleak after endograft placement, the delay can be 2 minutes.

COMPUTED TOMOGRAPHY ANGIOGRAPHY POSTPROCESSING

A large series of images is usually acquired during CTA. These images must be processed in order to best highlight the anatomy but also to allow complete evaluation of the images. There are multiple postprocessing techniques that can be used during CTA. The noncontrast and delayed acquisition images are evaluated at thicknesses of 2 to 5 mm. The arterially enhanced images are acquired at 0.625-mm to 1.25-mm slices and evaluated in the axial plane at 1-mm to 3-mm intervals. However, the 0.625-mm to 1.25-mm thin images are used to perform reconstructions and reformations. Coronal and sagittal reformations are usually performed automatically at the point of acquisition and are performed with the vessels and adjacent soft tissues. These reformations have become standard for all body CT examinations.

The thin images are then processed on a 3D workstation to perform the necessary maximal intensity projection (MIP) of the vessels. An MIP image displays the highest intensity value voxel from the acquired data in the evaluated projection. After removing the bony structures, this creates a 3D image of the contrast-enhanced arteries along with the associated calcium (**Fig 1**A). Because a single MIP image lacks depth and spatial details, a rotational evaluation of batched MIPs is required in order to assess the depth of the imaged volume. Volume-rendered (VR) reconstructions maintain all of the image's density information, which is converted to opacity values to allow for spatial relationships and depth between structures (**Fig 1**B). These images are the most visually pleasing but may hide subtle differences because some algorithms may smooth an image.[2] Furthermore, on a 3D workstation, curved planar reconstructions (CPR) can be performed to evaluate a vessel path as it travels along multiple planes by creating a single two-dimensional view of the vessel path (**Fig 1**C). A CPR can be rotated and allows evaluation of the vessel lumen as well as the vessel wall in order to assess for stenosis.[3]

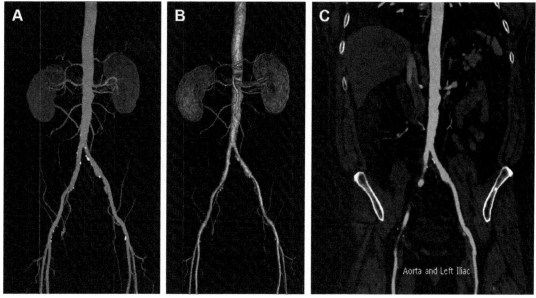

Fig. 1. Image reconstructions. (*A*) MIP shows a single two-dimensional (2D) representation of the highest pixel values along a projection. (*B*) Volume-rendered (VR) image uses color and shading to show the density of the structures within a volume. (*C*) Curved planar reconstruction (CPR) shows the course of a vessel's center path on a single 2D image, allowing evaluation of a vessel that may be in multiple planes on a single image.

ANATOMY OF THE AORTA

The aorta is composed of multiple segments, including the aortic root, sinotubular junction, ascending aorta, aortic arch, descending aorta, and abdominal aorta. The aorta is composed of 3 basic layers: the intima, media, and adventitia. The intima is the inner, single layer of endothelial cells. The media is the thickest and most variable layer of the aortic wall, composed of elastin sheets and collagen sheets with interspersed elastin fibers. The different elastin to collagen ratio and amount of smooth muscle cells gives the aorta the elastic and recoil properties that are needed for continued blood flow during diastole. The adventitia is the thin outer layer of the aorta, composed of connective tissue, fibroblasts, and the vasa vasorum. Acquired disease of the aorta predominantly involves certain aortic segments.

ATHEROSCLEROSIS

The primary acquired disease of the aorta is atherosclerosis. Atherosclerosis is a degenerative and inflammatory condition that affects the aorta and its branches, as well as other vessels such as the coronary, cerebral, and lower extremity arteries. Atherosclerosis is the leading cause of cardiovascular mortality and morbidity in Western countries. It is a complex and chronic process

that begins in the intima, likely during childhood. The hallmark of atheromatous formation involves fatty streaks composed of lipid-laden macrophages and smooth muscle cells located in the subendothelial space. There is formation of atheroma, or plaque, composed of these macrophages and smooth muscle cells along with cholesterol, triglycerides, and other cellular debris such as fibrin. These fatty depositions are covered by a fibrous cap. Some plaques rupture acutely, causing occlusion and symptoms, whereas more stable, chronic plaques result in inflammation, causing medial thinning, cellular necrosis, plaque growth, as well as plaque calcification. Plaque formation can be associated with arterial vessel narrowing and occlusion leading to symptoms.[4]

Atherosclerosis is the most common cause of occlusive disease of the aorta and iliac arteries. There are multiple cardiovascular risk factors for atherosclerotic disease. The modifiable risk factors include smoking, sedentary lifestyle, diabetes, hypertension, and hyperlipidemia. Patients' age (>40 years), sex (male), and genetics (including family history) are not modifiable risk factors. The most common portion of the aorta affected by atherosclerotic disease is the infrarenal segment, followed by the proximal descending thoracic aorta and the aortic arch along with its great vessel origins.

Aortoiliac disease is a spectrum of disease that starts with plaque formation, intraluminal stenosis, and eventually occlusion. CTA is an excellent modality for evaluation of the aorta as well as its branches. Non–contrast-enhanced images evaluate the degree of vessel calcification, a marker for chronic atherosclerotic disease. The contrast-enhanced images highlight the vessel lumen, allowing proper identification of plaque, ulceration, and degree of stenosis of the vessel lumen (Fig 2). The most severe form of aortoiliac disease is Leriche syndrome. These patients classically present with severe hip or buttock claudication, erectile impotence, and decreased femoral pulses caused by functional occlusion of the distal aorta and the iliac bifurcation. CTA is helpful not only in diagnosis but in treatment planning of this condition. It is uniquely able to identify the site of vascular occlusion, reconstitution, amount of underlying calcification, as well as the involvement and proximity to important vessels such as the renal artery, inferior mesenteric artery, hypogastric artery, and common femoral artery (Fig. 3). Involvement of the middle or visceral abdominal aorta by atherosclerotic disease is less common than the aortoiliac segment. It is usually identified in women smokers. Midaortic syndrome is the term used to describe this pattern of disease. Treatment of these patients is challenging because of the involvement of the visceral artery origins.

CTA can be used to assess both endovascular (Fig. 4) and surgical (Fig. 5) revascularization, particularly in patients with symptoms that may warrant intervention or in anatomic sites where ultrasonography evaluation can be limited.

Atherosclerotic occlusive disease of the thoracic aorta is extremely rare. Atherosclerotic disease is typically seen in the descending thoracic aorta with areas of calcified, noncalcified, or mixed plaque formation. These plaques may cause areas of irregularity along the vessel wall without significant narrowing of the vessel lumen. Plaque formation also occurs at the origins of the great vessel as well as along the inferior aspect of the aortic arch. Atherosclerotic disease in the thoracic aorta typically represents an area of plaque with vessel wall irregularity that is important if stiff wires or devices are going to be manipulated in this vessel.

AORTIC ANEURYSM

Aneurysmal disease is a common condition involving the aorta. The cause of aneurysmal disease involves the weakening of the aortic wall,

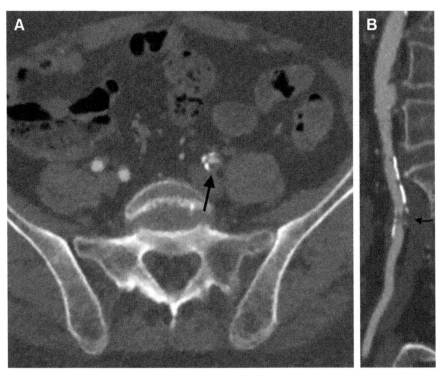

Fig. 2. Atherosclerotic disease. (*A*) Axial CTA image shows severe calcified and noncalcified plaque at the origin of the left external iliac artery (*black arrow*). (*B*) CPR image of the left iliac artery shows the extent of luminal narrowing (*black arrow*) caused by the atherosclerosis in the external iliac origin.

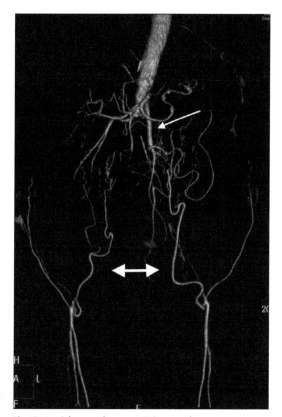

Fig. 3. Leriche syndrome. VR image shows severe aortoiliac disease. The CTA shows occlusion of the distal aorta and bilateral common and external iliac arteries with reconstitution of bilateral common femoral arteries. The examination shows an enlarged inferior mesenteric artery (*white arrow*) and bilateral inferior epigastric arteries (*double white arrow*).

primarily the media and adventitia, caused by the loss of elastin and collagen fibers. This process seems to be modulated by an inflammatory signal from recruited lymphocytes and macrophages that control the production of the metalloproteinases responsible for the proteolytic degradation, hence resulting in the breakdown of collagen and elastin. The biomechanical effects from the loss of elastin and collagen and the different ratio of elastin to collagen throughout the elastic segments may also explain the different patterns of expression identified within the different segments of the aorta. This process results in the reduction of tensile and radial strength as well as thickening of the aorta, which eventually leads to aneurysm dilatation.[5] Risk factors for aneurysmal disease include age, smoking, hypertension, and family history. Atherosclerosis is commonly seen in patients with aneurysmal disease and could be considered an independent risk factor for aneurysmal disease.[6]

Aneurysmal disease of the aorta is defined as a focal dilatation of the aorta greater than 1.5 times its normal diameter. However, the size of the aorta can vary with age, gender, and body size, making an arbitrary measurement criterion difficult to apply along a general population. By definition, a thoracic aortic aneurysm is dilatation of greater than 4.0 cm involving all 3 layers of the aortic wall, whereas an abdominal aortic aneurysm (AAA) is greater than 3.0 cm. A pseudoaneurysm is an aneurysm that does not involve all 3 layers of the aortic wall. There are several genetic conditions, such as Marfan, Loeys-Dietz, and Ehlers-Danlos syndromes, that are associated with aneurysm formation related to abnormal collagen or elastin content. In addition, bicuspid aortic valves are associated with thoracic aortic aneurysm (TAA). These conditions are important to recognize because early detection may lead to appropriate surveillance and properly timed surgical repair, reducing the risk of aortic dissection (AD), rupture, and death.[7]

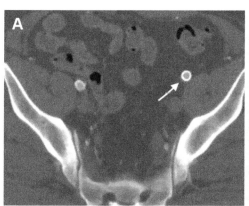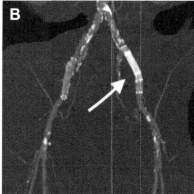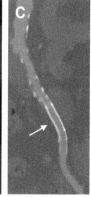

Fig. 4. Postendovascular revascularization. (*A*) Axial CT image of a left external iliac stent (*white arrow*). (*B*) MIP image of left iliac stents (*white arrow*) without the ability to assess patency. (*C*) CPR of a left iliac stent (*white arrow*) showing the ability to assess patency within the stent.

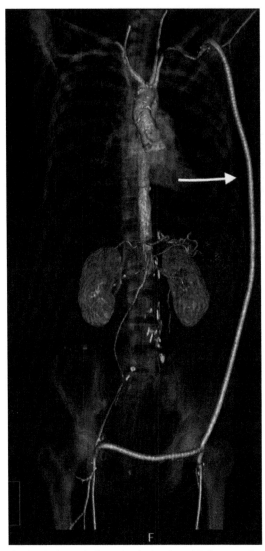

Fig. 5. Postsurgical revascularization. VR image of a left axillary to cross-femoral bypass (*white arrow*) for the treatment of aortoiliac occlusive disease.

Aneurysms of the aorta are incidentally discovered. Rarely, they present with symptoms from encroaching on nearby structures such as the airway, esophagus, or laryngeal nerve with large TAA or back pain from large AAA. AAA is 30 times more prevalent than TAA.[8] They are most common in the infrarenal position but can extend to involve the visceral artery origins in a juxtarenal, suprarenal, or thoracoabdominal location. The most significant complication of aortic aneurysms is rupture-related death. The rate of rupture is related to aneurysm size. A TAA with a diameter of greater than 6 cm has 7% risk of rupture per year, whereas an AAA greater than 7 cm has a 32.5% risk of rupture per year.[9] In the thoracic aorta, the ascending aorta and aortic root are affected most often, followed by the descending aorta and the aortic arch (**Fig. 6**). In TAA, maximal aneurysm diameters are also related to the risk of rupture. In addition, in TAA the increased diameter was thought to increase the risk of dissection; however, new long-term data seem to suggest otherwise.[10] Other complications of aortic aneurysms include distal embolization from the aortic sac thrombus.

CT angiography is an excellent modality for the evaluation of aortic aneurysms. The noncontrast phase of imaging shows wall calcifications as well as hemorrhage in an acute situation. The contrast-enhanced phase is helpful to assess the vessel diameter and the contrast-enhanced lumen as well as the extent of an aneurysm and its relationship with the great vessels in a TAA, and visceral arteries in both TAA and AAA (**Fig. 7**). The CTA and its reconstructions can be used to plan surgical, endovascular, or hybrid repairs by evaluation of the nature of the aneurysm, its branch vessel involvement, its angulation, and the access vessels.

AORTIC DISSECTION

AD is the most dangerous and difficult condition to treat in both the acute and chronic setting. The acute mortality from AD is high and increases with delayed diagnosis. An AD represents an intimal injury with subsequent separation of the inner third of the media from the outer third, which results in the entry of blood within this potential space, causing the space to expand along the aortic wall. Acute secondary complications include aortic rupture and proximal and/or distal extension to involve the aortic vessels, resulting in distal malperfusion.

An AD is classified anatomically by the most proximal aspect of the aorta that is involved. The classification is important because it has traditionally determined treatment. Two types of classification have been described: the Stanford and DeBakey classifications. Stanford type A or DeBakey type I and II ADs involve the ascending aorta (**Fig. 8**). This dissection type is traditionally treated with surgical replacement of the ascending aorta. Despite improvement in surgical techniques, perioperative mortality and neurologic complications remain high at 25% and 18%, respectively.[11] Stanford type B or DeBakey type IIIa/b AD involves the thoracic aorta, distal to the left subclavian artery. Type B AD can further be classified as complicated. The term complicated is reserved for those type B ADs with persistent pain, uncontrolled hypertension despite aggressive medical

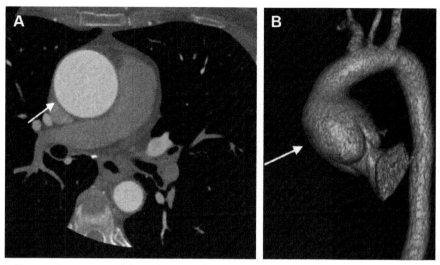

Fig. 6. Ascending aortic aneurysm. (*A*) Axial image of an ascending TAA (*white arrow*). (*B*) VR image of a 7.2-cm ascending aortic TAA (*white arrow*) in an asymptomatic man. The aortic valve was tricuspid. There is loss of the sinotubular ridge.

management, early aortic expansion, malperfusion, signs of rupture (increase in size of periaortic hematoma, hemothorax), and increasing false-lumen diameter. There has been some debate as to how to classify dissections involving the aortic arch, because they are type B but may require emergent therapy. However, AD management is challenging because AD can be a dynamic and evolving process, especially acutely.

Traditionally, uncomplicated type B AD is initially treated with medical management (pain and blood pressure control), whereas endovascular interventions are reserved for complicated type B AD. Endovascular interventions can focus on

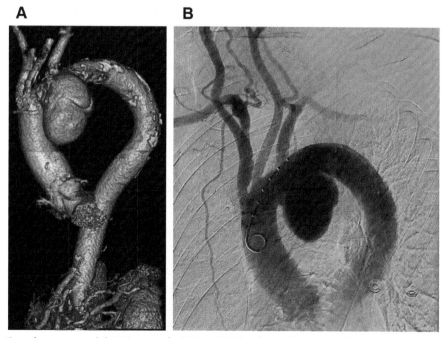

Fig. 7. Aortic arch aneurysm. (*A*) VR image of a 7.5-cm TAA involving the aortic arch, showing the relationship to the arch and great vessels. (*B*) Aortogram of the TAA involving the thoracic arch confirming CTA findings and relationship to great vessels.

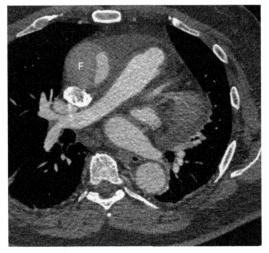

Fig. 8. Type A AD. Axial CTA image of an acute dissection involving the ascending aorta. There is diminished arterial flow appreciated in the false lumen (F). There is stranding surrounding the ascending aorta without rupture.

techniques to equalize the flow between the true and false lumens in order to improve malperfusion. Thoracic endovascular repair (TEVAR) can also be used with the goal of closure of the entry tear, redirecting blood flow into the true lumen and thrombosis of the false lumen, which in itself promotes vessel remodeling and stabilization (**Fig. 9**). There has been a transition to TEVAR in uncomplicated patients during the subacute phase (2–4 weeks after initial AD). The goal is to cause remodeling and lead to improved long-term survival.[12] Chronic AD (>3 months) shows thickening of the initial flap, making endovascular interventions more difficult. Also, in AD there is weakening of the aortic wall

causing long-term dilatation and aneurysmal change to the aortic lumens.

CT angiography is essential for evaluating AD. In the acute phase it allows rapid diagnoses and proper classification and subsequent triage. The non–contrast-enhanced phase of imaging evaluates acute hemorrhage, allowing identification of intramural hematoma as well as possible rupture or extravascular hemorrhage. The contrast-enhanced phase shows the intimal flap, dissection origin and extent, possible fenestrations between the true and false lumens, as well as an important assessment of the distal perfusion particularly to the vessels emanating distal to the dissection. In the subacute phase, CT imaging is used in order to assess small changes or evolution in the extent of the dissection, malperfusion, false-lumen expansion, or thrombosis that may prompt a change in treatment. In the chronic phase, there can be further dissection or extension but this usually presents clinically with an acute episode. Traditionally, patients with ADs are imaged to assess for further dilatation and aneurysm formation in the aorta that will require open surgical repair.

INFLAMMATORY DISEASE

Inflammatory disease of the aorta is a broad category, described by the term aortitis. These conditions should be thought of as conditions primary to the aortic wall, ranging from vasculitis to extrinsic processes indirectly affecting the vessel wall, such as radiation-induced arteritis or retroperitoneal fibrosis. When a vasculitis is considered, it is best to consider the patient's age and the size of the vessel involved. There are several

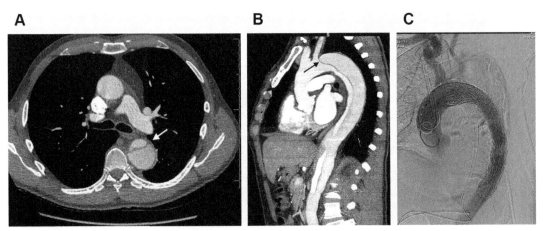

Fig. 9. Type B AD. (*A*) Axial image of a type B AD with an intimal flap (*white arrow*) within the descending aorta. (*B*) Sagittal oblique reconstruction showing the origin just distal to the left subclavian (*black arrow*). (*C*) Angiogram after placing a TEVAR showing exclusion of flow in the false lumen.

large vessel vasculitis affecting the aorta, including Takayasu arteritis (TA) and giant cell arteritis.[13] These vasculitides typically cause thickening of the vessel wall and can progress to segments of vessel narrowing and occlusion. Inflammatory arthritides are common conditions that can also manifest with a form of vasculitis. Although systemic rheumatoid vasculitis is the most common, systemic lupus, ankylosing spondylitis, Behçcet and Reiter arteritis can occur and may involve the aorta.

TA is a multifactorial, hereditary condition characterized by a necrotizing granulomatous obliterative subsegmental systemic inflammatory process that affects the aorta and its branches as well as the pulmonary artery. It was first described in 1908 by a Japanese ophthalmologist and commonly affects women less than 40 years of age. There is a higher predilection for patients of Asia and Latin American descent. There are 5 angiographic types of TA described, depending on the part of the aorta and its branches that are involved. The abdominal aorta is the most commonly involved aortic segment, followed by the descending thoracic aorta and the aortic arch (TA usually spares the ascending aorta) (**Fig. 10**). TA is a panarterial inflammatory process and commonly results in stenosis and vessel occlusions, causing clinical manifestations such as extremity claudication with a pulseless presentation and hypertension (as result of renal artery involvement). Giant cell arteritis is also a granulomatous disease but typically affects women more than men, of white descent, and more than 50 years of age. It primarily affects the subclavian and axillary arteries as well as the external carotid branches and vertebral arteries. Typical symptoms included headache, scalp tenderness, and jaw claudication. The aorta is typically affected in 15% of the patients and it primarily involves the ascending aorta and aortic arch, resulting in aneurysm. It is usually a more focal process and is more common than TA.[14]

Inflammatory changes of the aorta can be acute or chronic. In the acute phase, they usually show vessel wall enhancement, concentric wall thickening, and associated perivascular stranding that can be identified with CTA imaging. This finding

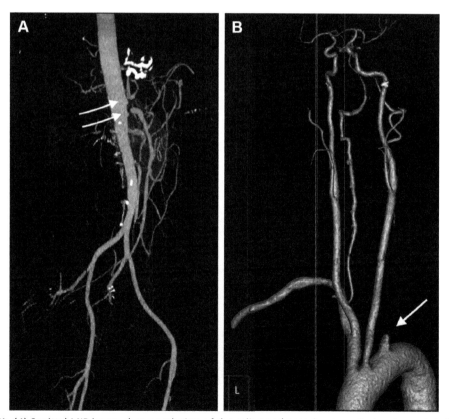

Fig. 10. TA. (*A*) Sagittal MIP image shows occlusion of the celiac and superior mesenteric artery origin (*white arrows*) in a patient with chronic TA. (*B*) VR image of the thoracic arch shows occlusion of the left proximal left subclavian artery (*white arrow*) in a patient with active TA.

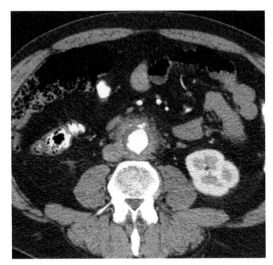

Fig. 11. Inflammatory aneurysm. Axial CTA image with an infrarenal AAA and circumferential periaortic soft tissue that enhances and is ill defined.

has been described as the double-ring appearance on CTA.[15] In the chronic phase, the enhancement is lost and the thickening becomes more of a fibrotic appearance. Occasionally, linear aortic wall calcifications can be seen (usually after 5 years of disease presentation).

An inflammatory aortic aneurysm is a rare and frequently misunderstood condition that is characterized by a circumferential thickened perianeurysmal tissue that enhances after contrast administration (**Fig. 11**). This entity should not be confused with an infectious aneurysm. The histology is typically a form of fibrosis. This process is almost exclusively seen in the abdominal aorta. Treatment of the aneurysm can be with an endovascular or open repair; however, the open repair

has been reported to have atypically higher mortality.[16]

INFECTIONS

Infectious diseases of the aorta are a cause of aortitis and are thought to be related to hematogenous spread from bacteria such as *Salmonella* and *Staphylococcus*, syphilis, mycobacterial tuberculosis, and viruses such as human immunodeficiency virus. Even though it may affect a healthy vessel wall by entering via the vasa vasorum, infection most commonly occurs at an area of atherosclerosis, aneurysm, or ulceration that may serve as a nidus. Contiguous seeding from a nearby infection, such as a diskitis or osteomyelitis, can also occur. An iatrogenic cause is the most common cause of infectious aortitis and usually occurs after a procedure. CT imaging can identify irregularity of the aortic wall or a periaortic mass with associated stranding into the surrounding perivascular fat that may be associated with adjacent fluid.[17] Infectious aortitis is a rapidly progressive process that destroys the vessel wall. Identification and prompt treatment are required (**Fig. 12**). Traditionally, this is treated with resection and surgical bypass.

Although rare today, tertiary syphilis can cause a particular form of infectious aortitis. This aortitis is a chronic process, usually seen 5 to 30 years after the primary infection, which results in inflammation and subsequent obliteration of the vasa vasorum, leading to fibrosis. It is thought that the resultant fibrosis in the adventitia leads to aneurysm formation, primarily affecting the ascending aorta and aortic arch. The chronic process results in thickening with layers of fibrosis in the aortic wall, which has been

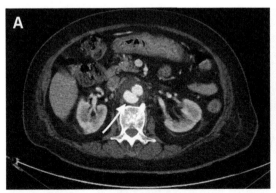
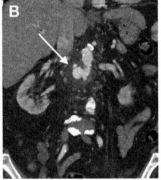

Fig. 12. Infectious aortitis. (*A*) Axial image with ulceration of the aortic lumen (*white arrow*). (*B*) Coronal CTA reconstruction shows an extensive, irregular ulcerative process involving the infrarenal aorta with perivascular stranding (*white arrow*) in a patient with progressive abdominal pain over 6 days and a positive culture for salmonella. The patient had a CT scan of the abdominal aorta that was unremarkable except for a minimal atherosclerotic calcification a year prior.

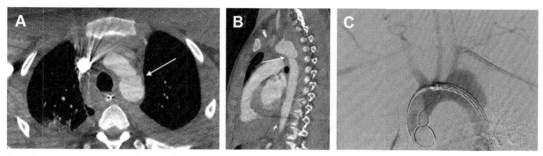

Fig. 13. Aortic transection. (*A*) Axial CTA image after motor vehicle crash showing aortic transection with pseudoaneurysm formation (*white arrow*). (*B*) Sagittal oblique reconstruction shows pseudoaneurysm at level of the proximal descending aorta (*white arrow*). (*C*) Aortogram shows pseudoaneurysm and aortic stent graft being positioned to repair the transection.

described by the term tree barking. Linear calcifications may occur within the layers of fibrosis. The slow and chronic dilatation may cause erosive changes to adjacent bony structures, particularly the right side of the manubrium and the medial end of the right clavicle.[18] Syphilitic aortic aneurysms commonly involve the ascending aorta and aortic arch.[16]

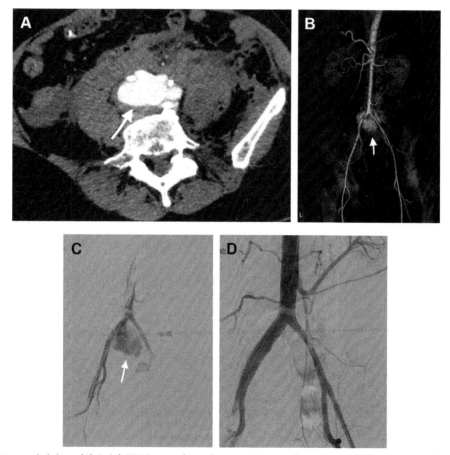

Fig. 14. Iatrogenic injury. (*A*) Axial CTA image shows large pelvic pseudoaneurysm (*white arrow*) with extravasation after attempted spinal procedure. (*B*) VR shows extent of the pseudoaneurysm (*white arrow*). (*C*) Retrograde right common femoral angiogram with a proximal aortic–right common iliac occlusion balloon in place confirms right common iliac injury and extravasation (*white arrow*). (*D*) Angiogram after placement of right common iliac covered stent with no further extravasation.

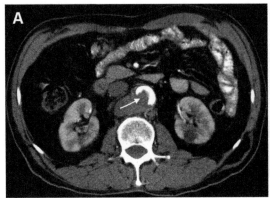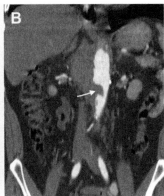

Fig. 15. Aortic neoplasm. (*A*) Axial CTA image shows an asymmetric soft tissue mass (*white arrow*) extending through the aortic wall as well as into the aortic lumen. (*B*) Coronal reconstruction showing intravascular and extramural extent of mass (*white arrow*). This mass was found to be a sarcoma on biopsy.

INJURIES

Injury to the aorta is common and can occur at any age or location. A traumatic transection of the thoracic aorta is a common example. These transections occur after a traumatic injury, causing a deceleration injury to the aorta at the level of the isthmus at the junction between the free and the fixed proximal descending thoracic aorta. Most patients with transection of the aorta die at the scene but a small percentage make it to a medical facility. Prompt diagnosis by CT imaging and subsequent repair are critical because the risk of rupture and death increases with time after the incident (**Fig. 13**). Other iatrogenic injuries to the aorta may occur during adjacent thoracic or abdominal procedures. CTA imaging is again helpful in the diagnosis and treatment planning for these unplanned events. Iatrogenic injury to the aorta typically presents as pseudoaneurysms or with contrast extravasation on CTA (**Fig. 14**). Pseudoaneurysms are focal dilated portions of the vessel wall that do not contain the usual 3 layers but contain nonlaminar vascular flow and are at high risk of rupture.

NEOPLASMS

Neoplasms of the aorta are rare and usually difficult to diagnose because they are initially clinically silent. Statistically, metastatic deposits are more common than primary neoplasms of the aorta. Primary neoplasms are usually muscular in origin (sarcomatous) and should be considered when there are changes that involve the vessel wall that are not typical of atherosclerosis or acute thrombus formation. Patients may have obstructive symptoms or arterial embolization from both tumor and thrombus that may be associated with

the tumor. These neoplasms can originate in the vessel wall (mural) or lumen (intimal), or extend out of the vessel. Enhancement may be identified by CT; however, the pattern of presentation on imaging is variable. CT can help to determine the extent of the neoplasm in order to plan tissue sampling and treatment resection if possible (**Fig. 15**). PET imaging has been helpful to confirm metabolic activity and serves as a noninvasive tool to suggest the diagnosis.[19]

SUMMARY

Acquired diseases of the aorta are extensive in their cause and appearance. CTA is a modality that allows rapid and dependable depiction of the aorta and its branches. Because conditions of the aorta can be significant and important to assess, the risk of renal dysfunction from the contrast material and the radiation exposure is usually outweighed by the potential benefits of the examination.

REFERENCES

1. Rubin GD, Leipsic J, Schoepf UJ, et al. CT Angiography after 20 years: a transformation in cardiovascular disease characterization continues to advance. Radiology 2014;271(3):633–52.
2. Rubin GD, Dake MD, Napel S, et al. Spiral CT of renal artery stenosis: comparison of three-dimensional rendering techniques. Radiology 1994;190(1):181–9.
3. Roos JE, Fleischmann D, Koechl A, et al. Multipath curved planar reformation of the peripheral arterial tree in the CT angiography. Radiology 2007;244(1):281–90.
4. Ross R. Atherosclerosis- an inflammatory disease. N Engl J Med 1999;340:115–26.

5. Satta J, Laurila A, Paakko P, et al. Chronic inflammation and elastin degradation in abdominal aortic aneurysm disease: an immunohistochemical and electron microscopic study. Eur J Vasc Endovasc Surg 1998;15:313–9.

6. Toghill BJ, Saratzis A, Bown MJ. Abdominal aortic aneurysm–an independent disease to atherosclerosis? Cardiovasc Pathol 2017;27:71–5.

7. Loughborough WW, Minhas KS, Rodrigues JC, et al. Cardiovascular manifestations and complications of Loeys-Dietz syndrome: CT and MR imaging findings. Radiographics 2018;38:275–86.

8. Golledge J, Norman PE. Atherosclerosis and abdominal aortic aneurysm: cause, response, or common risk factors? Arterioscler Thromb Vasc Biol 2010;30:1075–7.

9. Davies RR, Goldstein LJ, Coady MA, et al. Yearly rupture or dissection rates for thoracic aortic aneurysms: simple prediction based on size. Ann Thorac Surg 2002;73(1):17–27.

10. Evalgelista A, Isselbacher EM, Bossone E, et al. Insights from the International Registry of Acute Aortic Dissection: a 20-year experience of collaborative clinical research. Circulation 2018;137:1846–60.

11. Chiappini B, Schepens M, Tan E, et al. Early and late outcomes of acute type A aortic dissections: analysis of risk factors in 487 consecutive patients. Eur Heart J 2005;26:180–6.

12. Durham CA, Cambria RP, Wang LJ, et al. The natural history of medically managed acute type B aortic dissection. J Vasc Surg 2015;61:1192–9.

13. Jennette JC, Falk RJ, bacon PA, et al. 2012 Revised International Chapel Hill Consensus Conference nomenclature of vasculitides. Arthritis Rheum 2013; 65(1):1–11.

14. Broncano J, Vargas D, Bhalla S, et al. CT and MR imaging of cardiothoracic vasculitis. Radiographics 2018;38:997–1021.

15. Hayashi H, Katayama N, Takagi R. CT analysis of vascular wall during the active phase of Takayasu's aortitis [abstract]. Eur Radiol 1991;1(suppl):S239.

16. Restrepo CS, Ocazionez D, Suri R, et al. Aortitis: imaging spectrum of the infectious and inflammatory conditions of the aorta. Radiographics 2011;31: 435–51.

17. Macedo T, Stanson AW, Oderich GS, et al. Infected aortic aneurysms: imaging findings. Radiology 2004;231:250–7.

18. Bodhey NK, Gupta AK, Neelakandhan KS, et al. Early sternal erosion and luetic aneurysms of thoracic aorta: report of 6 cases and analysis of cause-effect relationship. Eur J Cardiothorac Surg 2005;28(3):499–501.

19. Restrepo CS, Betancourt SL, Martinez-Jimenez S, et al. Aortic tumors. Semin Ultrasound CT MR 2012;33:265–72.

Computed Tomography of Cardiac Valves: Review

Diana E. Litmanovich, MD[a],*, Jacobo Kirsch, MD, MBA[b]

KEYWORDS

• CT • Cardiac valves • Stenosis • Regurgitation • Prolapse

KEY POINTS

- Cardiac CT is a robust modality for qualitative and quantitative assessment of both morphology and function of cardiac valves.
- Quantitative CT assessment of cardiac valves is comparable to MR imaging and echocardiography measurements.
- Cardiac CT allows quantification of valvular calcification, thus providing crucial prognostic and treatment planning information.
- Cardiac CT plays an important role in the postsurgical assessment of prosthetic valves and complications of endocarditis.

INTRODUCTION

Valvular heart disease is a common clinical problem, with a reported prevalence of 2.5% in the United States.[1] Between 10% and 20% of cardiac surgical procedures in the United States are performed for treatment of valvular disease[2,3] Usually, echocardiography is the standard technique for the noninvasive evaluation of the cardiac valves, although high interobserver variability, low reliability in the measurement of the pulmonary valve (PV) and right heart function in transthoracic echocardiography, and the invasive nature of transesophageal echocardiography leave a role for other imaging modalities.[4] Cardiac CT is a noninvasive technique that may be used to characterize heart valve disease in patients with inconclusive findings at transthoracic echocardiography. Of even greater importance is the ability of CT imaging to provide ancillary data about cardiac chambers that may affect the management of cardiac valve disease in some patients.[5] Moreover, cardiac CT allows quantification of valvular calcification and characterization of valvular masses and

vegetations.[6,7] Often, cardiac valve pathology might be diagnosed in examinations performed for other indications. This review focuses on the growing role of ECG-gated multidetector (MD) CT in evaluating cardiac valvular pathology.

TECHNICAL CONSIDERATIONS AND ADVANCEMENTS IN CARDIAC COMPUTED TOMOGRAPHY
Native Valves

CT techniques for imaging the cardiac valves have changed with advancement of cardiac CT.[5] The scanning parameters for left heart valves are similar to those used in coronary CT angiography and vary with the scanner generation and vendor. Currently CT scanners with 64 channels or more are used.[8–10] The section thickness usually is 0.50 mm to 0.75 mm to obtain high spatial resolution image data sets with isotropic voxels. For most scanners, the pitch varies in keeping with the patient's heart rate, and the tube current–time product may vary with the patient's body habitus, whereas the voltage is usually near 120

[a] Radiology, Beth Israel Deaconess Medical Center, Harvard Medical School, FNASCI, 330 Brookline Avenue, Boston, MA 02215, USA; [b] Hospital Specialties, Department of Imaging, Cardiothoracic Imaging, Cleveland Clinic Florida, 2950 Cleveland Clinic Boulevard, Weston, FL 33331, USA
* Corresponding author.
E-mail address: dlitmano@bidmc.harvard.edu

Radiol Clin N Am 57 (2019) 141–164
https://doi.org/10.1016/j.rcl.2018.08.011
0033-8389/19/© 2018 Elsevier Inc. All rights reserved.

kilovolts (peak) (kV[p]). Patients with lower body mass index (<28–30) may benefit from 100 kV(p) .

Contrast material is typically injected as a bolus through an antecubital intravenous catheter, and either bolus tracking or bolus timing software is used to trigger contrast-enhanced acquisitions when the bolus reaches the ascending aorta. A variable volume of contrast material is used; a volume as low as 50 mL has been used with the intention of achieving opacification of only the left-sided cardiac chambers and aorta[9] but if a comprehensive evaluation of both sides of the heart is intended, intravenous contrast material volume is based on a patient's weight and is typically 100 mL to 120 mL. To achieve the optimal contrast opacification of the right heart, a modified split bolus protocol should be used, where 60 mL to 80 mL of nondiluted contrast material is injected at high rate (5–6 mL/s) followed by a slower infusion of 30 mL of nondiluted contrast (3 mL/s) and concluded with an injection of saline at the rate of 2 mL/s to 3 mL/s (saline flash) to achieve enhancement of pulmonary valves and tricuspid valves.[11,12]

Unenhanced prospectively ECG-gated acquisitions of the heart also may be performed if an assessment of calcification of the valvular or aortic calcification is needed to answer the clinical question.

Prosthetic Valves

Current ECG-gated MDCT technology, with its superior spatial and adequate temporal resolutions, minimizes beam-hardening and motion artifacts and thus is superior to echocardiography and cardiac MR imaging in terms of spatial resolution in examinations of prosthetic valves.[1,13–15] Initial unenhanced prospective ECG-gated scan for optimal assessment of valve calcifications, radiopaque suture material, and erroneously retained surgical objects is prudent, followed by a contrast-enhanced retrospective ECG-gated scan.

Postprocessing

Postprocessing reformations and measurements are performed at a dedicated 3-D workstation. Both native and postsurgical valvular anatomy are evaluated in multiple orthogonal planes in motionless diastolic and systolic volumetric data sets. A minimum of 2 perpendicular imaging planes of each prosthetic valve are created, including 1 positioned exactly in the plane of the evaluated valve ring and 1 set perpendicular to the prosthetic valve leaflets. Dynamic cine evaluation of the valves is performed with conventional short-axis and 2-chamber, 3-chamber, and 4-chamber long-axis reformations of the heart and in short-axis views positioned exactly in the plane of the evaluated valve and reconstructed over 10 or 20 phases of the MDCT volumetric data set at 10% or 5% intervals ranging from 0% to 90% or 95% of the R-R interval.[14] ECG-gated MDCT obtained through the entire cardiac cycle provides accurate measurements for assessing the opening and closing angles of mechanical prosthetic valves.[15] Retrospective ECG-gated MDCT with planimetry can be used to measure the effective orifice area in mechanical and biologic prosthetic valves as accurately as it can with transthoracic echocardiography and to assess for leaflet thickening, calcifications, and restricted motion.[14]

AORTIC VALVE
Normal Anatomy

The aortic valve complex consists of the aortic valve annulus, commissures, sinuses of Valsalva (SOVs), coronary ostia, and sinotubular junction. Three aortic valve cusps, left, right and noncoronary (posterior), are connected proximally to the wall of the left ventricular outflow tract (LVOT) by 3 anchor points at the nadir (hinge point) of each aortic cusp[16,17] (Fig. 1). Those nadir points, when virtually connected, form an oval-shaped, 3-pronged coronet—the virtual basal ring. The orientation of this virtual basal ring, or aortic annulus, is double oblique and does not correspond to conventional axial, coronal, or sagittal planes of MDCT. Multiple manipulations of the raw imaging data are required to create an image that would exactly correspond to the aortic annulus (virtual basal ring). The functional unit from the ventriculo-aortic junction (aortic valve ring) to the sinotubular junction constitutes the aortic root.[18,19]

The morphology of the aortic valve can be assessed using multiplanar reformation (MPR) and multiphasic cine movie loops at the midsystolic (open valve) and the mid-diastolic phase (closed valve).[5] Coverage can be extended to include the ascending aorta, which is frequently dilated in patients who have aortic valve disease. Aortic valve calcification can be measured on cardiac CT images in the same manner that coronary calcium scores are obtained. The amount of valvular calcification, expressed as an Agatston score, correlates with the severity of aortic stenosis (AS) and has been shown to provide prognostic information.[5]

Congenital Abnormalities of the Aortic Valve

Occasionally, rather than being a tricuspid valve, the aortic valve can have 1, 2, or even 4 or 5 cusps. Bicuspid aortic valve (2 cusps instead of 3) is the

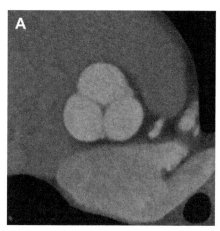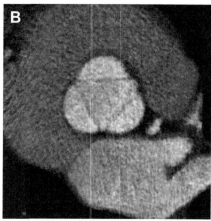

Fig. 1. Normal aortic valve. Axial images show a normal valvular anatomy with thin cusps in end diastole (*A*) and end systole (*B*).

most common congenital cardiovascular anomaly, with a prevalence of 1% to 2% in the general population (**Fig. 2**). The bicuspid aortic valve may be composed of 2 cusps, morphologically and functionally, or may present with 3 developmental anlagen of cusps and commissures. In the latter type, 2 adjacent cusps fuse to a single aberrant cusp with the development of a ridge or raphe, found in 75% of the bicuspid valves. The raphe may be developed partially or totally and often is thickened or calcified or both.[20,21] In 86% of this bicuspid aortic valve phenotype, the raphe was located between the right coronary cusp and left coronary cusp.[20,21]

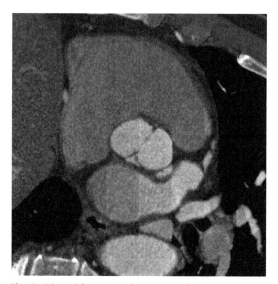

Fig. 2. Bicuspid aortic valve. Axial oblique maximum intensity projection images shows a noncalcified bicuspid aortic valve in diastole.

The presence of a bicuspid aortic valve is associated with an increased incidence of complications, such as stenosis, regurgitation, endocarditis, aneurysmal dilatation of the ascending aorta, and aortic dissection. These complications tend to manifest at an earlier age in patients with a bicuspid valve than in those with a normal valve (patients with a bicuspid aortic valve have an aortopathy similar to that seen in Marfan syndrome, with an increased propensity for dilatation, aneurysm, dissection, and rupture of the aorta).[22] ECG-gated MDCT is highly accurate for differentiation between bicuspid and tricuspid aortic valves. For bicuspid aortic valves without raphe, diastolic reconstructions are sufficient, whereas in those with a raphe, additional reconstructions in systole are required[20,23] and both systolic and diastolic data sets must be evaluated. Thus, when CT is performed to distinguish bicuspid from tricuspid aortic valves, retrospective ECG gating with acquisition of data throughout the entire cardiac cycle is necessary.[20,24]

Aneurysmal dilatation of 1 or more of the SOVs is rare but may occur congenitally as a result of focal weaknesses in fibroelastic tissue elements.[5] SOV aneurysms are frequently encountered in patients with connective-tissue disorders, such as Marfan and Loeys-Dietz syndromes or in association with AVR, a bicuspid aortic valve, or a ventricular septal defect. Possible causes of acquired SOV aneurysms include infection (endocarditis, syphilis, and tuberculosis), medial degeneration, hypertension, and trauma. Symptoms may result from local mass effect or from rupture of the aneurysm, which tends to produce an aortocardiac shunt and heart failure.[5,25,26]

Aortic Valve Stenosis

AS is defined as an obstruction of the LVOT at the subvalvular, supravalvular, or valvular level of the aortic valve. The valvular stenosis is the most frequent type and can be classified as congenital or acquired. In developed countries, AS is generally an acquired degenerative process with factors similar to those implicated in coronary atherosclerosis.[3,27,28] Rheumatic heart disease accounts for most cases of AS worldwide. In patients with rheumatic heart disease, inflammatory adherence of the cusps can lead to acquired fusion of the commissures, with resultant noncompliance of the cusps with subsequent stenosis, regurgitation, or a combination of the two.[5] Slowly progressive calcification and sclerotic thickening of the valve leaflets reduces valvular excursion and impedes left ventricular (LV) outflow (**Fig. 3**).

The pathophysiology of adult AS is characterized by a gradual decrease in valve area (normal values, 2.5–4.0 cm^2), in which initially nonhemodynamically relevant valve calcification progresses to a hemodynamically relevant obstruction of the LV outflow (<1 cm^2). The physiologic response is compensatory LV hypertrophy due to its increased afterload and dilatation of the aortic root.[29] A decreased LV ejection fraction and an increased LV mass have been associated with poor outcomes of AS in asymptomatic patients.[3,5]

Cardiac CT findings in AS may include thickening and calcification of the aortic valve cusps. The cardiac CT 3-D data set can also be reconstructed in the aortic valve plane in systole for planimetric measurements of the aortic valve area to classify the severity of AS. Even in patients with severe calcifications, planimetric measurements are not restricted as a result of artifacts and correlate significantly with transesophageal echocardiography findings and mean transvalvular pressure gradients.[30,31] Diagnostic accuracy of MDCT, compared with transthoracic echocardiography, in the identification of patients with moderate (100% sensitivity, specificity, and accuracy) or severe (91% sensitivity, 97% specificity, and 96% accuracy) AS is excellent. MDCT planimetric measurements of the aortic valve area are highly reproducible and correlate strongly with MR and TEE planimetric measurements of the aortic valve area. The main advantage of ECG-gated CT angiography compared with echocardiography is the more accurate measurement of the valve orifice area, which, in CT, is not limited by hemodynamic factors, such as low cardiac output.[30] CT gives a reproducible quantification of valve calcification that correlates with the severity of AS. In addition, compensatory LV hypertrophy and poststenotic dilatation of the ascending aorta can be seen.

Aortic Valve Calcifications

Age-related degenerative calcified AS is the most common cause of AS in adults and is associated with severe atherosclerosis of the aorta and the coronary arteries.[5] Presence of aortic valve calcifications (AVCs) has been proved as an indicator of atherosclerotic burden rather than just a degenerative change as shown by its strong association with atherosclerotic risk factors. In the recent Multi-Ethnic Study of Atherosclerosis population, AVCs were found in one-third of the study population and were independently associated with an increased severity of coronary artery calcification after controlling for demographic factors and cardiovascular risk factors.[3] Calcific aortic valve disease was shown to be a measure of subclinical atherosclerosis in a population free of known coronary artery disease and it is associated with

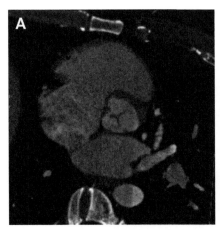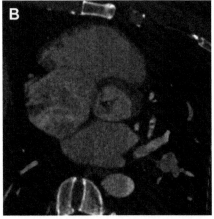

Fig. 3. AS. Axial oblique MPR images through the aortic valve during diastole (*A*) and during systole (*B*) show thickening of the valve leaflets and restricted opening of the aortic valve orifice resulting in significant stenosis.

coronary events and stroke as well as cardiovascular disease events in the general population.[32]

Large-scale, multicenter outcomes study of quantitative Doppler echocardiographic and MDCT assessment of AS showed that measuring AVC load provides incremental prognostic value for survival beyond clinical and Doppler echocardiographic assessment. Severe AVC independently predicts excess mortality after AS diagnosis, which is greatly alleviated by AVI.[33] All the 3 AVC load scores (Agatston score, calcium volume, and calcium mass) are highly correlated with aortic valve weight and with hemodynamic parameters of AS severity.[34]

For AS severity diagnostic purposes, interpretation of AVC load should be different in men and in women.[35] Currently proposed gender-specific CT-AVC thresholds for severe disease based on ECG-gated CT-AVC within 3 months of echocardiography (women 1377 Agatston units and men 2062 Agatston units or women 1274 Agatston units and men 2065 Agatston units) have been shown reproducible and generalizable in predicting severe AS and adverse effects.[36–38] Thus, in patients with a discordant grading severity of AS at Doppler echocardiography, or low flow–low gradient AS, AVC load seems to be an excellent surrogate marker of true AS severity, that is, truly severe AS or moderate AS.

For similar degrees of AS severity, bicuspid valves have higher absolute AVC scores in comparison with tricuspid valves but similar AVC density[38] (Fig. 4).

Aortic Valve Regurgitation

Aortic valve regurgitation (AVR) is characterized by blood reflux into the LV during diastole, caused by a failure of the aortic valve to close properly due to a malcoaptation of the valve cusps[5] (Fig. 5). A wide variety of disorders lead to aortic regurgitation by producing stiffened cusps that fail to coapt, by distorting the geometry of the aortic root, or by both mechanisms combined. Rheumatic heart disease is the most common cause of aortic regurgitation in the developing world; in developed nations, bicuspid aortic valve and ectasia of the aortic root are more prevalent causes.[39] Half of all patients with severe aortic valve regurgitation develop heart failure within a decade after receiving the diagnosis.[40]

AVR can be categorized by chronicity (acute vs chronic) and severity (mild to severe). Acute AVR is a rare condition that may be caused by endocarditis, Stanford type A aortic dissection, or thoracic trauma. Because there is inadequate time for the development of compensatory mechanisms, patients with this condition typically experience sudden heart failure or cardiogenic shock. Intrinsic, chronic AVR is commonly a result of atherosclerotic degeneration of a normal tricuspid aortic valve or is due to a congenital bicuspid or multicusp valve. The most common cause of AVR in older patients is idiopathic degeneration of the normal aortic valve, whereas aortic root dilatation secondary to Marfan syndrome is the most common cause in younger patients.[41–43]

The severity of aortic regurgitation is graded based on structural parameters; Doppler US assessment of regurgitant jets; or measurement of the regurgitant fraction, regurgitant volume, or regurgitant orifice area (ROA).[44]

Using cardiac CT, moderate to severe AI can be assessed qualitatively and quantitatively with a sensitivity and specificity higher than 95% compared with transesophageal

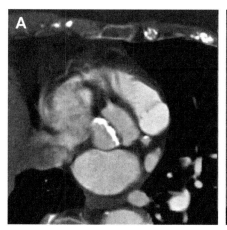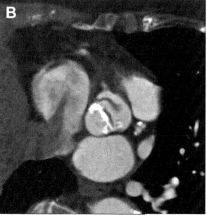

Fig. 4. Bicuspid aortic valve. Axial oblique MPR images during diastole (*A*) and systole (*B*) show a partially calcified bicuspid aortic valve with restricted opening of the valve orifice.

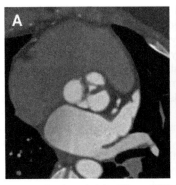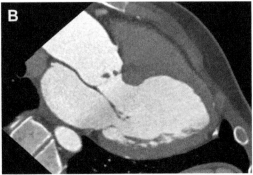

Fig. 5. Aortic regurgitation. Axial oblique MPR (*A*) and sagittal oblique MPR (*B*) images through the aortic valve show thickening and poor coaptation of the valve leaflets resulting in valve regurgitation.

echocardiography.[45] Prospective mode of scanning with reconstructions and measurements of AVR at 70% to 75% have been shown high sensitivity as well and were associated with substantial radiation dose savings.[46,47] During mid-diastole to end-diastole, planimetric CT measurements can be performed to evaluate the central valvular leakage area, which correlates with the severity of AI diagnosed with echocardiography.[42,43,48] In addition, the underlying disease can often be visualized by CT as shortened and thickened aortic cusps in intrinsic valve disease or a dilatation of the aortic root causing a malcoaptation of the valve cusps.[5]

On short-axis cross-sectional views of the aortic valve during diastole, presence of incomplete coaptation of the aortic cusps in the central area or in-between the commissures and its continuity from the aorta to the LVOT are markers of AVR. This visible incomplete coaptation of the aortic valve is referred to as ROA and is strongly associated with the severity of AVR. Studies have shown that the average anatomic area by MDCT is 0.04 cm^2 to 0.03 cm^2 for mild AVR, 0.09 cm^2 to 0.05 cm^2 for moderate AVR, and 0.27 cm^2 to 0.16 cm^2 for severe AVR.[47,49] Another study[50] suggested a cutoff ROA of 25 mm^2 to distinguish between mild and moderate AVR and a cutoff ROA of 75 mm^2 to distinguish between moderate and severe AVR.

Aortic regurgitant volume and fraction can be accurately quantified from differences in stroke volumes of the LVs and right ventricles (RVs) using CT in patients with isolated AVR.[50] The aortic regurgitant fraction can be obtained by dividing the aortic regurgitant volume by the LV stroke volume. This method of calculating the aortic regurgitant fraction, however, is inaccurate in the presence of multiple regurgitant heart valves and other cardiac anomalies.[51]

Infectious Endocarditis and Perivalvular Abscess in Native Aortic Valve

Bacterial endocarditis is on the rise currently primarily due to the nation-wide opioid crisis.[5] The aortic valve is involved in approximately one-half of cases. Infectious vegetations or nodular excrescences that form on the valve cusps, most commonly on the ventricular surface of the cusps, sometimes lead to embolism in patients with bacterial endocarditis. Progression with development of perivalvular abscesses or pseudoaneurysms is not infrequent[7] (**Figs. 6 and 7**).

Normal Postsurgical Appearance and Postsurgical Complications

Current ECG-gated MDCT technology, with its superior spatial and adequate temporal resolutions, minimizes beam-hardening and motion artifacts and thus is superior to other imaging modalities in examinations of prosthetic valves.[1,13–15,52,53] For most mechanical valves, image quality was excellent for leaflets and good to excellent for periprosthetic regions. Results for biological prostheses were less consistent.[54] Usually evaluation of postsurgical valvular abnormalities includes an initial unenhanced prospective ECG-gated scan for optimal assessment of valve calcifications, radiopaque suture materials, and retained surgical objects. Contrast-enhanced ECG-gated scan with the data acquired in the entire cardiac cycle is the second part of the examination. The postsurgical valvular anatomy is evaluated in at least 2 perpendicular imaging planes of each prosthetic valve are created, including 1 positioned exactly in the plane of the evaluated valve ring and 1 set perpendicular to the prosthetic valve leaflets. Dynamic cine evaluation of the valves is performed with conventional short-axis and 2-chamber, 3-chamber, and 4-chamber long-axis reformations of the heart and in short-axis views positioned exactly in the

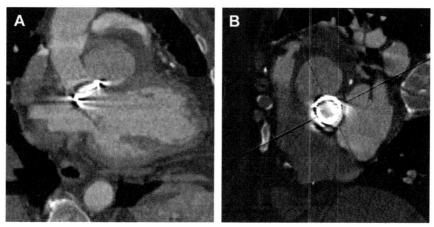

Fig. 6. Paravalvular pseudoaneurysm. Coronal oblique MPR (*A*) and sagittal oblique MPR (*B*) images through the aortic valve show the presence of a bioprosthetic aortic valve prosthesis with a large paravalvular pseudoaneurysm superior and anterior to the valve prosthesis.

plane of the evaluated valve and reconstructed over 10 or 20 phases of the MDCT volumetric data set.

Prosthetic valve obstruction, pannus, thrombus, prosthesis-patient mismatch, paravalvular regurgitation, infective endocarditis (IE), and pseudoaneurysm of the mitral-aortic intervalvular fibrosa are the most common indications for ECG-gated CT assessment of the replaced aortic valve[14] (Fig. 8).

Prosthetic valve obstruction is usually seen as restricted opening angles (ie, ≥20°) for the most commonly used valves (The SJM Regent™ mechanical heart valve) in aortic position and reduces aortic valve area[14] (Fig. 9). Pannus usually demonstrates itself as well-defined low-attenuation linear filling defect located directly underneath the valve ring that is contiguous with the adjacent LV

wall and can usually be differentiated from thrombus, which is seen as low-attenuation filling defect located on the aortic side of an aortic prosthetic valve (Figs. 10 and 11). Also, obstructive thrombi are imaged as hypodense masses with irregular anatomy directly attached to the leaflets and hinge points causing mechanical obstruction by leaflet restriction[55] (Fig. 12).

IE usually manifests itself as static or mobile low-attenuation filling defects consistent with vegetations abutting or distant from the prosthetic valve apparatus. If an enhancing periprosthetic cavity is detected, it would be consistent with abscess or pseudoaneurysm[14] (Figs. 13 and 14).

Paravalvular regurgitation is seen as contrast-filled gap between the native valve annulus and the prosthetic valve that is contiguous with the enhanced lumen of LV and aortic root in aortic

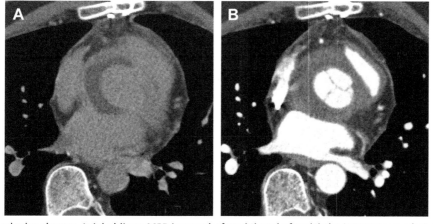

Fig. 7. Perivalvular abscess. Axial oblique MPR images before (*A*) and after (*B*) the intravenous administration of contrast show a perivalvular fluid collection.

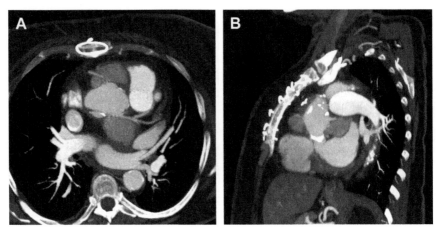

Fig. 8. Axial oblique MPR (*A*) and sagittal oblique MPR (*B*) images through the aortic valve show the presence of a bioprosthetic aortic valve prosthesis with 2 large paravalvular pseudoaneurysms anteriorly and posteriorly to the valve prosthesis.

valve paravalvular regurgitation. In patients with suspected prosthetic heart valve regurgitation, MDCT may be useful to rule out relevant abscess formation and to provide relevant information for treatment planning, but its role in regurgitation diagnosis was less prominent[48,56,57] (**Fig. 15**).

MITRAL VALVE

The mitral valve (MV) is a bicuspid valve that is critical for the unidirectional blood flow from the left atrium toward the LV.[58] The main components of the MV apparatus are the mitral annulus, MV leaflets (1 anterior and 1 crescentic posterior leaflet), chordae tendineae, and papillary muscles[45,58,59] (**Fig. 16**). The normal area of the valve ranges from 4.0 cm^2 to 6.0 cm^2.[59]

Mitral Stenosis

Mitral stenosis (MS) is defined as an obstruction of the LV inflow tract, which prevents proper filling of

the LV during diastole. The predominant cause of MS is rheumatic fever, especially in developing countries.[60] MS can also be caused by congenital anomalies, mitral calcifications, left atrial tumors, carcinoid syndrome, and an obstructive atrial thrombus[59,61]

This barrier between the left atrial and LV flow results in chronic elevation of left atrial pressure, which causes atrial dilatation and pulmonary vascular hypertension. Atrial fibrillation due to atrial dilatation and dyspnea due to pulmonary vascular hypertension are common symptoms of MS.[59,61,62]

Cardiac CT is particularly suited for the detection of leaflet, commissural, and annulus calcification, but it also may detect noncalcified leaflet thickening. For an evaluation of the valve components, a reconstruction at 65% to 75% of the R-R interval for the open MV and a reconstruction at 0% to 0% of the R-R interval are recommended for the closed MV.[62] Visual inspection of the entire

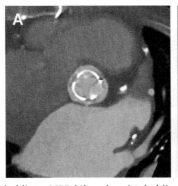
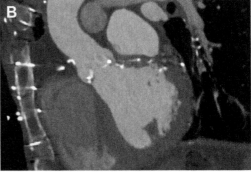

Fig. 9. Axial oblique MPR (*A*) and sagittal oblique MPR (*B*) images through the aortic valve prosthesis show star-like restricted opening of the valve leaflets with associated faint calcification.

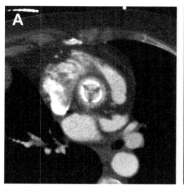
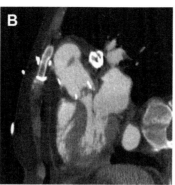
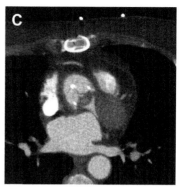

Fig. 10. Aortic valve prosthesis with pannus. Axial oblique MPR (*A*), sagittal oblique MPR (*B*), and axial (*C*) images through the aortic valve show the presence of a bioprosthetic aortic valve prosthesis with prominent pannus formation around the annulus and parts of the valve leaflets. The attenuation value of the pannus is 54 Hounsfield units compared with the attenuation of the enhanced blood pool of 355 HU.

mitral apparatus should be systematic. Assessment of extent of annular calcification (focal vs circumferential) and description of the presence and location of degenerative changes, their location according to the Carpentier nomenclature, and extent from base to coaptation line is recommended (**Figs. 17** and **18**). Understanding the severity of MS is important for determination of therapeutic options; therefore, whenever MS is suspected, careful quantitation of disease severity must be performed[63] and, although not recommended as the initial evaluation for severity assessment, CT provides accurate and reproducible planimetry of the MV orifice[18,64] (**Figs. 19** and **20**).

MS that is caused by rheumatic disease may have distinctive morphologic features unlike those of MS produced by other causes.[65,66] Restricted opening of the thickened valve from commissural fusion, valve calcification, or both results in a fish-mouth appearance on short-axis images.[62]

Additional information obtainable is that related to the aforementioned increased left atrial pressures such as left atrial size, left atrial appendage thrombus, RV hypertrophy, and radiographic evidence of pulmonary edema and pulmonary hypertension.[67]

Mitral Valve Regurgitation

Mitral valve regurgitation (MVR) is the most common manifestation of valve dysfunction in the United States, defined as retrograde blood flow from the LV to the left atrium during systole due to dysfunction of the MV complex (ie, annular dilatation, leaflet retraction, calcifications, anomalies of the chordae tendinae, and dysfunction of the papillary muscles).[27,45,62] MVR is typically classified as primary (degenerative) when a pathologic

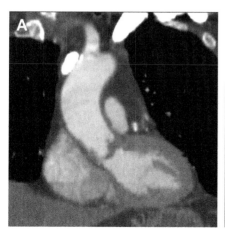
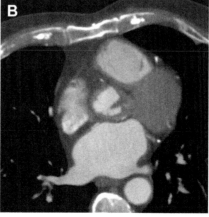

Fig. 11. Aortic valve endocarditis. Coronal MPR (*A*) and axial (*B*) images at the level of the aortic valve show prominent rind of soft tissue thickening circumferentially with extension to the valve leaflets.

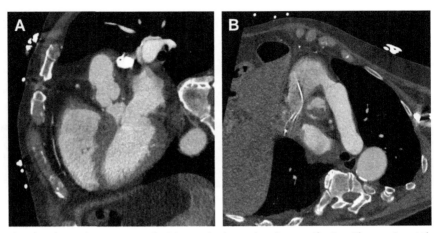

Fig. 12. Aortic valve shows the presence of a bioprosthetic aortic valve prosthesis with prominent thrombus formation within the left cusp (A). Thrombus attenuation of 44 Hounsfield units was measured (B).

abnormality of 1 or more of the components of the MV apparatus fail, leading to valvular incompetence, most commonly MV prolapse (MVP); or as secondary (functional), when MR occurs in the setting of LV remodeling (dilatation and/or global or regional dysfunction) that results in widening of the mitral annular circumference and failure of leaflet coaptation without a primary abnormality of the MV apparatus.[68,69]

The most common cause of MVR is MV prolapse caused by myxomatous valve degeneration. This congenital defect with abnormal fibroelastic connective tissue, causes an elongation and thickening of the MV complex with bowing of the mitral leaflet more than 2 mm beyond the annular plane into the atrium.[45,62]

Another cause of MVR is postrheumatic degeneration with diffuse fibrosis and thickening of the MV leaflets but without calcifications or commissural fusion.[45,70] Coaptation of the MV leaflets can also be affected by endocarditis, dilated cardiomyopathy, ischemic heart disease, or Marfan syndrome.[45]

As in AI, mitral regurgitation can be classified as acute or chronic.[45] Acute MVR is mainly caused by endocarditis or papillary muscle rupture. Papillary muscle rupture may occur in the clinical setting of acute myocardial infarction; however this is an uncommon finding. Chronic mitral regurgitation is often due to MV prolapse, dilated cardiomyopathy, or the result of the systolic anterior motion of the MV that is often seen in patients with hypertrophic cardiomyopathy with significant LVOT obstruction.[45,71]

Retrospective ECG gating can provide 4-D data sets, which are ideal to assess leaflet motion and

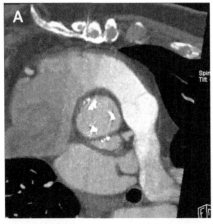
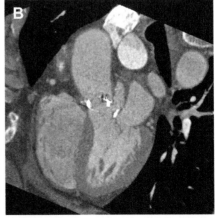

Fig. 13. Paravalvular pseudoaneurysm. Axial oblique MPR (A) and sagittal oblique MPR (B) images through the aortic valve show the presence of a bioprosthetic aortic valve prosthesis with a paravalvular pseudoaneurysm posteriorly to the valve prosthesis between the aorta and left atrium.

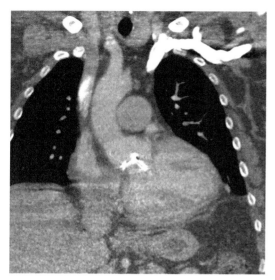

Fig. 14. AVR dehiscence. Coronal MPR image at the level of the aortic valve shows postoperative changes of aortic valve prosthesis, which appears malpositioned and partially migrated into the LV cavity with a large anastomotic defect laterally.

MR mechanism at the expense of contrast and radiation exposure. Although fast-moving structures like ruptured chordae may not be seen because of lower temporal resolution, previous studies showed overall good agreement between CT and echocardiography to detect MVP.[72–74] Two-chamber and 3-chamber views are preferred when assessing a MV prolapse; associated imaging findings include leaflet thickening (thickness of >5 mm) and a flail leaflet.[62]

CT can be used for the diagnosis of MVP with high sensitivity and specificity using transthoracic echocardiography as the reference standard. According to Shah and colleagues,[74] using the echocardiographic criteria of at least 2-mm single or bileaflet prolapse beyond the long-axis annular plane, prolapse can be detected with MDCT with a of sensitivity of 84.6% (**Fig. 21**). Alkadhi and colleagues[75] and Feuchtner and colleagues[76] demonstrated that MVP could be diagnosed with high accuracy regardless of the cardiac plane of imaging (ranging from 90% to 95%, depending on the plane analyzed).

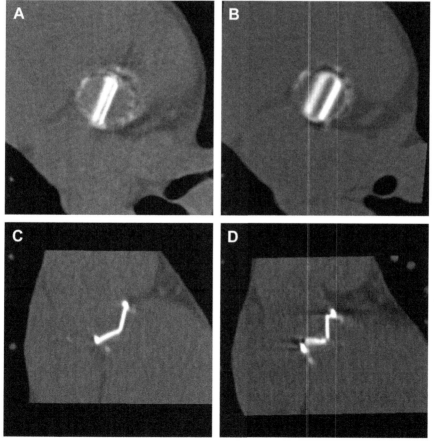

Fig. 15. Mechanical valve malfunction. Axial oblique MPR ([A] diastole and [B] systole) and coronal oblique MPR ([C] diastole and [D] systole) images show significant restricted motion of the mechanical valve leaflets resulting in severe stenosis.

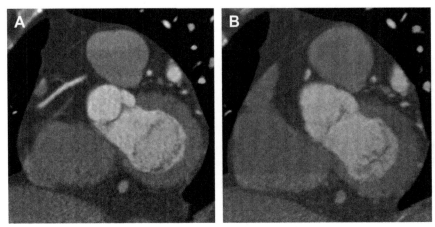

Fig. 16. Normal MV. Coronal oblique reformatted CT images show normal MV open leaflets during end diastole (*A*). A0 and closed MV leaflets during end systole (*B*).

In cases of isolated mitral regurgitation, cardiac CT is useful for grading the severity of mitral regurgitation, because its regurgitant fraction (RF) measurements, derived from RV and LV stroke volumes, correlate well with the results of 2-D transthoracic echocardiography. According to Lembcke and colleagues,[77] the severity of mitral regurgitation can be classified according to 4 grades: grade I (mild) RF of less than 20%; grade II (moderate) RF of 20% to less than 30%; grade III (moderately severe) RF of 30% to less than 44%; and grade IV (severe) RF of 44% or higher.

Infective endocarditis in native valve

In IE, CT is a modality of choice to demonstrate complications, such as abscesses or pseudoaneurysms, although the visualization of small vegetation is more challenging.[62,78]

Normal postsurgical appearance and postsurgical complications

MV repair is widely regarded as the procedure of choice for significant nonrheumatic mitral regurgitation requiring surgery. Recurrent mitral regurgitation is the most common cause of failure of MV repair, but MS is relatively rare after repair.[79] As seen in prosthetic aortic valve, MV pannus is believed a cause of limitation of motion of prosthetic valves, such as a fixed leaflet or valvular regurgitation, and elevation of transprosthetic PG.[80] MDCT has been shown more reliable than fluoroscopy for the assessment of leaflet motion and, importantly, can also depict periprosthetic masses that cause leaflet restriction (**Fig. 22**). In addition, MDCT may depict obstructive masses without restricted leaflet motion.[81] In contrast, the role of MDCT in (peri)prosthetic regurgitation detection is limited. Its strength

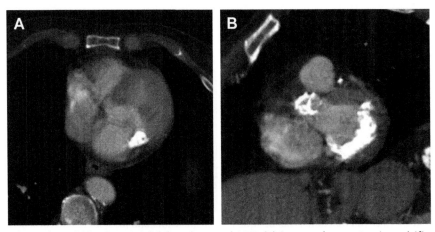

Fig. 17. Mitral annular calcification. Axial (*A*) and coronal MPR (*B*) images show extensive calcification of the mitral annulus.

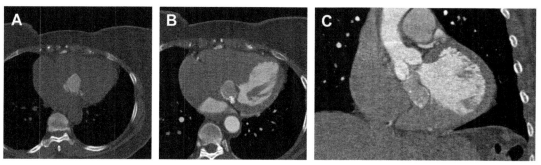

Fig. 18. Caseous mitral annular calcification. Axial nonenhanced (*A*) and enhanced (*B*) images and coronal MPR (*C*) image show a large bulky structure associated with the mitral annulus with central high-density material and capsular calcification consistent with caseous mitral annular calcification.

lies in ruling out complications or in detecting endocarditis complications and showing their relation to relevant anatomic structures, such as the coronary arteries[81] (**Figs. 23–25**).

PULMONARY VALVE

The semilunar pulmonary valve, with 3 semilunar leaflets (anterior, right, and left, with the left and the right leaflets adjacent to their synonymous aortic counterparts), is located between the RV and the pulmonary artery, anterior, and superior to the aortic valve at the level of the third intercostal space with a normal valve area of approximately 3 cm^2 (2 cm^2/m^2) (**Fig. 26**). Because of lower right heart pressures, the pulmonary valves and tricuspid valves are more delicate and

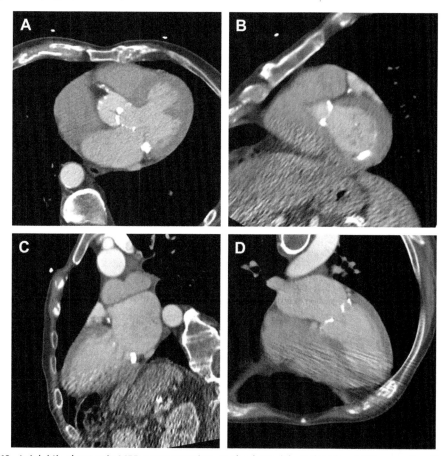

Fig. 19. MS. Axial (*A*), short-axis MPR reconstruction at the base (*B*), 2-chamber MPR reconstruction (*C*), and 4-chamber reconstruction MPR (*D*) images show calcification of the mitral leaflets with restricted opening of the valve at end-diastole resulting in valve stenosis. Mitral annular calcification also present.

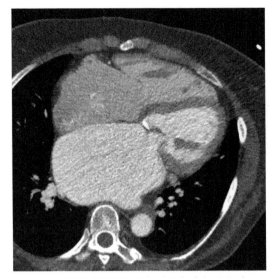

Fig. 20. MS. Axial image at the level of the MV shows calcification and thickening of the mitral leaflets with restricted opening of the valve at end-diastole resulting in valve stenosis.

cannot be easily seen on CT without ECG gating and adequate contrast opacification in the RV outflow tract (RVOT) and main pulmonary artery. In general, if the cusps of the right heart valves are easily visible, they are likely to be thickened.[5] For morphologic evaluation of the valve, prospective ECG-triggered acquisition is the default scanning mode to minimize radiation dose. If functional analysis of the valve or the RV is desired, however, retrospective ECG-gated multiphasic acquisition with tube current modulation is the ideal scanning mode.[82] Short-axis oblique images are ideal for optimal visualization of the leaflets.

Pulmonary Valve Congenital Abnormalities and Stenosis

PV atresia, bicuspid PV, and quadricuspid PV are rare congenital anomalies that are usually associated with other congenital cardiac anomalies, including tetralogy of Fallot spectrum.[83] Pulmonary stenosis (PS) is defined as an obstruction of the RVOT at the level of the pulmonary valve. Like AS, the stenosis can be subvalvular, supravalvular, or valvular, with valvular stenosis the most common (90%) and supravalvular associated with congenital abnormalities, such as patent ductus arteriosus or tetralogy of Fallot. The cause of PS is congenital heart disease in 95% of cases.[83,84] Acquired PS is a rare disease that may be caused by rheumatic fever or metastatic carcinoid syndrome.

Valvular PS results from thickening and fusion of the PV, leading to a decrease in the opening area, an increased pressure gradient across the valve and, often, dilated main and left pulmonary arteries. The degree of stenosis can be classifed as mild, moderate, or severe on the basis of the diameter of valve opening, velocity of jet leaving the RV outfow track, and amount of RV remodeling, which is not typically present unless there is signifcant concomitant PVR.[85]

CT findings may include PV thickening, decreased area of the valve, systolic interventricular septal shift to the left due to increased RV systolic pressure, RV hypertrophy, and dilatation (in the presence of coexisting PVR)[85] (**Fig. 27**). Because of the 90° angle origin of the right pulmonary artery, primarily the main and left pulmonary artery show dilatation in patients with PS, because the poststenotic turbulent flow is directed toward the left main pulmonary artery (**Fig. 28**).[5]

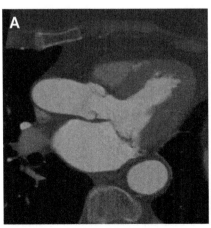
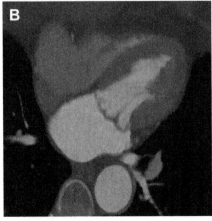

Fig. 21. MV prolapse; 3-chamber MPR reconstruction (*A*) and 4-chamber MPR reconstruction (*B*) images show thickening and bowing of the MV leaflets into the atrial chamber consistent with valve prolapse.

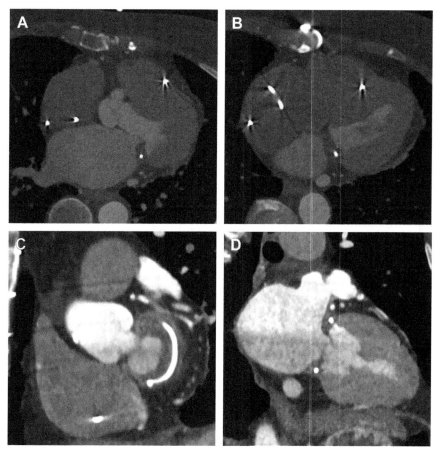

Fig. 22. MV annuloplasty with pannus. Two axial views at the superior margin (*A*) and inferior of the MV (*B*), a short-axis MPR reconstruction at the base of the heart (*C*) and a 2-chamber MPR reconstruction (*D*) images show soft tissue thickening surrounding the mitral annuloplasty ring consistent with pannus formation.

Pulmonary Valve Regurgitation

Pulmonary valve regurgitation (PVR) is defined as an incomplete closure of the pulmonary valve, which causes a blood leak backward into the RV.[86,87] Inadequate apposition of the leafets leads to regurgitation of deoxygenated blood back into the RV outfow tract during diastole. In progressive

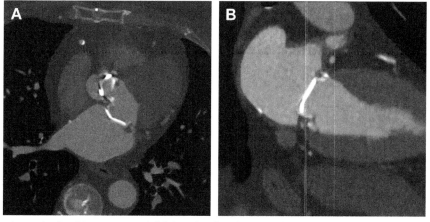

Fig. 23. Mitral prosthesis with pannus. Axial (*A*) and 2-chamber MPR (*B*) reconstruction images show soft tissue thickening surrounding the mitral prosthesis at its anastomotic edges consistent with pannus formation.

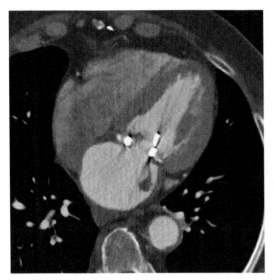

Fig. 24. MV prosthesis vegetation. Axial image at the level of the MV shows soft tissue thickening associated with the valve annulus and pedunculated soft tissue process associated with the mechanical leaflet.

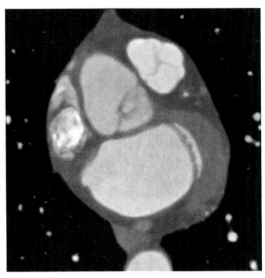

Fig. 26. Normal pulmonary valve. Axial CT maximum intensity projection image shows a normal pulmonary valve located anterior and to the left of the aortic valve.

disease, PVR leads to right-sided heart failure. The most common cause of PVR is dilatation of the valve ring, with resulting malcoaptation that is secondary to pulmonary hypertension or Marfan syndrome.

CT findings of moderate to severe PR might include a malcoaptation of the pulmonary valve cusps at end diastole, dilatation of the pulmonary

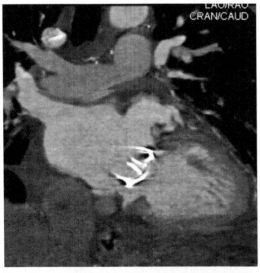

Fig. 25. MV prosthesis dehiscence; 2-chamber view MPR reconstruction shows separation of the inferior anastomotic edge of the valve prosthesis with direct communication between the left atrium and ventricle.

ring and pulmonary artery, RV dilatation, and hypertrophy[5] (Figs. 29–31).

Infective Endocarditis in Native and Prosthetic Valve

Among the cardiac valves, endocarditis of the PV is least common, most often associated with intravenous drug abuse, congenital heart disease, automatic implantable cardiac defbrillators, and central venous lines. Concomitant involvement of tricuspid valve is almost invariable. Friable vegetations of the valve that can be seen on echocardiography, CT, or MR imaging with macroscopic deposits randomly situated on all valve leafets as seen on pathologic inspection. These vegetations if larger than few millimeters can be seen on ECG-gated CT. Vegetations can also dislodge from the valve leaflets and embolize to the pulmonary vasculature and lung parenchyma, causing ischemia or spread of infection. Rheumatic heart disease after pharyngeal infection with *Streptococcus pyogenes* can also affect the PV. Approximately half of all patients with acute rheumatic fever develop infammation of the valvular endothelium (see Fig. 11). Such infammation may cause PVR or PS, or it may worsen the existing PV pathology. Rheumatic heart disease affecting the PV predisposes to recurrent IE.[88]

Thrombosis of the PV might be difficult to distinguish from vegetation, especially when it is small. Typically, on CT PV thrombus is seen as hypodense mass attached to the valve leaflets. It is

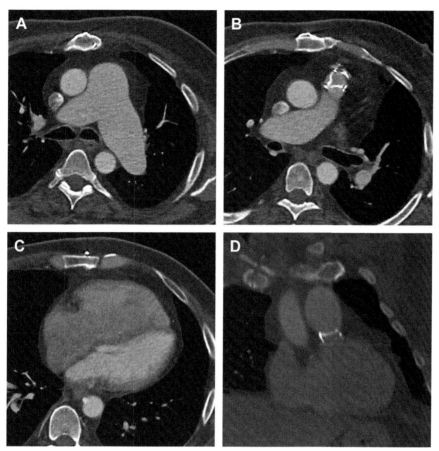

Fig. 27. Pulmonary valve prosthesis with stenosis. Three axial images (A–C) obtained in craniocaudal direction and a coronal MPR reconstruction (D) show postoperative changes of pulmonary valve prosthesis. Faint calcifications associated with the bioprosthetic valve leaflets present. Note the significant dilatation of the RV and main pulmonary artery.

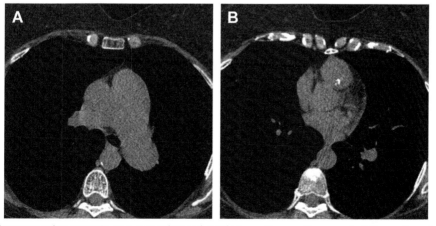

Fig. 28. Pulmonary valve stenosis. Two nonenhanced axial views show enlargement of the main pulmonary artery predominantly of the left branch (A) and pulmonary valve leaflet calcification (B) highly suggestive of underlying stenosis.

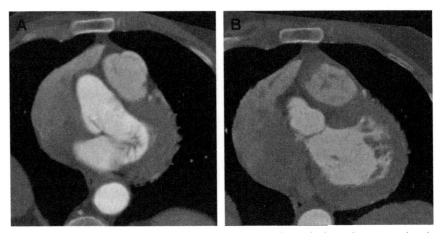

Fig. 29. Pulmonary valve regurgitation. Axial oblique MPR images through the pulmonary valve during systole (*A*) and during diastole (*B*) show mild thickening of the valve leaflets and poor coaptation of the valve during diastole resulting in significant regurgitation.

substantially more common but not exclusive in the setting of prosthetic PV. Thrombus may cause PV stenosis.[83,89,90]

TRICUSPID VALVE

The tricuspid valve is located between the right atrium and the RV. Similar to the MV, the tricuspid valve complex involves the tricuspid leaflets (septal anterior, superior, and inferior), the chordae tendinae, the papillary muscles, and the tricuspid valve annulus.[45] The normal leaflet area is often 3 cm^2 to 5 cm^2.[91]

Tricuspid valve dysfunction is seen in several primary and secondary abnormalities, both congenital and acquired. This can manifest as valvular stenosis, regurgitation, or both.[92,93]

CT is valuable in the evaluation of the tricuspid valve, particularly for providing morphologic information due to its good spatial and temporal resolutions and ability to do multiplanar reconstruction with isotropic resolution. The scan protocol has to be optimized to ensure adequate contrast opacification around the valve and minimize artifacts. Typically, a prospective ECG-triggered acquisition is used to minimize motion and radiation, but retrospective ECG gating is chosen if cine images are required. Intravenous administration of 50 mL to 70 mL of contrast agent, followed by a 50/50 mixture of contrast and saline, is used to reduce streak artifacts from the superior vena cava.[92]

Tricuspid Stenosis

In most cases, tricuspid stenosis is due to rheumatic heart disease, which is both stenotic and regurgitant. Other less common causes include

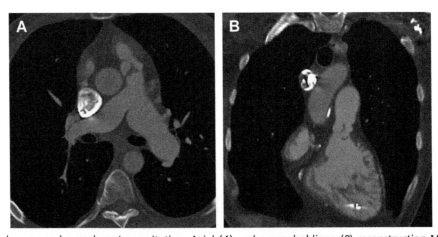

Fig. 30. Pulmonary valve prolapse/regurgitation. Axial (*A*) and coronal oblique (*B*) reconstruction MPR images show thickening and dysplasia of the valve leaflets with frank prolapse of a leaflet into the RV chamber.

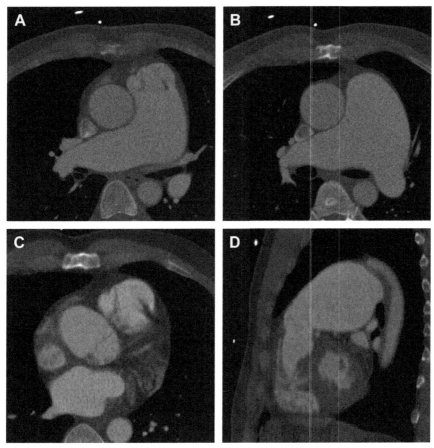

Fig. 31. Pulmonary valve regurgitation. Three axial images (A–C) and a sagittal MPR reconstruction (D) show pulmonary valve leaflet thickening and significant dilatation of the main pulmonary artery.

congenital disorders and infectious endocarditis, and rare etiologies, such as the presence of a mass, endomyocardial fibrosis, or systemic lupus erythematosus.[11,45,67]

CT findings include a narrowed valve annulus with a shortened and fused tricuspid valve complex, which can be difficult to assess depending on the quality of the images. Leaflet thickening

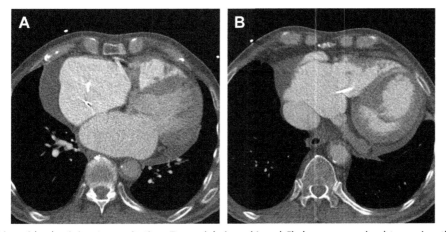

Fig. 32. Tricuspid valve injury/regurgitation. Two axial views (A and B) show a pacer lead traversing the medial tricuspid valve leaflet. Notice the resulting severe right atrial enlargement sequela of the underlying tricuspid regurgitation (A).

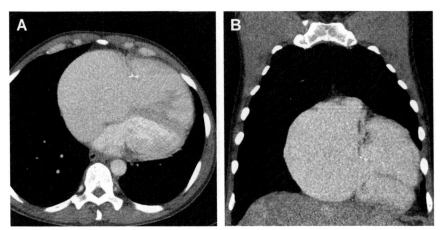

Fig. 33. Tricuspid regurgitation. Axial (*A*) and coronal MPR (*B*) show massive enlargement of the right-sided chambers, sequela of tricuspid regurgitation. Notice the calcifications associated with the tricuspid valve leaflet.

may be present. Secondary signs, such as signs of right heart failure with enlargement of the superior and inferior vena cava as well as dilated hepatic veins. should prompt close evaluation of the tricuspid valve apparatus.[11,45,67,69]

Tricuspid Regurgitation

Tricuspid regurgitation (TR) is the most common form of right-sided valvular heart disease and its prevalence is likely underestimated. Trace TR is seen in 80% to 90% of healthy individuals.[93] The pathophysiology is divided into 2 major categories: functional (associated with left or right heart pathology) and structural (from primary leaflet abnormalities). Functional TR often results from left-sided heart valve disease.[59,94] The most common cause (75%) of pathologic regurgitation is functional.[69,92,95]

As in tricuspid stenosis, secondary findings of TR can be present and should prompt close inspection of the valve itself. These include dilated RA, RV, hepatic veins, and inferior vena cava with systolic reflux of contrast into dilated hepatic veins and inferior vena cava.[3,4,92,93]

Measurements of tricuspid annulus diameter and assessment of lack of coaptation of leaflets are generally simple on good-quality 4-chamber cardiac CT images.[96] TR can be indirectly quantified using stroke volumes obtained from ventricular volumetric analysis in the absence of other valvular pathologies or intracardiac shunts. TR fraction = (RV stroke volume − LV stroke volume)/RV stroke volume × 100%. The accuracy of this technique is lower with arrhythmias.[92]

Some other potential benefits of CT scans are the detection of valvular calcifications, the evaluation of TV annuloplasty ring dislodgement, and the assessment of the spatial relationship between RV pacemaker leads and related TR[88,96] (**Figs. 32–34**).

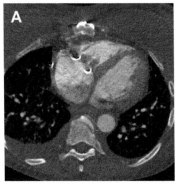 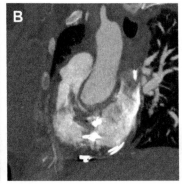 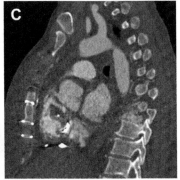

Fig. 34. Tricuspid valve prosthesis vegetation. Axial (*A*) and 2 sagittal oblique MPR reconstruction images (*B, C*) show extensive soft tissue thickening involving the prosthesis with large vegetation extending toward the RVOT.

SUMMARY

Cardiac CT is a useful tool in the evaluation of the valvular diseases. CT allows for improved quantification of valvular calcification due to its superior spatial resolution. CT also improves the detection of small valvular or perivalvular pathology or the characterization valvular masses and vegetations.

REFERENCES

1. Vogel-Claussen J, Pannu H, Spevak PJ, et al. Cardiac valve assessment with MR imaging and 64-section multi-detector row CT. Radiographics 2006; 26(6):1769–84.

2. Lloyd-Jones D, Adams R, Carnethon M, et al. Heart disease and stroke statistics–2009 update: a report from the American Heart Association Statistics Committee and Stroke Statistics Subcommittee. Circulation 2009;119(3):480–6.

3. Maganti K, Rigolin VH, Sarano ME, et al. Valvular heart disease: diagnosis and management. Mayo Clin Proc 2010;85(5):483–500.

4. Côté G, Denault A. Transesophageal echocardiography-related complications. Can J Anaesth 2008;55(9):622–47.

5. Bennett CJ, Maleszewski JJ, Araoz PA. CT and MR imaging of the aortic valve: radiologic-pathologic correlation. Radiographics 2012;32:1399–420.

6. Cueff C, Serfaty JM, Cimadevilla C, et al. Measurement of aortic valve calcification using multislice computed tomography: correlation with haemodynamic severity of aortic stenosis and clinical implication for patients with low ejection fraction. Heart 2011;97(9):721–6.

7. Gahide G, Bommart S, Demaria R, et al. Preoperative evaluation in aortic endocarditis: findings on cardiac CT. AJR Am J Roentgenol 2010;194(3):574–8.

8. Altiok E, Koos R, Schröder J, et al. Comparison of two-dimensional and three-dimensional imaging techniques for measurement of aortic annulus diameters before transcatheter aortic valve implantation. Heart 2011;97(19):1578–84.

9. Dashkevich A, Blanke P, Siepe M, et al. Preoperative assessment of aortic annulus dimensions: comparison of noninvasive and intraoperative measurement. Ann Thorac Surg 2011;91(3):709–14.

10. Li X, Tang L, Zhou L, et al. Aortic valves stenosis and regurgitation: assessment with dual source computed tomography. Int J Cardiovasc Imaging 2009;25(6):591–600.

11. Chen JJ, Manning MA, Frazier AA, et al. CT angiography of the cardiac valves: normal, diseased, and postoperative appearances. Radiographics 2009; 29(5):1393–412.

12. Kerl JM, Ravenel JG, Nguyen SA, et al. Right heart: split-bolus injection of diluted contrast medium for visualization at coronary CT angiography. Radiology 2008;247(2):356–64.

13. Habets J, Symersky P, van Herwerden LA, et al. Prosthetic heart valve assessment with multidetector- row CT: imaging characteristics of 91 valves 83 patients. Eur Radiol 2011;21:1390–6.

14. Ghersin E, Martinez CA, Singh V, et al. ECG-gated MDCT after aortic and mitral valve surgery. AJR Am J Roentgenol 2014;203(6):W596–604.

15. Konen E, Goitein O, Feinberg MS, et al. The role of ECG-gated MDCT in the evaluation of aortic and mitral mechanical valves: initial experience. AJR Am J Roentgenol 2008;191:26–31.

16. Litmanovich DE, Ghersin E, Burke DA, et al. Imaging in Transcatheter Aortic Valve Replacement (TAVR): role of the radiologist. Insights Imaging 2014;5(1): 123–45.

17. Piazza N, de Jaegere P, Schultz C, et al. Anatomy of the aortic valvar complex and its implications for transcatheter implantation of the aortic valve. Circ Cardiovasc Interv 2008;1:74–81.

18. Achenbach S, Delgado V, Hausleiter J, et al. SCCT expert consensus document on computed tomography imaging before transcatheter aortic valve implantation (TAVI)/transcatheter aortic valve replacement (TAVR). J Cardiovasc Comput Tomogr 2012;6:366–80.

19. Van Mieghem NM, Schultz CJ, van der Boon RM, et al. Incidence, timing, and predictors of valve dislodgment during TAVI with the Medtronic CoreValve System. Catheter Cardiovasc Interv 2012; 79(5):726–32.

20. Sabet HY, Edwards WD, Tazelaar HD, et al. Congenitally bicuspid aortic valves: a surgical pathology study of 542 cases (1991 through 1996) and a literature review of 2,715 additional cases. Mayo Clin Proc 1999;74:14–26.

21. Sievers HH, Schmidtke C. A classification system for the bicuspid aortic valve from 304 surgical specimens. J Thorac Cardiovasc Surg 2007;133: 1226–33.

22. Fedak PW, Verma S, David TE, et al. Clinical and pathophysiological implications of a bicuspid aortic valve. Circulation 2002;106:900–4.

23. Hiratzka LF, Bakris GL, Beckman JA, et al. 2010 ACCF/AHA/AATS/ACR/ASA/SCA/SCAI/SIR/STS/SVM guidelines for the diagnosis and management of patients with thoracic aortic disease: a report of the American College of Cardiology Foundation/American Heart Association Task Force on Practice Guidelines, American Association for Thoracic Surgery, American College of Radiology, American Stroke Association, Society of Cardiovascular Anesthesiologists, Society for Cardiovascular Angiography and Interventions, Society of Interventional Radiology, Society of Thoracic Surgeons,and Society for Vascular Medicine. J Am Coll Cardiol 2010;55(14):e27–129.

24. Alkadhi H, Leschka S, Pedro T, et al. Cardiac CT for the differentiation of bicuspid and tricuspid aortic valves: comparison with echocardiography and surgery. AJR Am J Roentgenol 2010;195(4): 900–8.

25. Maleszewski JJ, Miller DV, Lu J, et al. Histopathologic findings in ascending aortas from individuals with Loeys-Dietz syndrome (LDS). Am J Surg Pathol 2009;33(2):194–201.

26. Bricker AO, Avutu B, Mohammed TL, et al. Valsalva sinus aneurysms: findings at CT and MR imaging. Radiographics 2010;30(1):99–110.

27. Nkomo VT, Gardin JM, Skelton TN, et al. Burden of valvular heart diseases: a population-based study. Lancet 2006;368(9540):1005–11.

28. Brickner ME, Hillis LD, Lange RA. Congenital heart disease in adults. First of two parts. N Engl J Med 2000;342(4):256–63.

29. Weidemann F, Herrmann S, Störk S, et al. Impact of myocardial fibrosis in patients with symptomatic severe aortic stenosis. Circulation 2009;120(7): 577–84.

30. Pouleur AC, le Polain de Waroux JB, Pasquet A, et al. Aortic valve area assessment: multidetector CT compared with cine MR imaging and transthoracic and transesophageal echocardiography. Radiology 2007;244(3):745–54.

31. Nasir K, Katz R, Al-Mallah M, et al. Relationship of aortic valve calcification with coronary artery calcium severity: the Multi-Ethnic Study of Atherosclerosis (Mesa). J Cardiovasc Comput Tomogr 2010; 4(1):41–6.

32. Kälsch H, Lehmann N, Mahabadi AA, et al, Investigator Group of the Heinz Nixdorf Recall Study. Beyond Framingham risk factors and coronary calcification: does aortic valve calcification improve risk prediction? The Heinz Nixdorf Recall Study. Heart 2014;100(12):930–7.

33. Clavel MA, Pibarot P, Messika-Zeitoun D, et al. Impact of aortic valve calcification, as measured by MDCT, on survival in patients with aortic stenosis: results of an international registry study. J Am Coll Cardiol 2014;64(12):1202–13.

34. Boulif J, Gerber B, Slimani A, et al. Assessment of aortic valve calcium load by multidetector computed tomography. Anatomical validation, impact of scanner settings and incremental diagnostic value. J Cardiovasc Comput Tomogr 2017;11(5):360–6.

35. Aggarwal SR, Clavel MA, Messika-Zeitoun D, et al. Sex differences in aortic valve calcification measured by multidetector computed tomography in aortic stenosis. Circ Cardiovasc Imaging 2013;6: 40–7.

36. Pawade T, Clavel MA, Tribouilloy C, et al. Computed tomography aortic valve calcium scoring in patients with aortic stenosis. Circ Cardiovasc Imaging 2018; 11(3):e007146.

37. Clavel MA, Messika-Zeitoun D, Pibarot P, et al. The complex nature of discordant severe calcified aortic valve disease grading: new insights from combined Doppler echocardiographic and computed tomographic study. J Am Coll Cardiol 2013;62:2329–38.

38. Nguyen V, Cimadevilla C, Estellat C, et al. Haemodynamic and anatomic progression of aortic stenosis. Heart 2015;101:943–7.

39. Enriquez-Sarano M, Tajik AJ. Clinical practice. Aortic regurgitation. N Engl J Med 2004;351(15):1539–46.

40. Dujardin KS, Enriquez-Sarano M, Schaff HV, et al. Mortality and morbidity of aortic regurgitation in clinical practice: a long-term follow-up study. Circulation 1999;99(14):1851–7.

41. Bonow RO, Lakatos E, Maron BJ, et al. Serial long-term assessment of the natural history of asymptomatic patients with chronic aortic regurgitation and normal left ventricular systolic function. Circulation 1991;84(4):1625–35.

42. Feuchtner GM, Dichtl W, Muller S, et al. 64-MDCT for diagnosis of aortic regurgitation in patients referred to CT coronary angiography. AJR Am J Roentgenol 2008;191(1):W1–7.

43. Feuchtner GM, Dichtl W, Schachner T, et al. Diagnostic performance of MDCT for detecting aortic valve regurgitation. AJR Am J Roentgenol 2006; 186(6):1676–81.

44. Zoghbi WA, Enriquez-Sarano M, Foster E, et al. Recommendations for evaluation of the severity of native valvular regurgitation with two-dimensional and Doppler echocardiography. J Am Soc Echocardiogr 2003;16(7):777–802.

45. Ketelsen D, Fishman EK, Claussen CD, et al. Computed tomography evaluation of cardiac valves: a review. Radiol Clin North Am 2010;48:783–97.

46. Zeb I, Hamirani YS, Mao S, et al. Detection of aortic regurgitation with 64-slice multidetector computed tomography (MDCT). Acad Radiol 2010;17(8): 1006–11.

47. Jassal DS, Shapiro MD, Neilan TG, et al. 64-slice multidetector computed tomography(MDCT) for detection of aortic regurgitation and quantification of severity. Invest Radiol 2007;42(7):507–12.

48. Ko SM, Park JH, Shin JK, et al. Assessment of the regurgitant orifice area in aortic regurgitation with dual-source CT: comparison with cardiovascular magnetic resonance. J Cardiovasc Comput Tomogr 2015;9(4):345–53.

49. Alkadhi H, Desbiolles L, Husmann L, et al. Aortic regurgitation: assessment with 64-section CT. Radiology 2007;245:111–21.

50. Feuchtner GM, Spoeck A, Lessick J, et al. Quantification of aortic regurgitant fraction and volume with multi-detector computed tomography comparison with echocardiography. Acad Radiol 2011;18: 334–42.

51. Meng Y, Zhang L, Zhang Z, et al. Cardiovascular magnetic resonance of quinticuspid aortic valve with aortic regurgitation and dilated ascending aorta. J Cardiovasc Magn Reson 2009;11(1):28.

52. Chenot F, Montant P, Goffinet C, et al. Evaluation of anatomic valve opening and leaflet morphology in aortic valve bioprosthesis by using multidetector CT: comparison with transthoracic echocardiography. Radiology 2010;255(2):377–85.

53. Habets J, Budde RP, Symersky P, et al. Diagnostic evaluation of left-sided prosthetic heart valve dysfunction. Nat Rev Cardiol 2011;8:466–78.

54. Suchá D, Symersky P, Tanis W, et al. Multimodality imaging assessment of prosthetic heart valves. Circ Cardiovasc Imaging 2015;8(9):e003703.

55. Tanis W, Habets J, van den Brink RB, et al. Differentiation of thrombus from pannus as the cause of acquired mechanical prosthetic heart valve obstruction by non-invasive imaging: a review of the literature. Eur Heart J Cardiovasc Imaging 2014;15(2):119–29.

56. Suchá D, Symersky P, van den Brink RB, et al. Diagnostic evaluation and treatment strategy in patients with suspected prosthetic heart valve dysfunction: the incremental value of MDCT. J Cardiovasc Comput Tomogr 2016;10(5):398–406.

57. Habets J, Tanis W, Reitsma JB, et al. Are novel non-invasive imaging techniques needed in patients with suspected prosthetic heart valve endocarditis? A systematic review and meta-analysis. Eur Radiol 2015;25(7):2125–33.

58. Kim JH, Kim EY, Jin GY, et al. A review of the use of cardiac computed tomography for evaluating the mitral valve before and after mitral valve repair. Korean J Radiol 2017;18(5):773–813.

59. Manghat NE, Rachapalli V, Van Lingen R, et al. Imaging the heart valves using ECG-gated 64- detector row cardiac CT. Br J Radiol 2008;81(964):275–90.

60. Roberts WC, Perloff JK. Mitral valvular disease. A clinicopathologic survey of the conditions causing the mitral valve to function abnormally. Ann Intern Med 1972;77(6):939–75.

61. Braunwald E, Moscovitz HL, Amram SS, et al. The hemodynamics of the left side of the heart as studied by simultaneous left atrial, left ventricular, and aortic pressures; particular reference to mitral stenosis. Circulation 1955;12(1):69–81.

62. Morris MF, Maleszewski JJ, Suri RM, et al. CT and MR imaging of the mitral valve: radiologic-pathologic correlation. Radiographics 2010;30(6):1603–20.

63. Eleid MF, Foley TA, Said SM, et al. Severe mitral annular calcification. JACC Cardiovasc Imaging 2016;9(11):1318–37.

64. van Rosendael PJ, van Wijngaarden SE, Kamperidis V, et al. Integrated imaging of echocardiography and computed tomography to grade mitral regurgitation severity in patients undergoing transcatheter aortic valve implantation. Eur Heart J 2017;38(28):2221–6.

65. Messika-Zeitoun D, Serfaty JM, Laissy JP, et al. Assessment of the mitral valve area in patients with mitral stenosis by multislice computed tomography. J Am Coll Cardiol 2006;48(2):411–3.

66. Oh JK, Seward JB, Tajik AJ. The echo manual. 3rd edition. Philadelphia: Lippincott Williams & Wilkins; 2006. p. 202.

67. Rajani R, Khattar R, Chiribiri A, et al. Multimodality imaging of heart valve disease. Arq Bras Cardiol 2014;1–13. https://doi.org/10.5935/abc.20140057.

68. Levine RA, Hagége AA, Judge DP, et al. Mitral valve disease–morphology and mechanisms. Nat Rev Cardiol 2015;12(12):689–710.

69. Naoum C, Blanke P, Circulation JC. Cardiac computed tomography and magnetic resonance imaging in the evaluation of mitral and tricuspid valve disease: implications for transcatheter interventions. Circ Cardiovasc Imaging 2017;10(3) [pii:e005331].

70. Waller BF, Howard J, Fess S. Pathology of mitral valve stenosis and pure mitral regurgitation–Part II. Clin Cardiol 1994;17(7):395–402.

71. Luckie M, Khattar RS. Systolic anterior motion of the mitral valve–beyond hypertrophic cardiomyopathy. Heart 2008;94(11):1383–5.

72. Bouchard M-A, Côté-Laroche C, Beaudoin J. Multimodality imaging in the evaluation and treatment of mitral regurgitation. Curr Treat Options Cardiovasc Med 2017;19(12):91.

73. Moradi M, Nazari M, Khajouei AS, et al. Comparison of the accuracy of cardiac computed to- mography angiography and transthoracic echocardi- ography in the diagnosis of mitral valve prolapse. Adv Biomed Res 2015;4:221.

74. Shah RG, Novaro GM, Blandon RJ, et al. Mitral valve prolapse: evaluation with ECG-gated cardiac CT angiography. AJR Am J Roentgenol 2010;194:579–84.

75. Alkadhi H, Wildermuth S, Bettex DA, et al. Mitral regurgitation: quanti cation with 16-detector row CT initial experience. Radiology 2006;238(2):454–63.

76. Feuchtner GM, Alkadhi H, Karlo C, et al. Cardiac CT angiography for the diagnosis of mitral valve prolapse: comparison with echocardiography. Radiology 2010;254:374–83.

77. Lembcke A, Borges AC, Dushe S, et al. Assessment of mitral valve regurgitation at electron-beam CT: comparison with doppler echocardiography. Radiology 2005;236(1):47–55.

78. Asante-Korang A, O'Leary PW, Anderson RH. Anatomy and echocardiography of the normal and abnormal mitral valve. Cardiol Young 2006;16(Suppl 3):27–34.

79. Suh YJ, Chang BC, Im DJ, et al. Assessment of mitral annuloplasty ring by cardiac computed tomography: correlation with echocardiographic parameters and comparison between two different ring types. J Thorac Cardiovasc Surg 2015;150(5): 1082–90.

80. Chang S, Suh YJ, Han K, et al. The clinical significance of perivalvular pannus in prosthetic mitral valves: can cardiac CT be helpful? Int J Cardiol 2017;249(C):344–8.

81. Suh YJ, Lee S, Im DJ, et al. Added value of cardiac computed tomography for evaluation of mechanical aortic valve: emphasis on evaluation of pannus with surgical findings as standard reference. Int J Cardiol 2016;214:454–60.

82. Rajiah P, Nazarian J, Vogelius E, et al. CT and MRI of pulmonary valvular abnormalities. Clin Radiol 2014; 69(6):630–8.

83. Jonas SN, Kligerman SJ, Burke AP, et al. Pulmonary valve anatomy and abnormalities: a pictorial essay of radiography, Computed Tomography (CT), and Magnetic Resonance Imaging (MRI). J Thorac Imaging 2016;31(1):W4–12.

84. Sahn DJ. Accuracy of MRI evaluation of pulmonary blood supply in patients with complex pulmonary stenosis or atresia. Int J Card Imaging 2000;16: 479–80.

85. Snellen HA, Hartman H, Buis-Liem TN, et al. Pulmonic stenosis. Circulation 1968;38(suppl): 93–101.

86. Haddad F, Hunt SA, Rosenthal DN, et al. Right ventricular function in cardiovascular disease, part I: anatomy, physiology, aging, and functional assessment of the right ventricle. Circulation 2008;117: 1436–48.

87. Carabello BA. Valvular heart disease. In: Goldman L, Schafer AI, editors. Cecil medicine. Philadelphia: Saunders Elsevier; 2011.

88. Gopalan D. Right heart on multidetector CT. Br J Radiol 2011;84(3):S306–23.

89. Hatemi AC, Gursoy M, Tongut A, et al. Pulmonary stenosis as a predisposing factor for infective endocarditis in a patient with Noonan syndrome. Tex Heart Inst J 2010;37:99–101.

90. Gersony WM, Hayes CJ, Driscoll DJ, et al. Bacterial endocarditis in patients with aortic stenosis, pulmonary stenosis, or ventricular septal defect. Circulation 1993;87(suppl):I121–6.

91. Ramadan FB, Beanlands DS, Burwash IG. Isolated pulmonary valve endocarditis in healthy hearts: a case report and review of the literature. Can J Cardiol 2000;16:1282–8.

92. Franco A, Fernández-Pérez GC, Tomás-Mallebrera M, et al. Valvular heart disease: multidetector computed tomography evaluation. Radiologia 2014;56(3):219–28.

93. Shah S, Jenkins T, Markowitz A, et al. Multimodal imaging of the tricuspid valve: normal appearance and pathological entities. Insights Imaging 2016;7(5): 649–67.

94. Al-Bawardy R, Krishnaswamy A, Bhargava, et al. Tricuspid regurgitation in patients with pacemakers and implantable cardiac defibrillators: a comprehensive review. Clin Cardiol 2013;36(5):249–54.

95. Saremi F, Hassani C, Millan-Nunez V, et al. Imaging evaluation of tricuspid valve: analysis of morphology and function with CT and MRI. AJR Am J Roentgenol 2015;204(5):W531–42.

96. Huttin O, Voilliot D, Mandry D, et al. All you need to know about the tricuspid valve: tricuspid valve imaging and tricuspid regurgitation analysis. Arch Cardiovasc Dis 2016;109(1):67–80.

Transcatheter Aortic and Mitral Valve Replacements

Ryan Wilson, MB BCh[a], Charis McNabney, MB BCh[b],
Jonathan R. Weir-McCall, MBChB, PhD[b], Stephanie Sellers, PhD[b,c],
Philipp Blanke, MD[b,c], Jonathon A. Leipsic, MD, FRCPC[b,c,*]

KEYWORDS

- Computed tomography • Transcatheter aortic valve replacement • Transcatheter mitral valve repair
- Valve in valve

KEY POINTS

- Rapid growth in transcatheter valvular interventions over the past decade has been greatly helped by the integration of imaging, particularly computed tomography (CT).
- CT is a pivotal noninvasive imaging resource that can be used throughout many stages of the transcatheter heart valve process, enhancing procedural success and efficacy.
- CT affords a three-dimensional assessment of the aortic and challenging saddle-shaped mitral annulus, facilitating appropriate device selection, sizing, and preprocedural prediction angles for prosthetic deployment.
- Postprocedural imaging allows documentation of procedural success, evaluation of prosthesis positioning, and identifying asymptomatic complications.

INTRODUCTION

Over the last decade, the field of valvular heart disease has been disrupted by the introduction and maturation of transcatheter valvular interventions. Since the first transarterial transcatheter aortic valve replacement (TAVR) there has been a deluge of data supporting its role in the treatment of severe symptomatic aortic stenosis (AS) in an ever-growing group of patients. Although much of this progress has been owing to the advancement in the devices being deployed and procedural technique, the integration of advanced imaging, in particular computed tomography (CT), has also greatly helped with the evolution of the field and

in the reduction of procedural complications. Building on the lessons from TAVR, the integration of CT in transcatheter mitral valve replacement (TMVR) has been rapid and essential in the development of the technology. This article provides an overview of the role of CT in both TAVR and TMVR.

IMAGE ACQUISITION

Recent improvements in the temporal and spatial resolution of CT have enabled dynamic imaging of the heart and aortic root. This advance has been achieved by a combination of increased gantry rotation speed, broader Z-axis coverage, and improved detector sensitivity. Nonmodulated

Disclosure: J.A. Leipsic and P. Blanke provide corelab services to Edwards Lifesciences, Tendyne Holdings, Neovasc, and Medtronic and serve as consultants to Edwards Lifesciences, Neovasc, and Circle Imaging. This work was supported by an unrestricted grant from the Arnold and Anita Silber and Syd and Joanne Belzberg Foundations.

[a] Department of Radiology, Vancouver General Hospital, University of British Columbia, 899 West 12th Avenue, Vancouver, British Columbia V5Z1M9, Canada; [b] Department of Radiology, St Paul's Hospital, University of British Columbia, 899 West 12th Avenue, Vancouver, British Columbia V5Z1M9, Canada; [c] Centre for Heart Lung Innovation, St Paul's Hospital, University of British Columbia, 899 West 12th Avenue, Vancouver, British Columbia V5Z1M9, Canada
* Corresponding author. Department of Radiology, St. Paul's Hospital, 1081 Burrard Street, Vancouver, British Columbia V6Z 1Y6, Canada.
E-mail address: jleipsic@providencehealth.bc.ca

Radiol Clin N Am 57 (2019) 165–178
https://doi.org/10.1016/j.rcl.2018.08.001

CT axial acquisition of the aortic root and heart obtained at multiple phases throughout the cardiac cycle provides a four-dimensional isotropic dataset. When combined with electrocardiogram (ECG) synchronization, this dataset can be retrospectively manipulated to produce motion-free multiplanar reformatted images of the heart and aorta at any point of the cardiac cycle.

A quality contrast-enhanced study of the aortic root and left heart is essential for preprocedural assessment before TAVR and TMVR respectively. An optional adjunct noncontrast acquisition of the aortic or mitral valve with the same imaging parameters of a coronary artery calcium score can be performed before the angiographic study to quantify the extent of valve calcification. The calcium score of the aortic valve has been shown to correlate with the severity of AS.[1]

The contrast-enhanced CT can be obtained using prospective ECG triggering to obtain images in the optimal phase of the cardiac cycle or alternatively scanning throughout the cardiac cycle and using ECG synchronization to retrospectively reconstruct images in the desired phase. Scan timing is guided either by injecting a test bolus to determine transit time or bolus triggering with a region of interest (ROI), activated by a preselected minimum Hounsfield unit (HU), typically 150 HU. Preassessment TAVR scans are triggered from the ascending aorta giving maximal enhancement of the aortic root and left ventricular outflow tract (LVOT), whereas TMVR scans are triggered from the left ventricle, allowing optimal enhancement of the left heart and interatrial septum.

There is an increased prevalence of chronic kidney disease in patients undergoing TAVR because this patient population commonly has multiple comorbidities such as diabetic nephropathy.[2] The dose-effect relationship between administered contrast medium volume and incurring renal toxicity has been well cited,[3] therefore the decision to proceed with contrast-enhanced imaging should be balanced against clinical benefit.

Administration of less than 90 mL of intravenous contrast medium has been reported to reduce the incidence of contrast-induced acute kidney injury in patients undergoing CT before TAVR.[4]

TMVR preassessment studies usually benefit from a prolonged injection to ensure that the right heart does not wash out, to allow assessment of the interatrial septum. This outcome is usually achieved using a single breath-hold following injection of 80 to 110 mL of intravenous contrast medium at 4 to 5 mL/s and a biphasic injection (contrast and saline).[5]

For pre-TAVR studies, the proximal supra-aortic vessels and iliofemoral vasculature access routes can be assessed by subsequent non-ECG synchronized data acquisition of the chest, abdomen, and pelvis using the same contrast medium bolus. For pre-TMVR CT, an ECG-gated acquisition is limited to the heart. Should a transapical approach be considered, an additional nongated low-dose CT chest scan can be performed to aid apex localization and septal puncture.

VALVE ANATOMY
Aortic

Multidetector CT (MDCT) can quantify calcification and assess for patterns of calcification either on or below the valve, associated with adverse outcomes such as paravalvular aortic regurgitation (PAR) and annular rupture. These outcomes are presumed to be caused by bulky or nodular calcifications resulting in reduced expansion and poor apposition of the device with the native valve, as well as exerting excessive focal pressure on certain parts of the annulus.

With TAVR extending to a lower risk group, bicuspid aortic valve (BAV) disease is encountered with higher frequency.[6] High-resolution and functional cine assessment of valve morphology and movement with CT has led to a better understanding of BAV pathogenesis, enabling the development of a BAV classification based on the number of commissures and raphes (**Fig. 1**). From the unique CT features, there is mounting consensus that a large number of functionally bicuspid tricommisural aortic valves are congenital rather than acquired, as previously suggested.[7] Recently the TAVR-directed simplified BAV imaging (BAVi) classification of BAV morphology has been proposed, replacing now antiquated methods such as those of Sievers and the Bicuspid Aortic Valve Consortium.[8,9] Although initially associated with higher rates of PAR and root injury,[10] BAVs have been shown to be amenable to transcatheter heart valves (THVs) with better identification of patients with high-risk anatomy and a newer generation of devices.[11]

Displacement of the native aortic valve cusps during device deployment can result in occlusion of the coronary artery ostia with a reported incidence of 0.6% to 4.1%. Patients with increased aortic leaflet length and bulky leaflet calcifications are at increased risk of coronary occlusion. A reduced distance from the annular plane to the inferior margin of the coronary ostia of less than 10 to 12 mm along with shallow sinus of Valsalva (<30 mm) increase the risk of coronary occlusion.[12,13] Ribeiro and colleagues[13] created a multicenter registry to help better define the risk of coronary occlusion after TAVR. Through caliper

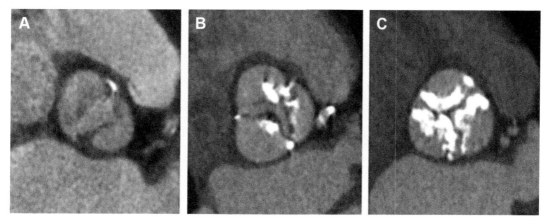

Fig. 1. Contrast-enhanced cardiac CT reconstructed in the systolic phase of the cardiac cycle using retrospective ECG gating. Multiplanar reformatted transverse images through the aortic valve of 3 different patients with severe AS showing BAV classification based on CT. (*A*) Bicommissural non–raphe-type bicuspid aortic valve; (*B*) bicommissural raphe-type bicuspid aortic valve; (*C*) tricommissural, functionally bicuspid aortic valve.

matching, they highlighted additional measures that are incremental to the previously established ones, including a sinus of Valsalva/annular ratio of 1.25.

The self-expanding CoreValve THV extends beyond the sinotubular junction (STJ) into the ascending aorta and therefore measurements of the diameter of the aorta at the STJ and 40 mm above the annulus are required to ensure anatomic eligibility. All of these features can be easily and reliably assessed with the high-resolution three-dimensional (3D) functionality of CT, therefore predicting and avoiding these complications associated with high morbidity and mortality.

Mitral

The mitral valve is a complex functional unit that depends on the integrity and harmonious interplay of each of its components. These components include the mitral annulus, mitral valve leaflets, the chordae, and left ventricular wall with its attached papillary muscles.[14–17]

An advantage of MDCT is its ability to interrogate landing zone calcification. It can determine not only severity but also whether it encroaches on the valve leaflets and whether it is localized or diffuse. Mitral annular calcification (MAC) can also present in various forms, ranging from dense nodular calcifications to soft caseous patterns.

Device selection often depends on the types and pattern of calcification. To date, classification of MAC is subjective and characterization of the various tissue properties of MAC is not able to be quantified, which makes it difficult to verify how these factors will affect complications and clinical outcomes. One way of standardizing segmentation of the annulus is to ignore protruding nodules of calcification, creating a smoothly marginated structure with better reproducibility.

For TMVR valves currently in production, severe MAC has been a relative contraindication, inhibiting device capture and ability to obtain adequate apposition with the native annulus. However, in the appropriate setting, MAC can also be a prerequisite for valve insertion. In the event of mitral stenosis, MAC greater than 75% of the circumference of all 4 quadrants can provide sufficient purchase and sustain enough radial force for an aortic THV to be inserted.[18]

ANNULAR SIZING
Aortic

An accurate evaluation of aortic annular size is critical for THV selection and sizing, with inappropriate sizing being associated with an increased risk of paravalvular regurgitation and annular rupture.[9,19,20]

Rather than being a true anatomic structure, the aortic valve annulus is a virtual ring defined by the plane immediately below the hinge points of the aortic valve cusps.[21] The isotropic nature of the CT dataset allows 3D assessment and measurement of this virtual annular ring in a reproducible manner with high intraobserver and interobserver correlation.[22,23]

This assessment is achieved by using a double-oblique multiplanar reformat (MPR) technique to align the sagittal plane with the long axis of the LVOT orthogonal to the annular plane to estimate the annular ring. The crosshairs can then be rotated perpendicular to the ring to transect the other hinge points and bring them into the plane of the annular ring. Standard annular measurements include short-axis and long-axis diameters, annular area, and perimeter (**Fig. 2**).[24]

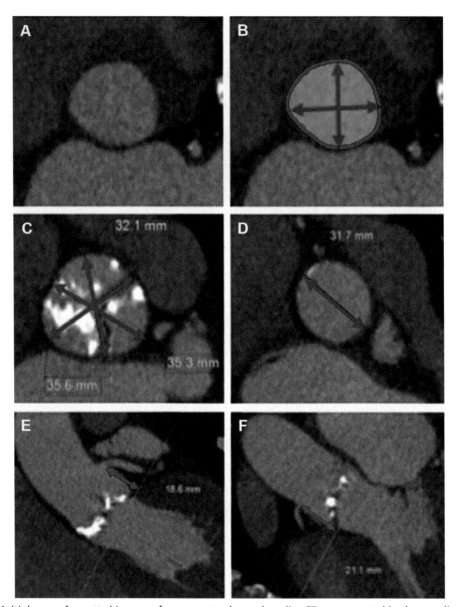

Fig. 2. Multiplanar reformatted images of a contrast-enhanced cardiac CT reconstructed in the systolic phase of the cardiac cycle using retrospective ECG gating. (*A*) A double-oblique transverse view of the aortic annular plane created by transecting the basal hinge points of the 3 aortic cusps. (*B*) The standard aortic annular dimensions; short and long-axis diameter (*blue arrows*), area (*green*) and perimeter (*red line*). The sinus of Valsalva (*C*) is measured as a mean of the distance (*blue arrows*) from the valve commissures to their opposite valve cusp. (*D*) The aortic diameter (*blue arrows*) at the level of the STJ. The left (*E*) and right (*F*) coronary ostial height is measured as a perpendicular line (*red arrows*) from the aortic annular plane to the coronary artery ostium.

Rather than circular, as originally thought, 3D techniques such as CT have shown that the aortic annulus is most commonly ovoid with short-axis and long-axis diameters that differ on average by 5.5 mm.[25] Moreover, the aortic annulus is a dynamic structure that changes in size and shape throughout the cardiac cycle, with annular flattening and increased eccentricity resulting in smaller size during diastole. The largest annular area is observed at end systole, most commonly at 20% of the R-R interval. Therefore, in order to minimize the risk of undersizing, the authors recommend measuring the annulus using the phase with the best image quality during 20% to 40% of the R-R interval or before mitral valve opening.[26]

The reproducibility of CT and the noninvasive nature of the technique have resulted in the emergence of CT as the first-line modality in the assessment of the annulus and in device selection.[27] This approach is supported by increasing evidence that the integration of MDCT enables improved clinical outcomes, reducing complications such as annular rupture and PAR as well as the overall morbidity and mortality associated with TAVR.[20,28]

Once annular measurements have been performed, the process of device selection and sizing can be multifactorial. In TAVR it is necessary to insert a THV that is larger than the native valve annulus to minimize PAR and risk of embolization; this has been termed oversizing. The degree of oversizing varies depending on which device is inserted and the measurement parameter used.

In the past, device sizing was based on two-dimensional (2D) transthoracic echocardiogram (TTE) measurements combined with 10% oversizing. TTE typically underestimated the annular long axis and leads to systematic device undersizing with high rates of PAR. With CT, clinicians can better assess the annular geometry and more accurately quantify its size. Because the aortic annulus is almost always noncircular, the percentage of oversizing required depends on the measurement parameter used. On average, the calculated percentage oversizing based on annular area is twice that of derived diameters or perimeter.[29] In clinical practice, sizing is calculated using either area or perimeter, and confusing the measurement parameter used can lead to complications. Because of the limited number of device size options, algorithms for THV sizing increase incrementally. Occasionally in borderline cases in which more than 1 valve size may be appropriate, consideration should be taken when oversizing and incorporating other adverse features. A patient-specific approach when choosing which device to use has also been suggested to produce the best results; that is, selecting a THV with a risk profile most compatible with the patient's particular annular size and adverse anatomic features.[30]

The percentage of oversizing that is appropriate also depends on the device deployed. Each device differs in design and in the extent of radial force exerted on the aortic root. Self-expanding devices exert less radial force and require a greater degree of oversizing, typically 10% to 25% based on perimeter, than balloon-expandable devices to prevent the same PAR.[31,32] Balloon-expandable devices exert more radial force and have increased risk of annular rupture, particularly when aggressive oversizing is combined with adverse patterns of annular calcification.[33] The next generation of balloon-expandable devices contain features such as an outer sealing skirt that reduce PAR and require less oversizing, offsetting the risk of rupture. The SAPIEN 3 THV requires 2% to 10% area oversizing compared with the past generation SAPIEN XT, which requires 5% to 20%[34] owing to the sealing skirt on this device. These next-generation devices have also shown improved results in BAVs, with comparable rates of PAR seen in BAV and tricuspid aortic valve (TAV) cohorts undergoing TAVR with a SAPIEN 3 valve.[35]

Mitral

The mitral annulus is a fibrous structure with a complex 3D geometry. It has a nonplanar saddle-shaped configuration consisting of 2 elevated peaks, or horns, that attach to the anterior and medial fibrous trigones of the aortomitral continuity. The aortomitral continuity forms the anterior mitral annulus and slopes upward in an atrial direction toward the left and the noncoronary cusps. The posterior mitral valve insertion/annulus is defined at the junction of the atrial and ventricular myocardium. This posterior component slopes in an atrial direction, resulting in the formation of a posterior peak.

Although the mitral valve has a complex saddle-shaped morphology, the true 3D annular geometry, area, and perimeter of the valve can be readily assessed using CT.[28] This assessment is achieved by using specialized software to systematically place seeding points at regular intervals along the mitral annulus. Another manual approach is to create a standardized 2D annular plane by truncating the anterior mitral valve at the level of the fibrous trigones; this is followed by identifying the posterior annular free edge insertion point. Hence, a D-shaped annulus is created that excludes the valve apparatus anterior to the medial and lateral trigones. Advantages of this technique are low interobserver variability and less risk of the implanted device protruding into the LVOT.[36]

Once the mitral valve annulus has been delineated, standard measurements include 2D area; perimeter; and intercommisural, septal-lateral, and intertrigonal distances (**Fig. 3**).[36,37] The relevance of each of these measurements varies across specific devices with different annular sizing methods integrated into the different manufacturers guidelines. As TMVR develops further, investigation will be required to create more tailored device selection and sizing algorithms.

PREVENTING COMPLICATIONS

CT has been shown to help inform device selection and procedural risk assessment for the last

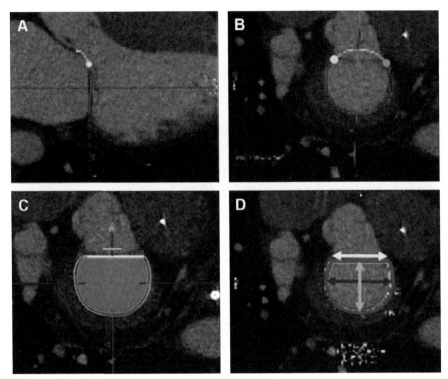

Fig. 3. Multiplanar reformatted contrast-enhanced cardiac CT reconstructed in end diastole. Three-chamber view (*A*) and mitral valve short-axis view (*B*) outline the anterior (*pink line*) and posterior (*red line*) mitral valve annulus as well as the identify the lateral (*yellow circle*) and medial (*green circle*) trigones. Short-axis views of the mitral annulus truncated at lateral and medial trigones showed the D-shaped annulus, (*C, D*). Standard measurements of the mitral annulus include area (*green*), perimeter (*red line*), intercommisural distance (*purple arrows*), septal-lateral distance (*blue arrows*), and intertrigonal distance (*yellow arrows*).

decade. Commonly these modifications are not only to the result of annular features but also ancillary root or LVOT findings that can directly affect procedural risk. Awareness of adverse features can aid proceduralists in adapting their technique in an attempt to minimize the risk of major complication.

Rupture

Balloon-expandable and self-expanding THVs carry different risk profiles owing to variability in exerted radial force and their structural design. The aortic annulus generally conforms to the circular shape of a balloon-expandable valve, whereas self-expanding valves conform more to the geometry of the aortic annulus. It is for this reason that balloon-expandable valves confer increased risk of annular rupture and are sized by area, which provides a more conservative measurement than perimeter when assessing a borderline noncircular annulus.[29,30]

Subannular calcification located within the upper LVOT is associated with increased incidence of rupture. Risk of aortic rupture is further increased with protruding nodular calcifications and calcification situated below the noncoronary cusp[33,38] (Fig. 4). Other nonanatomic factors linked to annular rupture, such as prior radiation therapy and female sex, also need to be taken into consideration.[33,39]

The mitral valve is less susceptible to annular rupture because TMVR valves are self-expandable, have larger annulus, and are more reliant on barbs for capture and sealing than radial force.

Coronary Occlusion

Although rare, coronary artery occlusion has a high risk of mortality (40.9% at 30 days).[13,40] As previously mentioned, there are 2 main factors to be considered when avoiding this rare complication. The largest series of patients with coronary obstruction following transcatheter aortic valve implantation (TAVI) to date showed that 86% who experienced this complication had a coronary artery height of less than 12 mm, although 26% of those who did not also had a coronary height of less than 12 mm. Most patients (71%) with

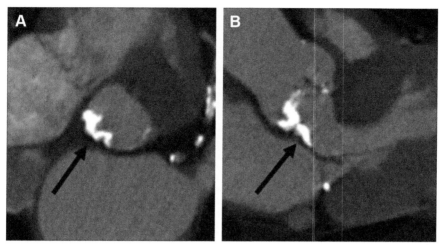

Fig. 4. Multiplanar reformatted contrast-enhanced cardiac CT reconstructed in end diastole. Short-axis views of the LVOT (A) and 3-chamber view (B) showing subannular nodular calcification (arrows) located immediately below the noncoronary cusp. This distribution of calcification places the patient at increased risk of annular rupture and should be taken into consideration during pre-TAVR work-up.

coronary obstruction had a sinus of Valsalva diameter less than 30 mm, with one-third of the control population having a sinus of Valsalva less than 30 mm. Only 13.3% of patients with a combination of these two adverse anatomic features did not have coronary occlusion, suggesting that they should be assessed in tandem when evaluating for potential risk of coronary occlusion.[13]

Heart Block

Left bundle branch block (LBBB) is a common complication of TAVI (5%–40%) caused by direct trauma to the left bundle branch of His at the time of the procedure.[41–43] These patients have a poorer prognosis, with an increased risk of complete atrioventricular (AV) block, heart failure, and sudden cardiac death. Implantation of a pacemaker is performed during follow-up in 13.9% to 20% of LBBBs after TAVI.[44] Low deployment of both balloon and self-expandable THV during TAVR is the biggest predictor of LBBB and is associated with a higher rate of permanent pacemaker (PPM) insertion.[45–50]

The bundle of His emerges onto the left ventricle surface just below the AV membranous septum. The longer the membranous septum (MS), the further the His bundle is from the aortic annulus and the less likely an implanted THV is to interfere with the conduction pathway. Hamdan and colleagues[51] showed that, when assessed using CT before TAVR, MS length was highly variable and reduced length was the strongest preprocedural predictor of AV block (odds ratio [OR], 1.35; 95% confidence interval [CI], 1.1–1.7; $P = .01$) as well

as the need for a PPM following the procedure (OR, 1.43; 95% CI, 1.1–1.8; $P = .002$). They also found that the difference between the MS length, on CT, and the THV implantation depth below the aortic annulus, on fluoroscopy, was inversely proportional to the rate of AV block. The difference between MS length and implantation depth in combination with calcification at the basal septum was the most powerful predictor of postprocedural PPM implantation (OR, 1.39; 95% CI, 1.2–1.7; $P<.001$; and OR, 4.9; 95% CI, 1.2–20.5; $P = .03$, respectively).

Left Ventricular Outflow Tract Obstruction in Transcatheter Mitral Valve Replacement and Mitral Valve in Valve

LVOT obstruction is a major complication of mitral valve interventions, resulting in high morbidity and mortality.[52,53] There are many factors that can contribute to a patient being at increased risk of LVOT obstruction. Increased angulation between the mitral outflow tract and the LVOT long axis (aortomitral angle) is associated with an increased risk of LVOT obstruction. Other anatomic variables associated with increased risk include reduced ventricular size, basal septal hypertrophy, and increased anterior mitral valve leaflet length. Procedural factors include device selection, intraoperative tilting, and an inability to deploy the valve in a coaxial plane.[54,55]

There are several mitral THV procedures for the treatment of a spectrum of mitral valve disease, including valve in MAC, valve in ring, valve in valve (ViV), and TMVR. Based on data from the Valve-in-Valve International Database (VIVID) registry, the relative risk and mechanism of LVOT obstruction is different for each of these procedures and each type of landing zone. Virtual implantation of device-specific stereolithographic files of the valve that is intended to be implanted can be superimposed on the CT dataset to model the deployed device, and this creates a neo-LVOT that is defined by the septum and the virtual implanted device. The neo-LVOT can then be assessed perpendicular to its long axis to determine the point of greatest narrowing (Fig. 5). Although few outcome data exist, a conservative threshold of 1.5 cm², based on hypertrophic cardiomyopathy data, has been suggested as the threshold for patients considered high risk of LVOT obstruction.[56] To date, late systole has been the favored imaging phase of the cardiac cycle because it provides assessment of the Neo-LVOT when the gradient is likely to be the highest.[57]

For valve-in-ring and valve-in-MAC procedures, CT can identify patients who may benefit from a more atrial deployment to reduce the risk of LVOT obstruction; however, this is not the case when placing a THV in a failed surgical valve because the THV effectively creates a covered stent within the LVOT and therefore a more atrial offset is of no benefit in a fashion similar to a deep implant in an aortic VIV deployment.

Note that a major factor in LVOT obstruction relates to distortion of the anterior mitral valve leaflet or rupture of the anterior cords, which cannot be reliably predicted with preprocedural simulation of device implantation.[54,55]

PREPROCEDURAL ANGLE PREDICTION FOR TRANSCATHETER AORTIC VALVE REPLACEMENT AND TRANSCATHETER MITRAL VALVE REPLACEMENT

THV implementation depends on periprocedural imaging, such as intraoperative transesophageal echocardiography (TOE) or fluoroscopy. It is relevant that fluoroscopic viewing angles depend on the 3D orientation of the valve complex. As with any planar structure, there are many projections that allow a coplanar view of the aortic or mitral annuli.[58] CT can provide information about aortic root orientation in relation to body axis.[59] Successful valve deployment relies on accurate positioning, with the use of fluoroscopy perpendicular to the native valve to ensure coaxial deployment of the implanted valve along the center line of the aorta. Preprocedural CT can provide interventionists with a map of equivalent views of what they can anticipate seeing at corresponding C-arm angle fluoroscopic projections. If stent orientation is inaccurate, there is a risk of inappropriate device positioning and therefore increased likelihood of procedural complications, such as stent embolization.[59,60]

Computed Tomography–Based Prediction of Angiographic Projection Angles for Transcatheter Aortic Valve Replacement

Given there is significant variation in patient anatomy, individuals' aortic root orientations can be extracted from CT datasets to predict appropriate angles of implementation, therefore reducing the need for repeat aortograms at the time of intervention and so reducing procedure time, contrast medium volume, and radiation exposure.[60,61] There

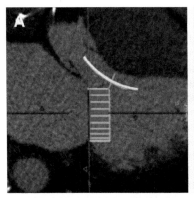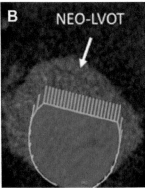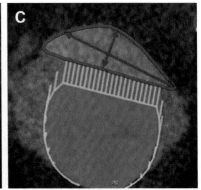

Fig. 5. Multiplanar reformatted contrast-enhanced cardiac CT reconstructed in late systole. Three-chamber view (A) with a simulated THV showing the neo-LVOT center line (*yellow line*) through the long axis of the neo-LVOT. Short-axis views of the narrowest part of the neo-LVOT (B) are obtained by scrolling perpendicular to the neo-LVOT center line. Standard measurements of the narrowest neo-LVOT (C) include area (*green*), perimeter (*red line*), as well as long-axis and short-axis diameters (*blue arrows*).

are numerous orthogonal projections of the native valve plane that follow a certain line of perpendicularity, meaning that any point in the right anterior oblique to left anterior oblique spectrum can be used as long as the correct degree of cranial and caudal angulation is matched.[62] Appropriate angulations are derived from CT angiographic datasets either manually by using the MPR function or modern work-flow platforms so long as angulations are reported by the software or specifically designed applications. To optimize results, it should be noted that angles predicted from CT are only transferable to a hybrid operating suite assuming the same position at the time of CT and TAVR.

Computed Tomography–Based Prediction of Angiographic Projection Angles for Transcatheter Mitral Valve Replacement

Likewise, coplanar angulation can also assist TMVR valve implantation. Following segmentation, coplanar fluoroscopic angles can be determined that allow optimal visualization of the mitral annulus according to the needed projection, to assist the interventionist guide the device in a perpendicular fashion to the mitral annulus.

VALVE IN VALVE

Placement of a THV within a failing surgical heart valve (SHV) is increasingly used as an alternative treatment option to repeat surgery in high-risk and inoperable patients. Although this ViV procedure has shown good technical success rates and short-term outcomes, it carries its own inherent risks.[63] Coronary obstruction is a major concern with the VIVID registry, revealing a 2.3% rate of coronary occlusion, 4 times that of native TAVR implantation.[64,65]

When the THV is deployed, its mesh displaces the SHV leaflets outward, effectively creating a covered stent within the aortic root. When leaflets come in contact with or close proximity to the coronary ostium, this results in obstruction. With CT, clinicians can virtually insert the cylindrical structure of the displaced SHV leaflets and anticipate the distance between the deployed THV and the coronary ostia. The virtual THV-to-coronary (VTC) distance has been shown to be the only independent predictor of coronary obstruction in ViV.[66] Riberio and colleagues[65] assessed 1612 patients from the multicenter VIVID and showed that a VTC threshold less than 4 mm was highly discriminatory for coronary occlusion with an AUC of 0.943. They also identified that stentless bioprosthetic valves and stented surgical valves with externally mounted leaflets were associated with a higher risk of coronary occlusion compared with stented valves with internally mounted leaflets.

To assess VTC, the authors use MPR to identify the basal ring of the SHV or create a plane that intersects the lowest points of the valve struts. The inside diameter of this ring is now the narrowest point to which the THV will be deployed and anchored, and thus should be used for device sizing. The true inside diameter is 1 to 2 mm less than this measurement in internally mounted leaflets.[67] If we fix an ROI the diameter of the THV device to be inserted in the basal ring, we can scroll superiorly in the same plane to the level of the ostia and measure the VTC (**Fig. 6**).[68]

If the SHV struts extent beyond the STJ and the virtual stent comes in contact with the aortic wall, it is possible to seal off the sinus and effectively eliminate flow to the coronary vessels; this can be assessed by scrolling the virtual ring upward to the superior margin of the SHV struts and ensuring it does not come in contact with the aortic wall.[68]

Other hostile features can be evaluated on CT that should also be considered and reported on. Bulky calcifications and valve thickening also potentially reduce the distance from the leaflets to the coronary ostium when the THV is deployed. Also of note is that SHVs with reduced internal area are associated with higher gradients and worse outcomes after ViV.[69]

HYPOATTENUATED LEAFLET THICKENING AND POSTIMPLANT ASSESSMENT

Cardiac CT offers limited value for routine postoperative TAVR recipients and as such there are no formal recommendations for its use following the procedure. Intraoperative TOE may confirm appropriate prosthetic position and function, as well as assessing for paravalvular regurgitation.[70,71] However, MDCT does serve as a complimentary imaging modality to TOE to suggest patient-specific mechanisms of PAR and in circumstances in which there are equivocal findings, suspicion of valvular thrombosis, infective endocarditis, and structural degeneration.[72]

A 2D postdeployment angiogram is technically limited to indicating prosthetic position and expansion only. Should the aforementioned conditions be deemed satisfactory, paravalvular regurgitation cannot be excluded. In contrast, postinterventional CT offers a 3D assessment of the aortic root, which affords the potential to assess for compromise to valve function and identify asymptomatic complications and underlying causes of paravalvular leak, and poor device

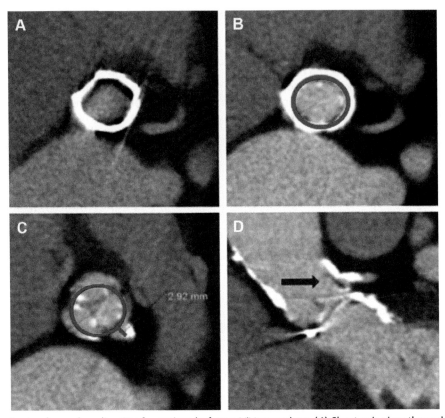

Fig. 6. Contrast-enhanced cardiac CT of a patient before a ViV procedure. (*A*) Short-axis view through the basal ring of a failing Metroflow (Sorin) SHV. (*B*) A 20-mm virtual ring (*red circle*) is placed within the neoannulus of the SHV, representing the diameter of the proposed TAVR valve. By scrolling up to the level of the left coronary ostium (*C*), the VTC distance (*red line*) can be measured. In this case the VTC distance is less than 3 mm, placing the patient at high risk of coronary occlusion. (*D*) A long-axis view through the aortic root shows the close proximity of the SHV radiolucent stent posts (*arrow*) to the left coronary ostium.

apposition caused by large subannular protruding nodules.[73–76]

Compromise to valve function may be caused by thrombus formation or early hypoattenuated leaflet thickening (HALT). Thrombus is a hypodense structure with an attenuation less than the ventricular septum that develops on the aortic side of the aortic valve.[77] HALT has been described as hypodense thickening of the prosthetic leaflets combined with reduced valve motion. It is thought to indicate thrombus formation because it resolves with anticoagulation.[72,75] Restricted leaflet motion is consistent with the presence of HALT.[74] With retrospective acquisition, cine CT images can allow assessment of valve motion and therefore identify limited leaflet opening.[78] Given the variety of balloon and self-expandable THVs, reporters should familiarize themselves with the different physical properties of the devices and therefore establish abnormal appearances associated with each device.[79]

SUMMARY

Advances in CT technology have led to it now being considered an essential tool in the work-up of patients undergoing TAVR and TMVR. It has emerged as the best modality for identifying hostile anatomy, instructing device selection, and providing intraprocedural guidance. As knowledge of these procedures increases, CT is also playing an increasing role in the follow-up of both TAVR and TMVR, with imagers becoming crucial adjudicators in the multidisciplinary team caring for these patients.

REFERENCES

1. Clavel MA, Messika-Zeitoun D, Pibarot P, et al. The complex nature of discordant severe calcified aortic valve disease grading: new insights from combined Doppler echocardiographic and computed tomographic study. J Am Coll Cardiol 2013;62(24): 2329–38.

2. Stevens PE, Farmer CK, Hallan SI. The primary care physician: nephrology interface for the identification and treatment of chronic kidney disease. J Nephrol 2010;23(1):23–32. Available at: http://www.ncbi.nlm.nih.gov/pubmed/20091483.

3. Raju R, Thompson AG, Lee K, et al. Reduced iodine load with CT coronary angiography using dual-energy imaging: a prospective randomized trial compared with standard coronary CT angiography. J Cardiovasc Comput Tomogr 2014;8(4):282–8.

4. Jochheim D, Schneider V-S, Schwarz F, et al. Contrast-induced acute kidney injury after computed tomography prior to transcatheter aortic valve implantation. Clin Radiol 2014;69(10):1034–8.

5. Naoum C, Leipsic J, Cheung A, et al. Mitral annular dimensions and geometry in patients with functional mitral regurgitation and mitral valve prolapse implications for transcatheter mitral valve implantation. JACC Cardiovasc Imaging 2016;9(3):269–80.

6. Rossi A, Dini FL, Faggiano P, et al. Independent prognostic value of functional mitral regurgitation in patients with heart failure. A quantitative analysis of 1256 patients with ischaemic and non-ischaemic dilated cardiomyopathy. Heart 2011;97(20):1675–80.

7. Jilaihawi H, Chen M, Webb J, et al. A bicuspid aortic valve imaging classification for the TAVR Era. JACC Cardiovasc Imaging 2016;9(10):1145–58.

8. Sievers HH, Schmidtke C. A classification system for the bicuspid aortic valve from 304 surgical specimens. J Thorac Cardiovasc Surg 2007;133(5):1226–33.

9. Michelena HI, Prakash SK, Della Corte A, et al. Bicuspid aortic valve: identifying knowledge gaps and rising to the challenge from the International Bicuspid Aortic Valve Consortium (BAVCon). Circulation 2014;129(25):2691–704.

10. Leon MB, Smith CR, Mack MJ, et al. Transcatheter or surgical aortic-valve replacement in intermediate-risk patients. N Engl J Med 2016;374(17):1609–20.

11. Yoon S-H, Bleiziffer S, De Backer O, et al. Outcomes in transcatheter aortic valve replacement for bicuspid versus tricuspid aortic valve stenosis. J Am Coll Cardiol 2017;69(21):2579–89.

12. Delgado V, Ewe S, Ng A, et al. Multimodality imaging in transcatheter aortic valve implantation: key steps to assess procedural feasibility. EuroIntervention 2010;6(5):643–52.

13. Ribeiro HB, Webb JG, Makkar RR, et al. Predictive factors, management, and clinical outcomes of coronary obstruction following transcatheter aortic valve implantation. J Am Coll Cardiol 2013;62(17):1552–62.

14. Delgado V, Tops LF, Schuijf JD, et al. Assessment of mitral valve anatomy and geometry with multislice computed tomography. JACC Cardiovasc Imaging 2009;2(5):556–65.

15. Naoum C, Blanke P, Cavalcante JL, et al. Cardiac computed tomography and magnetic resonance imaging in the evaluation of mitral and tricuspid valve disease: implications for transcatheter interventions. Circ Cardiovasc Imaging 2017;10(3) [pii:e005331].

16. Garbi M, Monaghan MJ. Quantitative mitral valve anatomy and pathology. Echo Res Pract 2015;2(3):R63–72.

17. Cheung A, Webb J, Verheye S, et al. Short-term results of transapical transcatheter mitral valve implantation for mitral regurgitation. J Am Coll Cardiol 2014;64(17):1814–9.

18. Eleid MF, Cabalka AK, Williams MR, et al. Percutaneous transvenous transseptal transcatheter valve implantation in failed bioprosthetic mitral valves, ring annuloplasty, and severe mitral annular calcification. JACC Cardiovasc Interv 2016;9(11):1161–74.

19. Masri A, Schoenhagen P, Svensson L, et al. Dynamic characterization of aortic annulus geometry and morphology with multimodality imaging: predictive value for aortic regurgitation after transcatheter aortic valve replacement. J Thorac Cardiovasc Surg 2014;147(6):1847–54.

20. Jilaihawi H, Kashif M, Fontana G, et al. Cross-sectional computed tomographic assessment improves accuracy of aortic annular sizing for transcatheter aortic valve replacement and reduces the incidence of paravalvular aortic regurgitation. J Am Coll Cardiol 2012;59(14):1275–86.

21. Piazza N, de Jaegere P, Schultz C, et al. Anatomy of the aortic valvar complex and its implications for transcatheter implantation of the aortic valve. Circ Cardiovasc Interv 2008;1(1):74–81.

22. Blanke P, Euringer W, Baumann T, et al. Combined assessment of aortic root anatomy and aortoiliac vasculature with dual-source CT as a screening tool in patients evaluated for transcatheter aortic valve implantation. AJR Am J Roentgenol 2010;195(4):872–81.

23. Gurvitch R, Webb JG, Yuan R, et al. Aortic annulus diameter determination by multidetector computed tomography: reproducibility, applicability, and implications for transcatheter aortic valve implantation. JACC Cardiovasc Interv 2011;4(11):1235–45.

24. Leipsic J, Gurvitch R, Labounty TM, et al. Multidetector computed tomography in transcatheter aortic valve implantation. JACC Cardiovasc Imaging 2011;4(4):416–29.

25. Willson AB, Webb JG, Labounty TM, et al. 3-dimensional aortic annular assessment by multidetector computed tomography predicts moderate or severe paravalvular regurgitation after transcatheter aortic valve replacement: a multicenter retrospective analysis. J Am Coll Cardiol 2012;59(14):1287–94.

26. Murphy DT, Blanke P, Alaamri S, et al. Dynamism of the aortic annulus: Effect of diastolic versus systolic

CT annular measurements on device selection in transcatheter aortic valve replacement (TAVR). J Cardiovasc Comput Tomogr 2016;10(1):37–43.

27. Leipsic JA, Blanke P, Hanley M, et al. ACR appropriateness criteria ® imaging for transcatheter aortic valve replacement. J Am Coll Radiol 2017;14(11): S449–55.

28. Binder RK, Webb JG, Willson AB, et al. The impact of integration of a multidetector computed tomography annulus area sizing algorithm on outcomes of transcatheter aortic valve replacement: a prospective, multicenter, controlled trial. J Am Coll Cardiol 2013;62(5):431–8.

29. Blanke P, Willson AB, Webb JG, et al. Oversizing in transcatheter aortic valve replacement, a commonly used term but a poorly understood one: dependency on definition and geometrical measurements. J Cardiovasc Comput Tomogr 2014;8(1):67–76.

30. Dvir D, Webb JG, Piazza N, et al. Multicenter evaluation of transcatheter aortic valve replacement using either SAPIEN XT or CoreValve: degree of device oversizing by computed-tomography and clinical outcomes. Catheter Cardiovasc Interv 2015;86(3): 508–15.

31. Buzzatti N, Maisano F, Latib A, et al. Computed tomography-based evaluation of aortic annulus, prosthesis size and impact on early residual aortic regurgitation after transcatheter aortic valve implantation. Eur J Cardiothorac Surg 2013;43(1):43–51.

32. Kasel AM, Cassese S, Bleiziffer S, et al. Standardized imaging for aortic annular sizing. JACC Cardiovasc Imaging 2013;6(2):249–62.

33. Barbanti M, Yang T-H, Rodes Cabau J, et al. Anatomical and procedural features associated with aortic root rupture during balloon-expandable transcatheter aortic valve replacement. Circulation 2013;128(3):244–53.

34. Blanke P, Pibarot P, Hahn R, et al. Computed tomography–based oversizing degrees and incidence of paravalvular regurgitation of a new generation transcatheter heart valve. JACC Cardiovasc Interv 2017;10(8):810–20.

35. Arai T, Lefèvre T, Hovasse T, et al. The feasibility of transcatheter aortic valve implantation using the Edwards SAPIEN 3 for patients with severe bicuspid aortic stenosis. J Cardiol 2017;70(3):220–4.

36. Blanke P, Dvir D, Cheung A, et al. A simplified D-shaped model of the mitral annulus to facilitate CT-based sizing before transcatheter mitral valve implantation. J Cardiovasc Comput Tomogr 2014; 8(6):459–67.

37. Achenbach S, Delgado V, Hausleiter J, et al. SCCT expert consensus document on computed tomography imaging before transcatheter aortic valve implantation (TAVI)/transcatheter aortic valve replacement (TAVR). J Cardiovasc Comput Tomogr 2012;6(6):366–80.

38. Hansson NC, Nørgaard BL, Barbanti M, et al. The impact of calcium volume and distribution in aortic root injury related to balloon-expandable transcatheter aortic valve replacement. J Cardiovasc Comput Tomogr 2015;9(5):382–92.

39. Barbanti M, Buccheri S, Rodés-Cabau J, et al. Transcatheter aortic valve replacement with new-generation devices: a systematic review and meta-analysis. Int J Cardiol 2017;245:83–9.

40. Ribeiro HB, Nombela-Franco L, Allende R, et al. Coronary obstruction following transcatheter aortic valve implantation for degenerative bioprosthetic surgical valves: a systematic literature review. Rev Bras Cardiol Invasiva (English Ed) 2013;21(4): 311–8.

41. Erkapic D, De Rosa S, Kelava A, et al. Risk for permanent pacemaker after transcatheter aortic valve implantation: a comprehensive analysis of the literature. J Cardiovasc Electrophysiol 2012;23(4):391–7.

42. Sinhal A, Altwegg L, Pasupati S, et al. Atrioventricular block after transcatheter balloon expandable aortic valve implantation. JACC Cardiovasc Interv 2008;1(3):305–9.

43. Akin I, Kische S, Paranskaya L, et al. Predictive factors for pacemaker requirement after transcatheter aortic valve implantation. BMC Cardiovasc Disord 2012;12(1):87.

44. Urena M, Webb JG, Cheema A, et al. Impact of new-onset persistent left bundle branch block on late clinical outcomes in patients undergoing transcatheter aortic valve implantation with a balloon-expandable valve. JACC Cardiovasc Interv 2014; 7(2):128–36.

45. Urena M, Mok M, Serra V, et al. Predictive factors and long-term clinical consequences of persistent left bundle branch block following transcatheter aortic valve implantation with a balloon-expandable valve. J Am Coll Cardiol 2012;60(18):1743–52.

46. Piazza N, Onuma Y, Jesserun E, et al. Early and persistent intraventricular conduction abnormalities and requirements for pacemaking after percutaneous replacement of the aortic valve. JACC Cardiovasc Interv 2008;1(3):310–6.

47. Franzoni I, Latib A, Maisano F, et al. Comparison of incidence and predictors of left bundle branch block after transcatheter aortic valve implantation using the CoreValve versus the Edwards valve. Am J Cardiol 2013;112(4):554–9.

48. Colombo A, Latib A. Left bundle branch block after transcatheter aortic valve implantation: inconsequential or a clinically important endpoint? J Am Coll Cardiol 2012;60(18):1753–5.

49. Calvi V, Conti S, Pruiti GP, et al. Incidence rate and predictors of permanent pacemaker implantation after transcatheter aortic valve implantation with self-expanding CoreValve prosthesis. J Interv Card Electrophysiol 2012;34(2):189–95.

50. Aktug Ö, Dohmen G, Brehmer K, et al. Incidence and predictors of left bundle branch block after transcatheter aortic valve implantation. Int J Cardiol 2012;160(1):26–30.

51. Hamdan A, Guetta V, Klempfner R, et al. Inverse relationship between membranous septal length and the risk of atrioventricular block in patients undergoing transcatheter aortic valve implantation. JACC Cardiovasc Interv 2015;8(9):1218–28.

52. Guerrero M, Dvir D, Himbert D, et al. Transcatheter mitral valve replacement in native mitral valve disease with severe mitral annular calcification: results from the first multicenter global registry. JACC Cardiovasc Interv 2016;9(13):1361–71.

53. Yoon SH, Whisenant BK, Bleiziffer S, et al. Transcatheter mitral valve replacement for degenerated bioprosthetic valves and failed annuloplasty rings. J Am Coll Cardiol 2017;70(9):1121–31.

54. Blanke P, Naoum C, Dvir D, et al. Predicting LVOT obstruction in transcatheter mitral valve implantation: concept of the Neo-LVOT. JACC Cardiovasc Imaging 2017;10(4):482–5.

55. Wang DD, Eng M, Greenbaum A, et al. Predicting LVOT obstruction after TMVR. JACC Cardiovasc Imaging 2016;9(11):1349–52.

56. Qin JX, Shiota T, Lever HM, et al. Impact of left ventricular outflow tract area on systolic outflow velocity in hypertrophic cardiomyopathy: a real-time three-dimensional echocardiographic study. J Am Coll Cardiol 2002;39(2):308–14.

57. Kim D-H, Handschumacher MD, Levine RA, et al. In vivo measurement of mitral leaflet surface area and subvalvular geometry in patients with asymmetrical septal hypertrophy: insights into the mechanism of outflow tract obstruction. Circulation 2010; 122(13):1298–307.

58. Blanke P, Dvir D, Naoum C, et al. Prediction of fluoroscopic angulation and coronary sinus location by CT in the context of transcatheter mitral valve implantation. J Cardiovasc Comput Tomogr 2015; 9(3):183–92.

59. Masson J-B, Kovac J, Schuler G, et al. Transcatheter aortic valve implantation: review of the nature, management, and avoidance of procedural complications. JACC Cardiovasc Interv 2009;2(9):811–20.

60. Kurra V, Kapadia SR, Tuzcu EM, et al. Pre-procedural imaging of aortic root orientation and dimensions. comparison between X-ray angiographic planar imaging and 3-dimensional multidetector row computed tomography. JACC Cardiovasc Interv 2010;3(1):105–13.

61. Gurvitch R, Webb JG, Yuan R, et al. Aortic annulus diameter determination by multidetector computed tomography. JACC Cardiovasc Interv 2011;4(11): 1235–45.

62. Gurvitch R, Wood DA, Leipsic J, et al. Multislice computed tomography for prediction of optimal angiographic deployment projections during transcatheter aortic valve implantation. JACC Cardiovasc Interv 2010;3(11):1157–65.

63. Landes U, Kornowski R. Transcatheter valve implantation in degenerated bioprosthetic surgical valves (ViV) in aortic, mitral, and tricuspid positions: a review. Struct Hear 2017;1–11. https://doi.org/10.1080/24748706.2017.1372649.

64. Ribeiro HB, Webb JG, Makkar RR, et al. Predictive factors, management, and clinical outcomes of coronary obstruction following transcatheter aortic valve implantation: insights from a large multicenter registry. J Am Coll Cardiol 2013;62(17):1552–62.

65. Ribeiro HB, Rodés-Cabau J, Blanke P, et al. Incidence, predictors, and clinical outcomes of coronary obstruction following transcatheter aortic valve replacement for degenerative bioprosthetic surgical valves: insights from the VIVID registry. Eur Heart J 2018;39(8):687–95.

66. Dvir D, Leipsic J, Blanke P, et al. Coronary obstruction in transcatheter aortic valve-in-valve implantation: preprocedural evaluation, device selection, protection, and treatment. Circ Cardiovasc Interv 2015;8(1) [pii:e002079].

67. Bapat VN, Attia R, Thomas M. Effect of valve design on the stent internal diameter of a bioprosthetic valve. JACC Cardiovasc Interv 2014;7(2):115–27.

68. Blanke P, Soon J, Dvir D, et al. Computed tomography assessment for transcatheter aortic valve in valve implantation: the Vancouver approach to predict anatomical risk for coronary obstruction and other considerations. J Cardiovasc Comput Tomogr 2016;10(6):491–9.

69. Dvir D, Webb JG, Blanke P, et al. Transcatheter aortic valve replacement for failed surgical bioprostheses: insights from the PARTNER II valve-in-valve registry on utilizing baseline computed-tomographic assessment. Struct Hear 2017;1(1–2): 34–9.

70. Leon MB, Piazza N, Nikolsky E, et al. Standardized endpoint definitions for transcatheter aortic valve implantation clinical trials: a consensus report from the Valve Academic Research Consortium. J Am Coll Cardiol 2011;57(3):253–69

71. Kapadia SR, Leon MB, Makkar RR, et al. 5-year outcomes of transcatheter aortic valve replacement compared with standard treatment for patients with inoperable aortic stenosis (PARTNER 1): a randomised controlled trial. Lancet 2015;385(9986): 2485–91.

72. Pache G, Schoechlin S, Blanke P, et al. Early hypoattenuated leaflet thickening in balloon-expandable transcatheter aortic heart valves. Eur Heart J 2016; 37(28):2263–71.

73. Leetmaa T, Hansson NC, Leipsic J, et al. Early aortic transcatheter heart valve thrombosis: diagnostic value of contrast-enhanced multidetector computed

tomography. Circ Cardiovasc Interv 2015;8(4) [pii: e001596].

74. Hansson NC, Grove EL, Andersen HR, et al. Transcatheter aortic valve thrombosis. J Am Coll Cardiol 2016;68(19):2059–69.

75. Makkar RR, Fontana G, Jilaihawi H, et al. Possible subclinical leaflet thrombosis in bioprosthetic aortic valves. N Engl J Med 2015;373(21): 2015–24.

76. Yanagisawa R, Hayashida K, Yamada Y, et al. Incidence, predictors, and mid-term outcomes of possible leaflet thrombosis after TAVR. JACC Cardiovasc Imaging 2017;10(1):1–11.

77. Chan J, Marwan M, Schepis T, et al. Images in cardiovascular medicine. Cardiac CT assessment of prosthetic aortic valve dysfunction secondary to acute thrombosis and response to thrombolysis. Circulation 2009;120(19):1933–4.

78. Tsai I-C, Lin Y-K, Chang Y, et al. Correctness of multidetector-row computed tomography for diagnosing mechanical prosthetic heart valve disorders using operative findings as a gold standard. Eur Radiol 2009;19(4):857–67.

79. Blanke P, Schoepf UJ, Leipsic JA. CT in transcatheter aortic valve replacement. Radiology 2013; 269(3):650–69.

Imaging of Pericardial Disease

Seth Kligerman, MD

KEYWORDS

- Pericardium • Pericarditis • Radiology • CT • MR imaging

KEY POINTS

- Pericardial effusions are a common manifestation of various pathologic conditions and can be classified as transudative, exudative, hemorrhagic, or malignant.
- Although cross-sectional imaging should not be the first technique to evaluate for tamponade, there are findings on computed tomography (CT) and MR imaging that can suggest this physiologic diagnosis.
- There are numerous causes of acute pericarditis, and although most are classified as idiopathic, they are thought to be viral in cause.
- There are many findings on CT and MR imaging to suggest constrictive pericarditis, but increased septal flattening during early inspiration on real-time MR imaging is one of the best clues to diagnosis.
- There are numerous primary benign and malignant pericardial tumors but metastatic disease to the pericardium is much more common.

IMAGING OF THE PERICARDIUM

Anatomy and Normal Appearance on Imaging

Enveloping the heart, the pericardium is a dual-layer fibroserous sac composed of the visceral pericardium and parietal pericardium. Composed of a very thin (<1 mm) layer of mesothelial cells, the visceral pericardium lines the epicardial surface of the heart but is separated from the epicardium by a layer of epicardial fat of various thickness.[1] The structure of the parietal pericardium is more complex as it is composed of an outer fibrous layer and an inner serous layer.[2] The outer fibrous layer serves to anchor the pericardium by attaching to the diaphragm, sternum, deep cervical fascia, and great vessels.[3] The inner serous layer of the parietal pericardium, similar to the visceral pericardium, is composed of a thin layer of mesothelial cells and these 2 layers form the serous pericardium. Where the visceral and parietal serous layers are not attached is called the pericardial cavity, which normally contains 15 to 35 mL of pericardial fluid secreted by the mesothelial cells.[1] The fibrous layer of the parietal pericardium is attached to the mesothelial layer of the parietal pericardium and is composed of various layers of collagen and elastic fibers.[4]

Although the normal pericardium cannot be visualized on chest radiography, it can be seen on computed tomography (CT) and MR imaging. On CT, the pericardium appears as a thin soft tissue band enveloping the heart. It extends superiorly from the great vessels inferiorly to the diaphragm (Fig. 1). Although there may be certain areas where it is poorly visualized, such as overlying the lateral surface of the left ventricle, it is present except for rare circumstances, which will be discussed later. The pericardium is often thin, measuring only 1 to 2 mm in thickness, although a thickness less than 4 mm is considered normal.[5] A small amount of fluid is often present between

The author has no disclosures.
Diagnostic Radiology, University of California San Diego, 200 West Arbor Drive, San Diego, CA 92103, USA
E-mail address: skligerman@ucsd.edu

Radiol Clin N Am 57 (2019) 179–199
https://doi.org/10.1016/j.rcl.2018.09.001

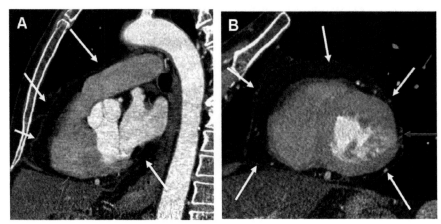

Fig. 1. (A, B) Normal pericardium on CT. Three millimeter thick ray-sum sagittal image of the thorax (A) and 3-mm thick ray-sum short axis image through midcavity of the left ventricle (B) shows the extend of the pericardium that encloses the heart (*white arrows*). Although portion of the pericardium is not well seen, such as that along the diaphragmatic surface (*red arrow*, see **Fig. 1**A) and along the lateral aspect of the left ventricle (*red arrow*, see **Fig. 1**B), the pericardium is present. Up to 35 mL of fluid is normally found in the pericardial sac and it is important not to confuse a small amount of physiologic fluid with pericardial thickening. (© 2018 Seth Kligerman.)

the layers of the pericardium. In addition, fluid is often present in various pericardial sinuses and recesses, as discussed later and should not be mistaken for pathology.

On MR imaging, the serous pericardium will appear low signal on steady-state free precession, T1- and T2-weighted sequences (**Fig. 2**)[6,7] and is outlined by the high signal of surrounding epicardial and mediastinal fat. Additional sequences can be used to visualize the pericardium, especially when certain diseases are suspected. Spatial modulation of magnetization (tagging), free-breathing nongated cine, T1-weighted post-contrast sequences, and delayed enhancement sequences can all be used to assess for various pathologic processes and will be discussed later.

The portion of the visceral pericardium that covers the vessels is arranged in the form of 2 short tubes.[8–10] The arterial mesocardium encloses the proximal portions of the ascending aorta and pulmonary trunk, whereas the venous mesocardium encloses the superior vena cava (SVC) and inferior vena cava (IVC) and the 4 pulmonary veins. The oblique sinus of the pericardium is formed where the venous mesocardium attaches to the serous layer of the parietal pericardium posterior to the left atrium and between the pulmonary veins (**Fig. 3**).[3,8,9] The oblique sinus is contiguous with the subcarinal region and forms a posterior pericardial recess.

The transverse sinus is a second tunnel between the arterial and venous mesocardium, lying superior to the left atrium and posterior to the aorta and main pulmonary artery (see **Fig. 3**). The

transverse sinus communicates with several recesses including the superior aortic, inferior aortic, right pulmonic, and left pulmonic recesses.[11] The pulmonary recesses form the lateral extents of the transverse sinus and lie inferior to their respective pulmonary arteries. The inferior aortic recess represents the inferior extent of the transverse sinus and is located between the aortic root and right atrium and extends inferior to the level of the aortic annulus.[12] The superior aortic recess is the superior extent of the transverse sinus that extends upward along the ascending aorta and is often visible on CT.[9] The superior aortic recess is divided into anterior and posterior portions given their relation to the ascending aorta. The anterior portion of the superior aortic recess lies anterior to the ascending aorta and pulmonary artery and often has a triangular shape but may be quite variable in appearance and extent. The posterior aspect of the superior aortic recess normally has a crescentic-shaped fluid collection posterior of the ascending aorta. When these recesses are prominent or "high riding," they can also be mistaken for pathology such as mediastinal cysts or lymphadenopathy (**Fig. 4**).[12]

There are 3 additional recesses of the pericardial cavity proper: the postcaval recess, the left pulmonary vein recess, and the right pulmonary vein recess.[9,13] The postcaval recess is posterior and right lateral to the SVC. The left and right pulmonary venous recesses are located between the superior and inferior pulmonary veins on each side.[11] These recesses are often quite small and rarely mistaken for pathology. However, as the right

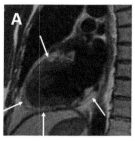
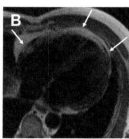
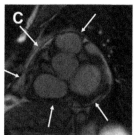
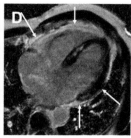

Fig. 2. (A–D) Normal appearance of pericardium on MR imaging. Two-chamber T2-weighted (A) and 4-chamber T1-weighted (B) short axis images from a steady-state free precession sequence (C) and 4-chamber delayed enhancement image (D) in a 38-year-old man, which shows a normal pericardium (arrows) that is isointense to hypointense to adjacent myocardium on all sequences. Similar to CT, the pericardium is best seen when outlined by hyperintense mediastinal fat and may not be visible in certain areas but is almost always present. (© 2018 Seth Kligerman.)

inferior pulmonary veins extend through the fibrous pericardium to drain into the left atrium, a serosal sleeve of pericardium invests the vein.[14] Fluid within this sleeve surrounding the right inferior pulmonary vein can mimic adenopathy or a tumor (Fig. 5). The characteristic location and presence of curvilinear fluid attenuation partially surrounding but not invading or significantly compressing the vein can help differentiate this normal finding from pathology.

Congenital Anomalies of the Pericardium

Pericardial cyst and diverticulum

Pericardial cysts are rare benign mesothelial line cysts occurring in 1 in 100,000 patients.[15] The majority occur at the cardiophrenic angles, on the right greater than the left.[16] A minority occur in other parts of the mediastinum usually related to

the pericardium. Most patients are asymptomatic but up to one-third may present with chest pain, dyspnea, or cough, particularly if the cyst compresses adjacent structures.

Imaging features of pericardial cysts are often characteristic. On chest radiography, the cyst typically manifests as a rounded density that contacts the hemidiaphragm and anterior chest wall (Fig. 6).[16] On CT and MR imaging, pericardial cysts typically appear as thin-walled round or ovoid lesions with homogenous internal attenuation or signal, respectively (see Fig. 6; Fig. 7).[17] Because of the presence of proteinaceous material, on CT pericardial cysts can have increased attenuation measuring that of soft tissue although the attenuation remains homogeneous.[18] If the diagnosis of a cyst cannot be definitively made on CT, MR imaging can help with the diagnosis

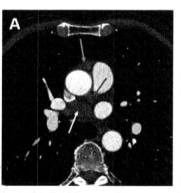
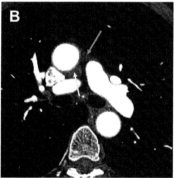
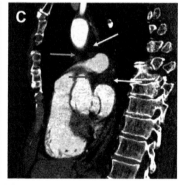

Fig. 3. (A–C) Oblique and transverse sinuses anatomy in a 44-year-old man. (A) Axial CT image demonstrates fluid within the oblique sinus (white arrow), which is located superior to the left atrium and anterior to the transverse sinus (red arrow). Fluid is also present in the superior aortic recess (blue arrow) that communicates with the transverse sinus. (B) Axial image more superiorly shows crescentic fluid in the posterior aspect of the superior aortic recess (yellow arrow). Fluid is also seen in the anterior aspect of the superior aortic recess (blue arrow). (C) Sagittal oblique image shows that the more posterior oblique sinus (white arrow) does not communicate with the more anterior transverse sinus (red arrow). Fluid within the anterior (blue) and posterior (yellow) portions of the superior aortic recess are also seen. Fluid in these locations is common and should not be confused with adenopathy or other pathology. (© 2018 Seth Kligerman.)

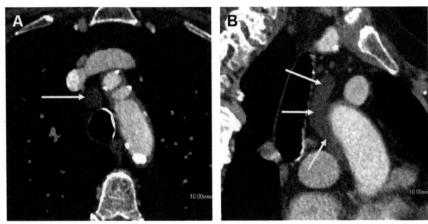

Fig. 4. (*A, B*) A 71-year-old woman with a history of breast cancer with "high-riding" superior pericardial recess mimicking lymphadenopathy. (*A*) Axial image at the level of the aortic arch vessels shows a rounded lesion in the right paratracheal region that measures fluid attenuation (*arrow*). (*B*) Sagittal image shows that this fluid collection (*white arrow*) communicates with the posterior (*yellow arrow*) aspect of the superior aortic recess, consistent with a "high-riding superior aortic recess." This anatomic variant can be easily confused with lymphadenopathy or cystic mass, which could lead to unnecessary intervention. Diagnosis can be made by its fluid attenuation and characteristic location best seen on multiplanar reformats. (© 2018 Seth Kligerman.)

(see **Fig. 7**). Although many cysts will have homogenous low signal on T1-weighted imaging and high signal on T2-weighted imaging, this can greatly vary depending on the degree of proteinaceous material. Cysts with a large degree of proteinaceous material can have low to intermediate signal on T2-weighted imaging and intermediate to high signal on T1-weighted imaging.[19] However, on both MR imaging and CT, the signal or attenuation will be homogenous throughout the lesion and internal septations should be minimal or absent. Although the rim of the cyst may enhance, no internal enhancement should be seen on first-pass perfusion or postcontrast imaging. On MR imaging, cysts will not restrict diffusion.

Internal enhancement, areas of discrete fat or soft tissue signal (MR imaging) or attenuation (CT) (**Fig. 8**), a thickened wall, mass effect, or thickening or enhancing septations (**Fig. 9**) should raise the possibility of a cystic tumor.

Unlike a pericardial cyst, a pericardial diverticulum retains a small communication with the pericardial space (**Fig. 10**).[20] Although it is often difficult to differentiate between the 2 at any single point in time, fluid within a pericardial diverticulum can change over studies due to its connection with the pericardial cavity. Most pericardial cysts and diverticula do not undergo treatment but symptomatic cysts may require aspiration or surgery.[21–23]

Pericardial defect

Congenital absence of the pericardial is an uncommon abnormality that can be defined as partial or complete. Left-sided defects are more common.[24] Although the cause is unclear, one hypothesis is that early regression of embryonic left common cardiac vein leads to a defect.[25,26] In most instances, the defect is an incidental finding in an asymptomatic patient. In extremely rare instances, portions of the left atrium can herniate through a partial defect leading to incarceration, left atrial infarction, and with subsequent syncope and sudden death.[27] Although these defects usually occur in isolation, 30% to 50% of patients have associated congenital anomalies, including atrial septal defect, patent ductus arteriosus, bicuspid aortic valve, or pulmonary abnormalities.[28,29]

On radiography, absence of the pericardium most often appears as leftward and posterior rotation of the heart given that most defects are left-sided. Another good clue to the diagnosis on radiograph is the sharp delineation of the main pulmonary artery and transverse aorta due to interposition of lung between these 2 structures (**Fig. 11**).[25] In some cases of partial absence, a bulge in the region of the left atrial appendage may be the only radiographic finding.[28]

On CT or MR imaging, the appearance depends on whether the abnormality is partial or complete. In both partial and complete left-sided defects, there is usually leftward rotation of the heart into the left chest, with interposition of the lung between the aorta and pulmonary artery.[18] If the defect is partial, the heart often bulges leftward in the region of the left atrial appendage (**Fig. 12**). The actual defect in partial absence of the

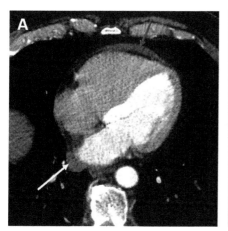
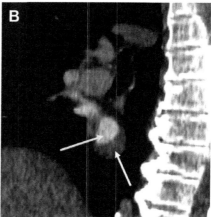

Fig. 5. (*A, B*) Four-chamber (*A*) and sagittal oblique multiplanar reformat (*B*) in a 45-year-old man with melanoma shows fluid in a serosal sleeve (*white arrows*) that surrounds the right inferior pulmonary vein (*yellow arrow,* see Fig. 5B). This fluid attenuation collection has a characteristic location and appearance that should prevent it from being confused for pathology. A normal amount of fluid in the pericardium anteriorly is also present (*A, red arrow*). (© 2018 Seth Kligerman.)

pericardium may be difficult to visualize over the lateral aspect of the left ventricle because even the normal pericardium can be difficult to see in this area.[7] It the left-sided defect is complete, the entire heart is typically displaced to the left and lung is interposed between its inferior margin of the heart and the diaphragm. On functional cine imaging, excessive motion of the cardiac apex has been observed in individuals with complete absence of the pericardium.[30]

Acquired Pericardial Diseases

Pericardial effusion

Pericardial effusions are a common manifestation of various pathologic conditions. Fluid within the pericardium may be characterized as transudative, exudative, hemorrhagic, or malignant.[31,32] Common findings of transudative effusions include congestive heart failure or other conditions that cause increased right-heart filling pressures (**Fig. 13A**).[33] Exudative effusions are common in multiple conditions including, autoimmune disorders (**Fig. 13B**), malignancy (**Fig. 13C**), infection (**Fig. 13D**), chronic renal disease, and pericardial trauma. Although uncommon, in pyopericardium frank pus fills the pericardial space and is associated with a high mortality rate (**Fig. 13E**).[34] Hemopericardium can occur after surgery, trauma, or aortic dissection (**Fig. 13F**).

On radiograph, large effusions can often be suggested if the heart has an enlarged, "water-bottle" morphology on posteroanterior (PA) imaging

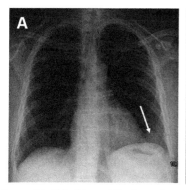
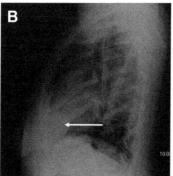
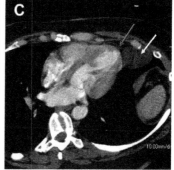

Fig. 6. (*A–C*) Incidental finding of a pericardial cyst on preoperative radiograph in a 33-year-old woman. Posteroanterior (PA) (*A*) and lateral (*B*) radiographs demonstrate a rounded mass (*arrow*) at the left cardiophrenic angle that contacts both the diaphragm and chest wall. (*C*) Axial oblique image shows the fluid attenuation mass (*white arrow*) contiguous with the pericardium (*red arrow*). Although this is a benign lesion, the patient requested surgical resection, which confirmed a pericardial cyst. (© 2018 Seth Kligerman.)

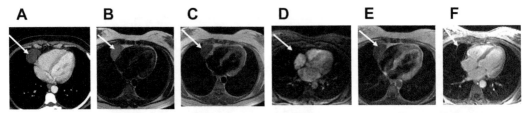

Fig. 7. (*A–F*) CT and MR imaging of a pericardial cyst incidentally discovered in a 39-year-old woman. (*A*) Four-chamber reconstruction from a chest CT shows a homogenous low attenuation mass (*arrow*) in the right cardiophrenic sulcus with an internal attenuation of 30 HU. (*B, C*) Four-chamber T2-weighted (*B*) and T1-weighted (*C*) images show homogenously high (*B*) and intermediate (*C*) signal within the mass (*arrows*), respectively. Because of the varying degree of proteinaceous material within any mediastinal cyst, the signal on T1- and T2-weighted sequences can vary significantly. (*D*) First-pass perfusion imaging shows no perfusion in the mass (*arrow*). (*E*) T1-weighted postcontrast sequence through the mass shows no appreciable enhancement (*arrow*). (*F*) Delayed enhancement image obtained with an inversion time of 600 msec shows mild enhancement of the wall of the cyst (*arrow*) but not internal enhancement. Homogenous signal, lack of evidence of internal soft tissue components, thin smooth rim, lack of perfusion, and lack of enhancement all help to characterize this lesion as a benign cyst. (© 2018 Seth Kligerman.)

(**Fig. 14**). On the lateral radiograph, a fat pad sign composed of pericardial fluid outlined by lower attenuation mediastinal and epicardial fat can help make the diagnosis.[35] Another imaging manifestation of a pericardial effusion is a rapid increase in the size of the cardiac silhouette over a short period of time.[36]

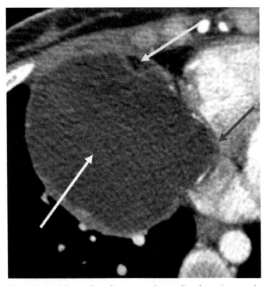

Fig. 8. Incidentally discovered cardiophrenic angle mass in a 23-year-old woman after a motor vehicle accident. Axial CT image shows that the mass is predominantly fluid attenuation (*white arrow*), although the attenuation seems slightly heterogeneous. However, there is a very subtle focus of macroscopic fat (*yellow arrow*) within the mass anteriorly. In addition, the mass demonstrates rim calcification and has mass effect on the right atrium (*red arrow*). These findings are atypical for a cyst. The lesion was resected, which revealed a cystic teratoma. (© 2018 Seth Kligerman.)

Echocardiography is often the first technique in the evaluation of pericardial effusion and/or tamponade physiology due to its availability, lack of ionizing radiation, ability to assess physiologic changes, low cost, and portability.[37] However, echocardiogram can be limited by poor acoustic windows, the location of an effusion, and its ability to adequately characterize a pericardial collection.[32]

On CT, increased attenuation within a pericardial effusion may indicate an exudative or hemorrhagic process, although there can be overlap.[38] If pericardial inflammation if present, the pericardium will often enhance after the administration of intravenous contrast as discussed in further detail later in this article (see **Fig. 13**B, D, E). Nodularity along the pericardium or the development of a pericardial effusion in a patient with known malignancy should raise the concern for a malignant pericardial effusion (see **Fig. 13**C).

High attenuation fluid suggests hemopericardium, especially in patients with a history of trauma, surgery, or aortic dissection (see **Fig. 13**F; **Fig. 15**).

MR imaging is an excellent modality to characterize a pericardial effusion. Most effusions are high in signal on steady-state free precession (SSFP) and T2-weighted sequences (**Fig. 16**), although areas of intermediate and/or low signal due to blood products or proteinaceous material can lead to a heterogenous appearance (see **Fig. 15**). On T1-weighted sequences, simple transudative effusions typically display low signal intensity (see **Fig. 16**), whereas proteinaceous, exudative or hemorrhagic effusions are more likely to demonstrate intermediate to high signal intensity (see **Fig. 15**).[39,40] However, pericardial fluid characterization can be difficult, especially in

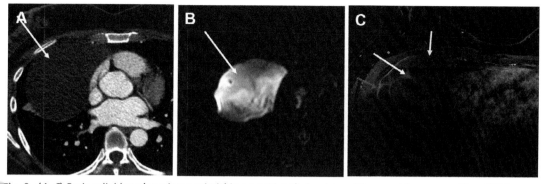

Fig. 9. (*A–C*) Pericardial lymphangioma mimicking a pericardial cyst in a 34-year-old woman with a BRCA mutation. (*A*) Axial image from a chest CT shows a large homogenous, fluid attenuation mass in the right cardiophrenic angle. The CT was obtained for presurgical planning. (*B, C*) The mass was incidentally discovered during breast MR imaging. (*B*) Axial T2-weighted sequence shows a heterogeneous, high signal mass with multiple internal septations. (*C*) T1-weighted postcontrast image shows enhancement of these septations (*white arrow*). In addition, the wall of the lesion is thin and imperceptible in some areas (*yellow arrow*) and thick and enhancing in other areas (*red arrow*). The findings are consistent with a cystic mass, which was confirmed to be a pericardial lymphangioma after resection. (© 2018 Seth Kligerman.)

cases of larger effusions because the nonlinear motion of pericardial fluid during cardiac motion can lead to a falsely elevated high signal on T1-weighted imaging, even in the presence of a simple transudate (see **Fig. 16**).[6]

On delayed enhancement imaging, the signal of pericardial fluid differs depending on whether the images are reconstructed using a magnitude or phase sensitive inversion technique (PSIR). Because the magnitude reconstruction represents an absolute value of transverse magnetization, both fat and fluid demonstrate high signal on magnitude imaging when the inversion time is set to null normal myocardium. This can make it difficult to differentiate epicardial fat from pericardial fluid (see **Fig. 16**). However, PSIR preserves the information about the polarity of the longitudinal relaxation. Therefore, using a PSIR reconstruction when the inversion time is set to null normal myocardium, material with a relatively rapid T1 relaxation time, such as fat, will seem bright, whereas material with a long T1 relaxation time, such as pericardial fluid, will seem very dark (see **Fig. 16**). Thus, PSIR is a useful tool to not only elucidate pathology such as in the case of pericardial thickening or adjacent myocardial inflammation

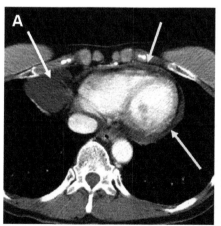
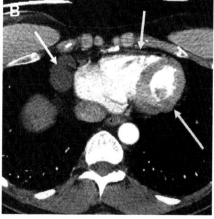

Fig. 10. (*A, B*) Pericardial diverticulum in a 63-year-old woman with a history of metastatic breast cancer. (*A*) Axial image obtained during routine screening shows a homogeneous, fluid attenuation lesion in the right cardiophrenic angle, which suggests a pericardial cyst (*white arrow*). A small pericardial effusion (*yellow arrows*) is also present. (*B*) A few months later, the pericardial effusion has resolved (*yellow arrows*) and the fluid in the pericardial diverticulum has decreased in size (*white arrow*). Unlike a pericardial cyst, a pericardial diverticulum retains a small connection with the pericardial cavity proper and can increase and decrease in size. (© 2018 Seth Kligerman.)

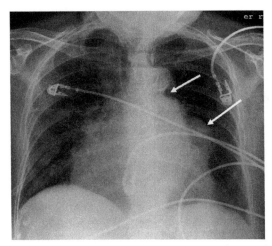

Fig. 11. PA radiograph shows findings of partial absence of the pericardium with herniation of the left atrial appendage (*white arrow*) and air extending between the aorta and main pulmonary artery (*yellow arrow*). Although left atrial herniation can occasionally lead to strangulation and infarction of the left atrial appendage, this patient was asymptomatic. (© 2018 Seth Kligerman.)

but to also help differentiate between normal types of tissue.

Pericardial tamponade

Pericardial tamponade occurs when increased intrapericardial pressures compress the chambers of the heart, most notably the right ventricle.[41] Because of decreased right ventricular filling, tamponade can lead to hemodynamic compromise and rapid death. The development of tamponade depends on the distensibility of the pericardium and rapidity in the accumulation of the pericardial fluid.[1] In patients with a distensible pericardium and a slow accumulation of pericardial fluid, a large effusion can be present without tamponade. However, in the setting of a rapidly developing effusion, especially if the pericardium is less compliant due to inflammation or scarring, tamponade can develop with as little as 100 to 200 mL of fluid.[42–44]

It is important to remember that pericardial tamponade is a clinical and physiologic diagnosis and cross-sectional imaging should not be the first technique used to evaluate for tamponade.[37] The diagnosis is usually made based on clinical criteria in combination with characteristic cardiac findings on echocardiography, notably diastolic collapse of the right ventricular free wall, right atrial collapse, paradoxic motion of the interventricular septum, and a swinging motion of the heart in the pericardial sac.[32] During inspiration, there will be an increase in flow across the tricuspid and pulmonic valves and decreased flow across the mitral and aortic valves, termed "flow velocity paradoxus."[45] Additional findings outside of the heart include dilation of the SVC and IVC and IVC plethora, all of which are due to increased right atrial pressure.[46]

Although CT should not play a primary role in the diagnosis of acute tamponade, given the common use of CT imaging in patients with chest pain or dyspnea, one should be aware of findings that can suggest the diagnosis. A common finding on

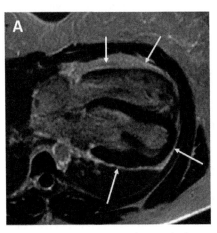
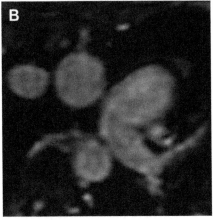

Fig. 12. (*A, B*). Incidental discovery of partial absence of the pericardium in a 55-year-old woman with an abnormal echocardiogram. (*A*) Four-chamber image from a delayed enhancement sequence shows leftward deviation of the heart. Most of the pericardium is absent (*yellow arrows*). Faint linear signal anterior to the free wall of the right ventricle may represent a small amount of pericardium (*white arrow*). (*B*) Axial image from an MR angiography shows the lung extending between the pulmonary artery and aorta into the aortic pulmonary window, a finding seen with absence of the pericardium. (© 2018 Seth Kligerman.)

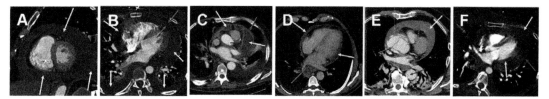

Fig. 13. Types of material in pericardial effusions on CT. (*A*) Short axis image from a CT in a 36-year-old man with hypoalbuminemia demonstrates a large transudative effusion (*yellow arrows*). The pericardium is not visibly thickened. Large pleural effusions are also present (*white arrow*). (*B*) Axial CT shows a sterile exudative effusion in a 26-year-old woman with lupus-related pleural (*white arrows*) and pericardial (*yellow arrows*) effusions. There is mild enhancement of the serous pericardium (*red arrows*). (*C*) Axial CT in a 27-year-old man with acute tuberculous pericarditis shows a multiloculated effusion (*yellow arrows*) with prominent pericardial thickening and enhancement (*red arrows*). Draining showed bloody and purulent fluid that grew out acid-fast bacilli. (*D*) Pyopericardium in a 44-year-old man with methicillin-resistant *Staphylococcus aureus* sepsis status post-pericardiocentesis shows a small pericardial effusion with pericardial thickening and enhancement (*yellow arrows*). There was associated necrotic subcarinal and hilar lymphadenopathy (*red arrow*), although the possibility of malignancy was (*E, yellow arrow*). Axial CT in a 50-year-old man with acute type A dissection (*red arrows*) shows a high attenuation pericardial effusion due to hemopericardium (*red arrows*). (*F*) Four-chamber reformat from a chest CT with contrast in a 47-year-old woman with metastatic lung cancer shows a moderate-sized pericardial effusion (*yellow arrows*), which was new from the prior study. Multiple pulmonary metastases are present (*red arrows*). Although no pericardial nodularity or enhancement was present, the findings were concerning for a malignant pericardial effusion. Pericardiocentesis showed bloody fluid with numerous malignant cells. (© 2018 Seth Kligerman.)

CT is a pericardial collection causing compression or flattening of the right atrium and/or right ventricular free wall (**Fig. 17**).[7,43] Bowing of the interventricular septum toward the left can also occur but is again nonspecific because it can be seen with any condition leading to severe pressure or volume overload of the right ventricle.[43] Other nonspecific findings of increased right atrial pressure can be seen, including dilation of the SVC, IVC, and azygous vein, as well as reflux of contrast into the hepatic veins (see **Fig. 17**).

Like CT, MR imaging is also not recommended to evaluate for acute tamponade, but the diagnosis can be made in the presence of a moderate to large effusion with diastolic chamber collapse, a "swinging heart" (**Fig. 18**), or an inspiratory septal bounce.

Inflammation of the Pericardium

Acute pericarditis

Acute inflammation of the pericardium can be classified as infectious, noninfectious, and idiopathic causes. Although 80% to 90% of cases in Western Europe and North America are classified as "idiopathic" after workup, most are presumed

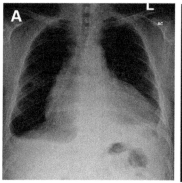
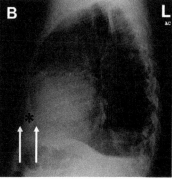
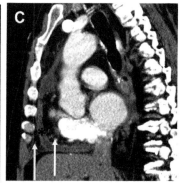

Fig. 14. (*A–C*) Diagnosis of a pericardial effusion on radiograph. (*A*) PA radiograph in a 52-year-old man with chronic renal insufficiency who presented to the emergency department with chest pain shows an enlarged cardiac silhouette that has a globular shape. There is no pulmonary edema. Small pleural effusions are present. (*B*) Lateral radiograph shows higher attenuation fluid (*asterisk*) outlined by epicardial fat centrally (*white arrow*) and mediastinal fat peripherally (*yellow arrow*). (*C*) Corresponding sagittal CT image shows the pericardial effusion (*asterisk*) outlined by epicardial (*white arrow*) and mediastinal (*yellow arrow*) fat. There is mild associated pericardial enhancement consistent with uremic pericarditis. (© 2018 Seth Kligerman.)

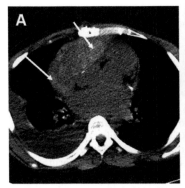
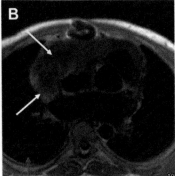
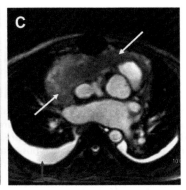

Fig. 15. (*A–C*) Hemopericardium after cardiac surgery in a 66-year-old man. (*A*) Axial CT image shows a heterogeneous attenuation collection with areas of high attenuation due to blood products (*white arrows*). (*B*) Axial T1-weighted image at the same level shows areas of intermediate (*yellow arrow*) and high signal (*white arrow*) due to blood products. (*C*) Axial SSFP image at the same level shows the heterogeneity of the hemopericardium (*white arrow*). This is in comparison with the simple transudative pleural effusions that are low and high in signal on T1-weighted (*B, red arrow*) and SSFP (*C, red arrow*) sequences, respectively. (© 2018 Seth Kligerman.)

to be viral in etiology.[47,48] Most cases of viral pericarditis occur weeks after a viral infection and it is thought that the pericardial inflammation is secondary to an immune-mediated process that is elicited by the virus.[48,49] Although less common, other infectious causes include bacterial, fungal, and parasitic infections. Of all the bacterial infections, mycobacterium tuberculosis is the most common, counting for approximately 4% of cases in the Western world but can be the causative organism in up to 70% of cases in certain developing countries (see **Fig. 13**D).[47]

Other causes of acute pericarditis include post-cardiac injury syndromes such as those that occur from autoimmune and systemic inflammatory disorders (systemic lupus erythematosus [SLE] [see **Fig. 13**B], rheumatoid arthritis [RA], scleroderma), drug reaction, radiation, metabolic conditions (chronic renal disease [see **Fig. 14**]), pericardial trauma, surgical manipulation, and malignancy.[47,50]

In addition, pericarditis can occur after myocardial infarction and can occur either immediately after infarct or have a delayed appearance. Although still rare, postinfract pericarditis occurs in the first few days after myocardial injury and is associated with a bigger infarct size.[51,52] However, a massive pericardial effusion can occur secondary to bleeding from the infarcted wall. The presence of

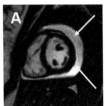
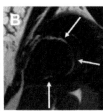
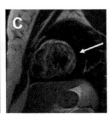
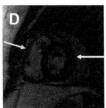
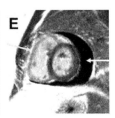

Fig. 16. (*A–E*) MR imaging of a transudative pericardial effusion in a 19-year-old woman with hypothyroidism, bipolar disorder, and chest pain. (*A*) Short axis SSFP image through the midcavity level of the left ventricle shows a moderate-sized pericardial effusion that is homogenously high in signal (*white arrows*). (*B*) T1-weighted dark blood imaging at the same level shows a relatively homogenous low-signal pericardial effusion (*white arrows*). An area of intermediate signal adjacent to the lateral segments (*yellow arrow*) is a common finding in moderate to large effusions due to the nonlinear motion of the pericardial fluid but can lead to the misdiagnosis of an exudative effusion. (*C*) T1-weighted postcontrast image at the same level shows no enhancement within the effusion or along the pericardium (*white arrow*). (*D, E*) Short axis magnitude (*D*) and phase sensitive inversion recovery (*E*) delayed gadolinium enhancement images set at an inversion time of 290 msec to null myocardium demonstrate the different appearance of the pericardial effusion between the 2 images. Because the magnitude reconstruction uses an absolute value of longitudinal magnetization (Mz), both fluid (*white arrow*) and epicardial fat (*yellow arrow*) seem similar in intensity. However, by preserving information about the polarity of Mz, pericardial fluid seems very dark (*white arrow*) because T1 relaxation is longer than myocardium time, whereas adjacent pericardial fat (*yellow arrow*) seems bright because its T1 relaxation time is shorter than myocardium. (© 2018 Seth Kligerman.)

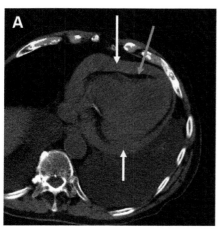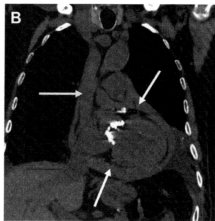

Fig. 17. (*A, B*) Cardiac tamponade in an 87-year-old patient after attempted minimally invasive cardiac surgery. (*A*) Axial CT shows hemopericardium (*white arrows*) and compression of the free wall of the right ventricle (*blue arrow*). (*B*) Coronal image again shows hemopericardium (*white arrows*) and dilation of the SVC (*yellow arrow*) and IVC (*red arrow*). These findings are concerning for but not diagnostic for pericardial tamponade, which was confirmed on echocardiogram. (© 2018 Seth Kligerman.)

massive pericardial effusion is associated with an increased mortality, usually secondary to tamponade and/or myocardial rupture.[53] Less commonly, pericarditis occurs a few weeks after a myocardial infarct (Dressler syndrome) and is more likely to be symptomatic with fever and a pericardial friction rub (**Fig. 19**). The cause of delayed pericardial inflammation is thought to be secondary to an immune response to cardiac proteins.[51]

Although the cause may differ, mesothelial response injury is limited. Acute inflammation releases various amounts of fluid, fibrin, and/or cells depending on the cause and severity of the insult,[54] similarly, the healing response depending on the cause and severity of injury. Patients with acute tuberculous pericarditis or pericarditis secondary to radiation, chronic renal failure, or collagen vascular disease are more likely to develop chronic pericardial fibrosis, adhesions, and calcification compared with patients with viral or drug-related pericarditis.[10]

Echocardiography is often the first imaging tool used when pericarditis is suspected. However, CT or MR imaging should be considered with inconclusive echocardiographic findings, if a patient fails to quickly respond to appropriate therapy, if

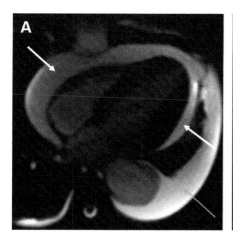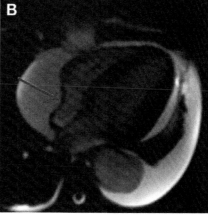

Fig. 18. (*A, B*) Cardiac tamponade in a 59-year-old man. (*A*) Four-chamber SSFP image during early systole demonstrates a large pericardial effusion (*white arrows*) and a large left pleural effusion (*yellow arrow*). (*B*) Four-chamber image obtained at the same level during early systole demonstrates collapse of the right atrium (*red arrow*), a finding that highly suggests cardiac tamponade, which was subsequently confirmed with echocardiogram. (© 2018 Seth Kligerman.)

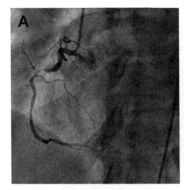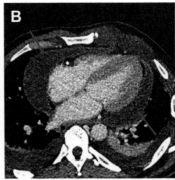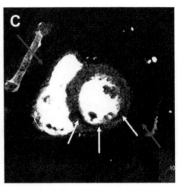

Fig. 19. (*A–C*) Dressler syndrome in a 62-year-old man with a right coronary artery (RCA) territory acute myocardial infarction (AMI). (*A*) C-view image of the RCA from cardiac catheterization shows a severe proximal stenosis (*arrow*) leading to the AMI. The RCA was stented and the patient was discharged 4 days later. (*B*) Axial CT image obtained 10 days after discharge shows a large pericardial effusion and mild pericardial enhancement (*arrows*). (*C*) Short axis 10-mm thick minimum intensity projection image (MinIP) shows subendocardial hypoperfusion in the inferoseptal, inferior, and inferolateral walls (*white arrows*) consistent with RCA territory infarct. The large effusion (*red arrows*) is difficult to see on this MinIP projection. (© 2018 Seth Kligerman.)

the clinical presentation is atypical, if there is a suspicion for constrictive pericarditis (CP) or effusive CP, or if there is a concern for malignancy or coexistent pulmonary infection, in the setting of chest trauma or possible dissection, and in the setting of a recent myocardial infarction.[37]

Pericardial thickening (>4 mm) and enhancement are classic CT findings in acute pericarditis (see **Fig. 13**B, D, E, **14**, and **19**; **Fig. 20**) but the absence of these findings does not exclude the diagnosis.[55] In addition, pericardial enhancement may be less conspicuous during arterial phase on intravenous contrast compared with a portal venous phase (see **Fig. 20**). Although associated pericardial effusions are common, one does not need to be present, especially if the pericardium is thickened and the cavity has been obliterated by prior pericardial injury.[10]

The imaging of pericarditis on MR imaging varies depending on severity of disease and pulse sequence used (**Fig. 21**). Thickening can be seen on T1-weighted, T2-weighted, and SSFP sequences, and the pericardium will often seem intermediate in signal intensity.[7] In some instances, fluid sensitive sequences will show pericardial edema and inflammation of the surrounding fat.[7,39,56] First-pass perfusion, postcontrast T1-weighted and delayed contrast-enhanced sequences will show pericardial enhancement.[39] In some cases, severe exudative inflammation can lead to the deposition of large amounts of fibrin and leukocytes, called fibrinous pericarditis (see **Fig. 21**). It is important to evaluate the adjacent myocardium because patients with associated myocardial inflammation, termed "myopericarditis," have a higher incidence of complications

(**Fig. 22**).[47] Follow-up imaging may show complete or near complete resolution of the pericardial inflammation while other patients may go on to develop irreversible pericardial scarring.

Fibrous and calcific pericarditis
Although the pericardium may return to normal after injury, in some instances the deposition of fibrous tissue causes permanent pericardial thickening and/or adhesions (**Fig. 23**).[10,37] Pericardial calcium deposition represents an end-stage reaction to pericardial injury.[54] Adhesions and calcification may be focal but extensive involvement can lead to obliteration of the pericardial space.

Although fibrous pericarditis can occur after any cause of pericardial injury, patients with recurrent episodes of pericardial inflammation, such as those with chronic renal disease and certain collagen vascular diseases, such as SLE (see **Fig. 23**), RA (**Fig. 24**), and scleroderma, are more like to develop fibrous pericarditis. Other causes of fibrous pericardial disease include radiation, infections (most notably tuberculosis [**Fig. 25**]), and pericardial injury due to cardiac surgery or trauma.[10]

On CT, fibrous pericarditis manifests as pericardial thickening with a variable-sized effusion (see **Fig. 24**). Pericardial enhancement with areas of calcification can be seen. On MR imaging, the pericardium will seem thickened and irregular with variable early enhancement (see **Figs. 23–25**).[7] Delayed enhancement is present secondary to the deposition of fibrous tissue (see **Fig. 24**). A MR imaging tagging sequence creates dark bands or grids across the heart and surrounding structures (see **Fig. 25**).[57] Normally,

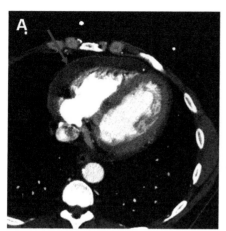
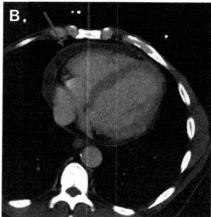

Fig. 20. (*A*, *B*) Viral pericarditis in a 69-year-old man with recent upper respiratory tract infection. Axial postcontrast CT images obtained during arterial (*A*) and portal venous phases (*B*) show a small pericardial effusion with pericardial thickening and enhancement (*arrows*) characteristic of pericarditis. The degree of enhancement seems more conspicuous on the portal venous phase likely due to decreased concentration of contrast in the blood. (© 2018 Seth Kligerman.)

these grid lines break during the cardiac cycle as the pericardial layers slip past one another. When the visceral and parietal pericardium are adherent to one another, the grid lines where adhesions are present will remain intact. Adhesions may occur in areas of normal pericardial thickness. Pericardial calcifications may be difficult to see on MR imaging but appear as areas of low signal on all sequences and do not enhance.[6,7] Although at increased risk for developing CP, the presence of pericardial fibrosis, adhesions, and calcification does not equate to this physiologic abnormality.

Calcium deposition in the pericardium represents an end-stage reaction to pericardial injury.[54] Although deposits may be focal (see **Fig. 23**E), extensive calcification can occur that

can lead to encasement of the entire heart (**Fig. 26**). The cause of calcific pericarditis is the same as those that lead to fibrous pericarditis. Calcifications are best visualized on CT although extensive pericardial calcifications can be seen on chest radiography (see **Fig. 26**). Calcification is not well seen on MR imaging but appears as linear areas of low signal on all sequences. Although fibrinous and or calcific pericarditis can be asymptomatic, it can lead to a constrictive physiology.

Constrictive pericarditis

CP is a condition in which reduced compliance of the pericardium leads to elevated ventricular diastolic pressures. Similar to tamponade, the heart

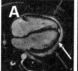
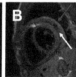
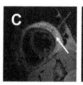
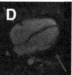
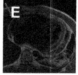
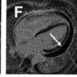
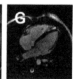

Fig. 21. (*A–G*) Idiopathic fibrinous pericarditis in a 21-year-old man with chest pain. (*A–C*) Four-chamber SSFP image (*A*), short axis T1-weighted image (*B*), and Spectral Adiabatic Inversion Recovery (SPAIR) T2-weighted image (*C*) from a cardiac MR imaging shows a large, complex pericardial effusion with septations (*white arrow*) and marked pericardial thickening (*red arrows*). The pericardial thickening is isointense to myocardium on the T1-weighted and SSFP sequences but high in signal on the SPAIR sequence, likely due to inflammation. (*D*) First-pass perfusion image shows enhancement of the pericardium (*red arrows*). (*E*) Four-chamber T1-weighted post-contrast imaging shows pericardial enhancement although the fluid does not demonstrate any significant enhancement. (*F*) Phase-sensitive inversion recovery (PSIR) delayed gadolinium enhancement imaging set at an inversion time of 300 msec shows enhancement of both the parietal (*red arrow*) and visceral (*white arrow*) pericardium. The pericardial fluid seems very low in signal on PSIR sequences. (*G*) Four-chamber SSFP image 2 months after pericardial window and antiinflammatory therapy shows complete resolution. Although some patients with fibrinous pericarditis may develop permanent pericardial thickening and fibrosis, others may show resolution without permanent dysfunction. (© 2018 Seth Kligerman.)

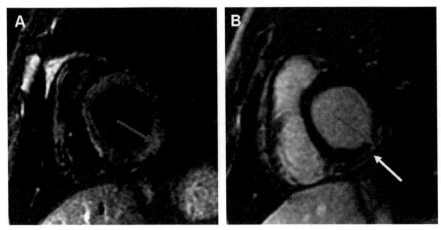

Fig. 22. (*A, B*) Myopericarditis in a 23-year-old man with elevated troponin levels but normal coronary arteries on cardiac catheterization. (*A*) Short axis (short tau inversion recovery) STIR image shows myocardial edema in a subepicardial location (*red arrow*). (*B*) Delayed gadolinium enhancement imaging set at an inversion time of 270 msec shows linear subepicardial enhancement (*red arrow*) consistent with myocarditis. In addition, there is adjacent pericardial enhancement (*white arrow*) with a small pericardial effusion consistent with pericarditis. (© 2018 Seth Kligerman.)

is forced to operate in a noncompliant space, leading to elevated systemic and pulmonary venous pressures that are required to maintain cardiac filling.[37] The noncompliant space also leads to ventricular interdependence as the increased volume in one ventricle leads to decreased volume in the other ventricle.

CP typically manifests with symptoms of low cardiac output, which particularly affects the right side of the heart.[58] Echocardiography is often obtained initially and can demonstrate equalization of pressures during diastole. In addition, the increased excursion velocity of the medial mitral annulus compared with the lateral mitral annulus (annulus paradoxus) and the decrease or reversal of blood flow in the hepatic venous during expiration can be measured using Doppler and highly suggest CP.[59] However, in some instances the echocardiogram is of limited diagnostic yield or the results are equivocal and additional imaging may aid in the diagnosis.

CT and MR imaging are additional techniques used to diagnose CP. Thickening of the pericardium is well visualized with both techniques. However, the absence of pericardial thickening does not exclude the diagnosis because up to 28% of

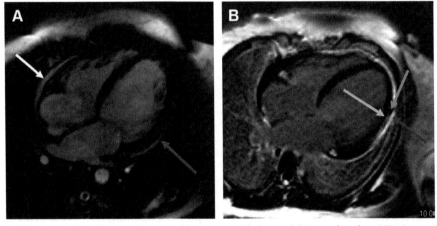

Fig. 23. (*A, B*) Fibrous pericarditis in a 41-year-old woman with lupus. (*A*) Four-chamber SSFP image shows pericardial thickening (*red arrow*) and a small pericardial effusion (*white arrow*). (*B*) PSIR delayed enhancement image shows enhancement of the parietal (*red arrow*) and visceral (*yellow arrow*) pericardium leading to obliteration of the pericardial space in certain areas (*blue arrow*). (© 2018 Seth Kligerman.)

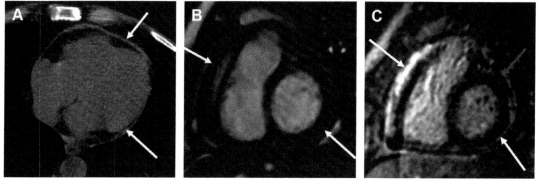

Fig. 24. (*A–C*) Fibrinous pericarditis in a 58-year-old woman with RA. (*A*) Axial CT image show a thickened pericardium encasing the heart (*white arrows*). (*B*) Short axis SSFP image shows circumferential pericardial thickening (*white arrows*). (*C*) Short axis delayed enhancement image at the same level as (*B*) shows intense enhancement of the pericardium (*white arrows*) due to the deposition of fibrous tissue. Only a small amount of pericardial fluid is present (*red arrow*). Despite the degree of thickening, the patients were relatively asymptomatic and constrictive pericarditis was absent. (© 2018 Seth Kligerman.)

patients with CP demonstrate normal pericardial thickness on CT and 18% had normal thickness on histology.[60] Moreover, patients with end-stage CP are more likely than those with reversible CP to have a normal diameter of the pericardium.[61,62] However, delayed enhancement of the pericardium is usually present due to fibrosis.

If pericardial effusions are present in CP, they are usually small in size. In rare instances, a patient with large pericardial effusion is superimposed on a stiff, noncompliant pericardium. This syndrome is referred to as effusive CP and is a rare entity occurring in less than 7% of patients presenting with pericardial tamponade.[63]

Other morphologic features may be visible on CT or MR imaging. Poor compliance of the pericardium causes morphologic changes to the cardiac chambers. The ventricles may have a conical appearance, right-sided chambers may be compressed, and the atria can be dilated.[19] Findings of elevated right-sided pressures are common including dilation of the IVC and azygous

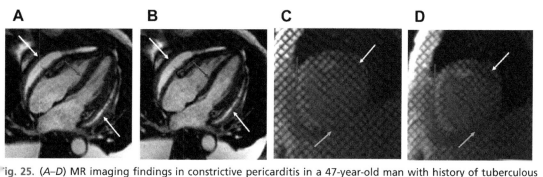

Fig. 25. (*A–D*) MR imaging findings in constrictive pericarditis in a 47-year-old man with history of tuberculous pericarditis. (*A, B*) Four-chamber SSFP images obtained during early diastole (*A*) and mid-diastole (*B*) show a septal bounce, which is characteristic of constrictive pericarditis. During early diastole, increased right ventricular (RV) pressures from early RV filling causes bowing of the septum to the left (*red arrow, A*). During mid-diastole, increased left ventricular (LV) pressures due to later LV filling causes the septum to bounce back to the right (*red arrow, B*), creating the characteristic bounce of constrictive pericarditis. There is pronounced pericardial thickening (*A, B, white arrows*) and the heart has a conical shape. (*C, D*) Images from a gradient echo tagging sequence in the short axis plane obtained during diastole (*C*) and systole (*D*) shows multiple grid lines. During diastole, the grid lines along the lateral wall of the LV (*white arrow*), inferior wall of the LV (*blue arrow*), and free wall of the RV (*red arrow*) are intact. (*F*) During systole, many of the grid lines along the LV (*white arrow*) and RV (*red arrow*) remain intact signifying that pericardium is scarred down and adherent to the underlying epicardium. Only the grids tags along the inferior wall of the left ventricle break (*blue arrow*), signifying a lack of adhesions in this area. Although pericardial adhesions are common in constrictive pericarditis, the presence of adhesions does not make this diagnosis. (© 2018 Seth Kligerman.)

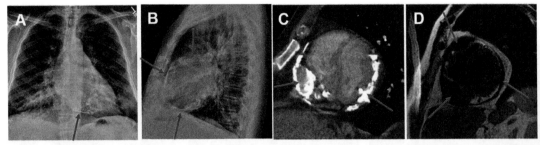

Fig. 26. (A–D) Diffuse pericardial calcification in a 44-year-old man with a history of tuberculous pericarditis and signs of constrictive pericarditis. (A, B) PA (A) and lateral (B) radiographs demonstrate extensive pericardial calcification, which is better seen on the lateral radiograph (*arrows*). (C) Short axis image from a contrast-enhanced CT shows the extensive pericardial calcification (*red arrows*), which is squeezing the heart. (D) Short axis T1-weighted image at the same level as (C) shows circumferential low signal due to calcification. (© 2018 Seth Kligerman.)

vein, ascites, pleural effusions, and peripheral edema. However, these findings are nonspecific.

On retrospectively gated cine MR imaging or cardiac CT angiography, ventricular interdependence leads to a classic septal bounce. In CP, rapid ventricular filling in early diastole is followed by abrupt termination of diastolic flow across the atrioventricular valves due to the noncompliant pericardium.[1] Because right ventricular filling occurs slightly before left ventricular filling, this early increase in right ventricular pressures leads to paradoxic leftward motion of the septum in early diastolic filing. The septum will then rebound back toward the right during left ventricular filling and increased left ventricular pressures creating a septal bounce (see **Fig. 25**). Although this early diastolic bounce can be seen in other conditions, the septal bounce in CP tends to be more pronounced.

One of the best methods to make the diagnosis of CP on MR imaging is to demonstrate respiratory variation of the diastolic bounce using nongated, free-breathing cine MR imaging sequences (**Fig. 27**).[64] In patients with CP, during inspiration the negative intrathoracic pressure increases venous return to the right heart. However, since the right ventricular motion is limited by the noncompliant pericardium, the increased right ventricular pressures lead to pronounced flattening or inversion of the interventricular septum. On expiration, the opposite occurs because positive intrathoracic pressure increases pulmonary return, resulting in a more normal appearance of the septum.[65] This technique is helpful not only in making the diagnosis of CP but also in differentiating between CP and restrictive cardiomyopathy.[64]

Epipericardial fat pad necrosis

Epipericardial fat necrosis, also called pericardial fat necrosis, is one of many causes of acute chest pain that can mimic other conditions.[66,67] The cause is unknown but pathologic findings can resemble that seen with epiploic appendagitis.[68] On CT, it most commonly appears as an encapsulated fatty lesion with focal inflammation centered in the juxtapericardial fat[66] (**Fig. 28**). Associated pleural and pericardial effusions are common. Epipericardial fat pad necrosis is a self-limited process and correct identification can prevent unnecessary testing and intervention.

Pericardial tumors

Primary pericardial tumors are quite rare and unlike their cardiac counterparts are more likely to be malignant. As the serous layers of the pericardium are layered by mesothelial cells, it is not surprising that primary pericardial mesothelioma accounts for 50% of primary pericardial neoplasms.[69] However, it is still extremely rare and in a necropsy series of 500,000 cases, the incidence was less than 0.0022%.[70] The association between asbestos exposure and pericardial mesothelioma is unclear. However, in approximately one-third of cases, patients have had a known exposure to asbestos. Early in the disease, CT and MR imaging demonstrates complex pericardial effusions and pericardial thickening that early in the disease may be mistaken for acute or chronic pericarditis. As the disease progresses, masses fill the pericardium, often invading surrounding structures including the heart and vasculature (**Fig. 29**).[71] Prognosis is poor and few patients survive longer than 12 months after diagnosis.[69]

In addition to mesothelioma, primary pericardial malignancies include sarcomas (**Fig. 30**), lymphoma, and germ cell tumors. Primary pericardial sarcomas can have a numerous histologic subtypes and the imaging appearance is often similar to that of other aggressive pericardial tumors.[71] Although most lymphomas that involve the pericardium represent part of a systemic disease, primary pericardial lymphoma can occur. Its

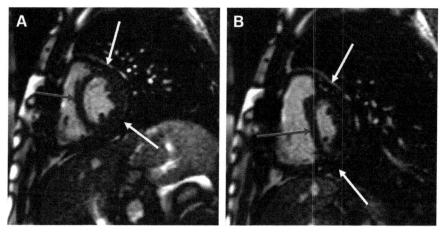

Fig. 27. (*A*, *B*) Constrictive pericarditis in a 70-year-old man with previous median sternotomy. Free-breathing, nongated short axis cine images obtained during expiration (*A*) and inspiration (*B*) show the respiratory variation in septal morphology in constrictive pericarditis. During expiration, LV pressures exceed RV pressures and the septum has a normal appearance (*A*, *red arrow*). On early inspiration, rapid increase of RV pressures due to increased right-sided venous return leads to dramatic flattening of the septum (*B*, *red arrow*). Notice the low signal surrounding the heart due to pericardial calcification (*A*, *B*, *white arrows*). (© 2018 Seth Kligerman.)

appearance is widely variable because it can appear as a diffusely infiltrative process or a solitary mass that can mimic other tumors. Primary effusion lymphoma is an extremely rare malignancy usually occurring in patients with human immunodeficiency virus. The main findings are large pleural and/or pericardial effusions filled with monoclonal B or T cells without associated soft tissue masses.[72] Although most intrapericardial germ cell tumors are benign teratomas, malignant germ cell tumors do occur and should be considered in any pediatric patient with a heterogenous intrapericardial mass.[73]

There are a wide variety of benign intrapericardial tumors. If the lesion is composed entirely of fat, the diagnosis of a lipoma can be made (**Fig. 31**). Other benign pericardial tumors include lymphangiomas (see **Fig. 9**) and hemangiomas. On noncontrast imaging, lymphangiomas and hemangiomas both appear as localized or serpiginous masses primarily of fluid attenuation on CT.[74] They may be infiltrative around structures but are not invasive. Septations that are usually

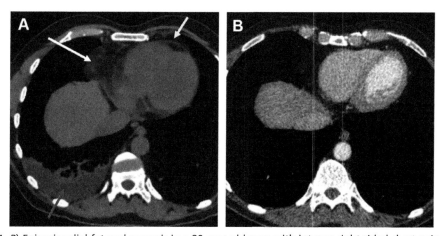

Fig. 28. (*A*, *B*) Epipericardial fat pad necrosis in a 39-year-old man with intense right-sided chest pain. (*A*). Axial image shows inflammatory changes in the pericardial fat (*white arrow*) There is a moderate right-sided pleural effusion (*red arrow*) and a small pericardial effusion (*yellow arrow*). (*B*) Three weeks later, repeat CT shows complete resolution of all the abnormalities. Recognition of this benign and self-limited entity is necessary to prevent unnecessary intervention. (© 2018 Seth Kligerman.)

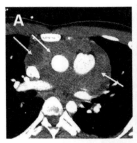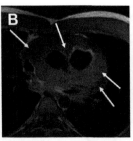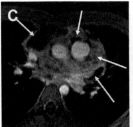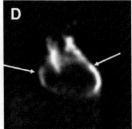

Fig. 29. (*A–D*) Pericardial mesothelioma in a 23-year-old man with shortness of breath. (*A*) Axial CT image shows confluent, enhancing soft tissue throughout the pericardium (*white arrows*). A small amount of fluid is present (*yellow arrows*). (*B*) T1-weighted precontrast image (*B*) at the same level as (*A*) shows predominantly intermediate signal (*white arrows*) with a few areas of low signal (*yellow arrows*). (*C*) T1-weighted postcontrast image shows intense enhancement of the pericardial soft tissue (*white arrows*). A few pockets of fluid (*yellow arrows*) correspond to the areas of lower signal on (*B*). (*D*) Coronal PET image shows circumferential fludeoxyglucose uptake. Biopsy confirmed pericardial mesothelioma, which is the most common primary pericardial tumor. (© 2018 Seth Kligerman.)

absent with pericardial cysts may be present and can show enhancement. On MR imaging, they are high-signal T2-weighted images but can vary from low signal to high signal on T1-weighted images. The administration of contrast can help distinguish between the 2 because lymphangiomas show no internal enhancement, whereas hemangiomas show nodular enhancement with progressive filling over time.[71] Other benign pericardial tumors include paragangliomas, fibromas, and teratomas.

Compared with primary pericardial tumors, secondary involvement of the pericardium is much more common and can occur by lymphatic extension, hematogenous spread, or direct invasion (**Fig. 32**).[75,76] Many tumors such as breast cancer and lymphoma seed the pericardium through lymphatic channels. Hematogenous melanoma and renal cell carcinoma pericardial metastases often show intense enhancement and are usually associated with extensive disease. Direct extension most commonly occurs from lung cancer

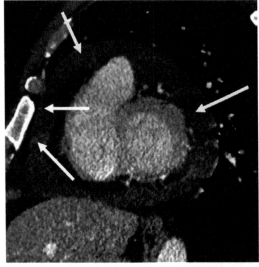

Fig. 30. Short axis image shows in a 50-year-old man with chest pain a lobulated, circumferential pericardial effusion (*yellow arrows*) with a few, very subtle enhancing pericardial nodules (*white arrows*). Initially, the patient was thought to have a pericarditis. However, after appropriate medical therapy, the effusion did not resolve, and the patient underwent pericardiocentesis, which showed a primary pericardial angiosarcoma. (© 2018 Seth Kligerman.)

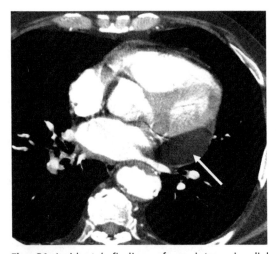

Fig. 31. Incidental finding of an intrapericardial lipoma in a 71-year-old man. Axial CT shows a fatty mass (*arrow*) located within the pericardium. Lipomas are benign lesions and are located in the pericardium, heart, or mediastinum. (© 2018 Seth Kligerman.)

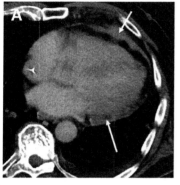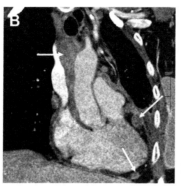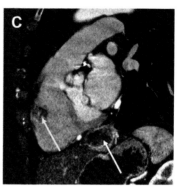

Fig. 32. (A–C) Pericardial metastases. (A) Four-chamber reconstruction from a contrast-enhanced CT shows nodular pericardial thickening (*white arrows*) in a 38-year-old man with lymphoma. Subsequent pericardiocentesis showed lymphomatous cells. (B) Coronal oblique image in a 58-year-old woman with metastatic lung cancer shows multiple enhancing pericardial masses (*white arrows*). Pleural metastases were also present. (C) Sagittal image in a 25-year-old man with metastatic fibrosarcoma shows large pericardial metastases (*white arrow*) and right ventricular metastases (*yellow arrow*). Pericardial metastases are much more common than primary pericardial tumors. (© 2018 Seth Kligerman.)

but can be seen with esophageal cancer, mediastinal lymphoma, or even breast cancer.[75]

Symptoms of pericardial metastases are variable. Nonspecific symptoms of chest pain and shortness of breath are frequent.[39] Effusions are often hemorrhagic and can be quite large, leading to tamponade in 16% of patients.[76] Diffuse involvement can encase the heart leading to pericardial constriction. CT and MR imaging may show the primary site of disease as well as the extent of pericardial involvement. Although pericardial tumor deposits or nodularity may be visible, in some cases the only finding is a pericardial effusion (see **Fig. 13**C). Enhancement of portions of the pericardium may be present after contrast administration using either CT or MR imaging.

SUMMARY

Although the pericardium is simply a 2-layered membrane enveloping the heart and great vessels, there are numerous anatomic variations, congenital anomalies, and pathologic conditions that can occur. Although echocardiography is still the first imaging modality used to assess the pericardium, CT and MR imaging are frequently being used to aid in diagnosis and assess response to therapy. Therefore, detailed knowledge of the pericardium in both its normal and diseased states is important to best direct patient care and potentially improve patient outcomes.

REFERENCES

1. Little WC, Freeman GL. Pericardial disease. Circulation 2006;113:1622–32.

2. Peebles CR, Shambrook JS, Harden SP. Pericardial disease–anatomy and function. Br J Radiol 2011; 84(Spec No 3):S324–37.

3. Spodick DH. Macrophysiology, microphysiology, and anatomy of the pericardium: a synopsis. Am Heart J 1992;124:1046–51.

4. Ishihara T, Ferrans VJ, Jones M, et al. Histologic and ultrastructural features of normal human parietal pericardium. Am J Cardiol 1980;46:744–53.

5. Bull RK, Edwards PD, Dixon AK. CT dimensions of the normal pericardium. Br J Radiol 1998;71:923–5.

6. Bogaert J, Francone M. Cardiovascular magnetic resonance in pericardial diseases. J Cardiovasc Magn Reson 2009;11:14.

7. Rajiah P. Cardiac MRI: part 2, pericardial diseases. AJR Am J Roentgenol 2011;197:W621–34.

8. Choe YH, Im JG, Park JH, et al. The anatomy of the pericardial space: a study in cadavers and patients. AJR Am J Roentgenol 1987;149:693–7.

9. Groell R, Schaffler GJ, Rienmueller R. Pericardial sinuses and recesses: findings at electrocardiographically triggered electron-beam CT. Radiology 1999; 212:69–73.

10. Roberts WC. Pericardial heart disease: its morphologic features and its causes. Proc (Bayl Univ Med Cent) 2005;18:38–55.

11. Kodama F, Fultz PJ, Wandtke JC. Comparing thin-section and thick-section CT of pericardial sinuses and recesses. AJR Am J Roentgenol 2003;181: 1101–8.

12. Truong MT, Erasmus JJ, Gladish GW, et al. Anatomy of pericardial recesses on multidetector CT: implications for oncologic imaging. AJR Am J Roentgenol 2003;181:1109–13.

13. Vesely TM, Cahill DR. Cross-sectional anatomy of the pericardial sinuses, recesses, and adjacent structures. Surg Radiol Anat 1986;8:221–7.

14. Truong MT, Erasmus JJ, Sabloff BS, et al. Pericardial "sleeve" recess of right inferior pulmonary vein mimicking adenopathy: computed tomography findings. J Comput Assist Tomogr 2004;28: 361–5.

15. Hynes JK, Tajik AJ, Osborn MJ, et al. Two-dimensional echocardiographic diagnosis of pericardial cyst. Mayo Clin Proc 1983;58:60–3.

16. Feigin DS, Fenoglio JJ, McAllister HA, et al. Pericardial cysts. A radiologic-pathologic correlation and review. Radiology 1977;125:15–20.

17. Pugatch RD, Braver JH, Robbins AH, et al. CT diagnosis of pericardial cysts. AJR Am J Roentgenol 1978;131:515–6.

18. Wang ZJ, Reddy GP, Gotway MB, et al. CT and MR imaging of pericardial disease. Radiographics 2003; 23(Spec No):S167–80.

19. Verhaert D, Gabriel RS, Johnston D, et al. The role of multimodality imaging in the management of pericardial disease. Circ Cardiovasc Imaging 2010;3: 333–43.

20. Maier HC. Diverticulum of the pericardium with observations on mode of development. Circulation 1957;16:1040–5.

21. Akiba T, Marushima H, Masubuchi M, et al. Small symptomatic pericardial diverticula treated by video-assisted thoracic surgical resection. Ann Thorac Cardiovasc Surg 2009;15:123–5.

22. Carretta A, Negri G, Pansera M, et al. Thoracoscopic treatment of a pericardial diverticulum. Surg Endosc 2003;17:158.

23. Sharma R, Harden S, Peebles C, et al. Percutaneous aspiration of a pericardial cyst: an acceptable treatment for a rare disorder. Heart 2007;93:22.

24. Nasser WK. Congenital diseases of the pericardium. Cardiovasc Clin 1976;7:271–86.

25. Tubbs OS, Yacoub MH. Congenital pericardial defects. Thorax 1968;23:598–607.

26. Faridah Y, Julsrud PR. Congenital absence of pericardium revisited. Int J Cardiovasc Imaging 2002; 18:67–73.

27. Abbas AE, Appleton CP, Liu PT, et al. Congenital absence of the pericardium: case presentation and review of literature. Int J Cardiol 2005;98:21–5.

28. Shah AB, Kronzon I. Congenital defects of the pericardium: a review. Eur Heart J Cardiovasc Imaging 2015;16(8):821–7.

29. Scheuermann-Freestone M, Orchard E, Francis J, et al. Images in cardiovascular medicine. Partial congenital absence of the pericardium. Circulation 2007;116:e126–9.

30. Psychidis-Papakyritsis P, de Roos A, Kroft LJ. Functional MRI of congenital absence of the pericardium. AJR Am J Roentgenol 2007;189:W312–4.

31. Alter P, Figiel JH, Rupp TP, et al. CT, and PET imaging in pericardial disease. Heart Fail Rev 2013;18: 289–306.

32. Maisch B, Seferovic PM, Ristic AD, et al. Guidelines on the diagnosis and management of pericardial diseases executive summary; the Task force on the diagnosis and management of pericardial diseases of the European society of cardiology. Eur Heart J 2004;25:587–610.

33. Natanzon A, Kronzon I. Pericardial and pleural effusions in congestive heart failure-anatomical, pathophysiologic, and clinical considerations. Am J Med Sci 2009;338:211–6.

34. Cracknell BR, Ail D. The unmasking of a pyopericardium. BMJ Case Rep 2015;2015 [pii: bcr2014207441].

35. Carsky EW, Mauceri RA, Azimi F. The epicardial fat pad sign: analysis of frontal and lateral chest radiographs in patients with pericardial effusion. Radiology 1980;137:303–8.

36. Eisenberg MJ, Dunn MM, Kanth N, et al. Diagnostic value of chest radiography for pericardial effusion. J Am Coll Cardiol 1993;22:588–93.

37. Klein AL, Abbara S, Agler DA, et al. American Society of Echocardiography clinical recommendations for multimodality cardiovascular imaging of patients with pericardial disease: endorsed by the Society for Cardiovascular Magnetic Resonance and Society of Cardiovascular Computed Tomography. J Am Soc Echocardiogr 2013;26:965–1012.e15.

38. O'Leary SM, Williams PL, Williams MP, et al. Imaging the pericardium: appearances on ECG-gated 64-detector row cardiac computed tomography. Br J Radiol 2010;83:194–205.

39. Bogaert J, Francone M. Pericardial disease: value of CT and MR imaging. Radiology 2013;267:340–56.

40. Frank H, Globits S. Magnetic resonance imaging evaluation of myocardial and pericardial disease. J Magn Reson Imaging 1999;10:617–26.

41. Spodick DH. Acute cardiac tamponade. N Engl J Med 2003;349:684–90.

42. Rienmuller R, Groll R, Lipton MJ. CT and MR imaging of pericardial disease. Radiol Clin North Am 2004; 42:587–601, vi.

43. Restrepo CS, Lemos DF, Lemos JA, et al. Imaging findings in cardiac tamponade with emphasis on CT. Radiographics 2007;27:1595–610.

44. Shabetai R, Meaney E. Proceedings: haemodynamics of cardiac restriction and tamponade. Br Heart J 1975;37:780.

45. Leeman DE, Levine MJ, Come PC. Doppler echocardiography in cardiac tamponade: exaggerated respiratory variation in transvalvular blood flow velocity integrals. J Am Coll Cardiol 1988;11:572–8.

46. Chong HH, Plotnick GD. Pericardial effusion and tamponade: evaluation, imaging modalities, and management. Compr Ther 1995;21:378–85.

47. Imazio M, Gaita F, LeWinter M. Evaluation and treatment of pericarditis: a systematic review. JAMA 2015;314:1498–506.

48. Kyto V, Sipila J, Rautava P. Clinical profile and influences on outcomes in patients hospitalized for acute pericarditis. Circulation 2014;130:1601–6.

49. Gold RG. Post-viral pericarditis. Eur Heart J 1988; 9(Suppl G):175–9.

50. LeWinter MM. Clinical practice. Acute pericarditis. N Engl J Med 2014;371:2410–6.

51. Indik JH, Alpert JS. Post-myocardial infarction pericarditis. Curr Treat Options Cardiovasc Med 2000; 2:351–6.

52. Lador A, Hasdai D, Mager A, et al. Incidence and prognosis of pericarditis after ST-elevation myocardial infarction (from the Acute Coronary Syndrome Israeli Survey 2000 to 2013 Registry Database). Am J Cardiol 2018;121:690–4.

53. Figueras J, Barrabes JA, Serra V, et al. Hospital outcome of moderate to severe pericardial effusion complicating ST-elevation acute myocardial infarction. Circulation 2010;122:1902–9.

54. Waller BF, Taliercio CP, Howard J, et al. Morphologic aspects of pericardial heart disease: part I. Clin Cardiol 1992;15:203–9.

55. Hammer MM, Raptis CA, Javidan-Nejad C, et al. Accuracy of computed tomography findings in acute pericarditis. Acta Radiol 2014;55:1197–202.

56. Yared K, Baggish AL, Picard MH, et al. Multimodality imaging of pericardial diseases. JACC Cardiovasc Imaging 2010;3:650–60.

57. Axel L. Assessment of pericardial disease by magnetic resonance and computed tomography. J Magn Reson Imaging 2004;19:816–26.

58. Myers RB, Spodick DH. Constrictive pericarditis: clinical and pathophysiologic characteristics. Am Heart J 1999;138:219–32.

59. Welch TD, Ling LH, Espinosa RE, et al. Echocardiographic diagnosis of constrictive pericarditis: Mayo Clinic criteria. Circ Cardiovasc Imaging 2014;7: 526–34.

60. Talreja DR, Edwards WD, Danielson GK, et al. Constrictive pericarditis in 26 patients with histologically normal pericardial thickness. Circulation 2003; 108:1852–7.

61. Feng D, Glockner J, Kim K, et al. Cardiac magnetic resonance imaging pericardial late gadolinium enhancement and elevated inflammatory markers can predict the reversibility of constrictive pericarditis after antiinflammatory medical therapy: a pilot study. Circulation 2011;124:1830–7.

62. Zurick AO, Bolen MA, Kwon DH, et al. Pericardial delayed hyperenhancement with CMR imaging in patients with constrictive pericarditis undergoing surgical pericardiectomy: a case series with histopathological correlation. JACC Cardiovasc Imaging 2011;4:1180–91.

63. Sagrista-Sauleda J, Angel J, Sanchez A, et al. Effusive-constrictive pericarditis. N Engl J Med 2004; 350:469–75.

64. Francone M, Dymarkowski S, Kalantzi M, et al. Assessment of ventricular coupling with real-time cine MRI and its value to differentiate constrictive pericarditis from restrictive cardiomyopathy. Eur Radiol 2006;16:944–51.

65. Francone M, Dymarkowski S, Kalantzi M, et al. Real-time cine MRI of ventricular septal motion: a novel approach to assess ventricular coupling. J Magn Reson Imaging 2005;21:305–9.

66. Giassi KS, Costa AN, Bachion GH, et al. Epipericardial fat necrosis: who should be a candidate? AJR Am J Roentgenol 2016;207(4):773–7.

67. Pineda V, Caceres J, Andreu J, et al. Epipericardial fat necrosis: radiologic diagnosis and follow-up. AJR Am J Roentgenol 2005;185:1234–6.

68. Fred HL. Pericardial fat necrosis: a review and update. Tex Heart Inst J 2010;37:82–4.

69. Burazor I, Aviel-Ronen S, Imazio M, et al. Primary malignancies of the heart and pericardium. Clin Cardiol 2014;37:582–8.

70. Suman S, Schofield P, Large S. Primary pericardial mesothelioma presenting as pericardial constriction: a case report. Heart 2004;90:e4.

71. Restrepo CS, Vargas D, Ocazionez D, et al. Primary pericardial tumors. Radiographics 2013;33: 1613–30.

72. Jeudy J, Kirsch J, Tavora F, et al. From the radiologic pathology archives: cardiac lymphoma: radiologic-pathologic correlation. Radiographics 2012;32: 1369–80.

73. Cohen R, Mirrer B, Loarte P, et al. Intrapericardial mature cystic teratoma in an adult: case presentation. Clin Cardiol 2013;36:6–9.

74. Shaffer K, Rosado-de-Christenson ML, Patz EF Jr, et al. Thoracic lymphangioma in adults: CT and MR imaging features. AJR Am J Roentgenol 1994;162: 283–9.

75. Chiles C, Woodard PK, Gutierrez FR, et al. Metastatic involvement of the heart and pericardium: CT and MR imaging. Radiographics 2001;21:439–49.

76. Thurber DL, Edwards JE, Achor RW. Secondary malignant tumors of the pericardium. Circulation 1962; 26:228–41.

Computed Tomographic Imaging of Cardiac Trauma

Demetrios A. Raptis, MD*, Sanjeev Bhalla, MD, Constantine A. Raptis, MD

KEYWORDS

- Cardiac trauma • Blunt cardiac injury • Penetrating cardiac injury • Myocardial contusion
- Myocardial rupture

KEY POINTS

- Although it is infrequent for a radiologist to be requested to specifically evaluate a patient for cardiac injury, findings of cardiac injury may be encountered on routine posttrauma multidetector row computed tomography.
- The right heart, specifically the right ventricle, is the most common location of cardiac injury in both blunt and penetrating trauma.
- Direct signs of cardiac injury include decreased myocardial attenuation (typically best appreciated in the portal venous phase), active extravasation of contrast, or a focal outpouching/defect in the myocardium.
- Indirect signs of cardiac injury include pulmonary edema, cardiac chamber enlargement, pneumopericardium, hemopericardium, and wound path/trajectory.

INTRODUCTION

Cardiac trauma occurs in the setting of blunt or penetrating traumas and results in significantly adverse outcomes. The incidence of blunt cardiac injury is unknown with a wide range of reported incidences varying from as low as 20% when accounting for all blunt traumas to as high is 76% in the setting of blunt trauma with severe thoracic injury.[1–3] It has been estimated that 25% of deaths in the setting of blunt cardiac trauma are secondary to cardiac-related injuries.[4] Scenarios most closely associated with cardiac injury include motor vehicle collisions, falls, explosions, crush injuries, and cardiovascular resuscitation. There are several proposed mechanisms of cardiac injury from blunt trauma, including direct precordial impact, crush injury from compression between the sternum and spine, deceleration or torsion, hydraulic effect, and blast injury.[5] Penetrating cardiac trauma has grave consequences as well,

with survival rates reported between 19% and 73%.[6] Common mechanisms of penetrating injury to the heart include stab wounds, gunshot wounds, and sternal fractures.

The clinical presentation of thoracic trauma is variable and depends on the mechanism and magnitude of injury. Patients can present with nonspecific clinical symptoms including chest pain, dyspnea, and cardiac arrhythmia. Patients with minor injuries may be nearly asymptomatic, whereas more severe injury can present with a complex clinical picture. Physical examination may demonstrate a chest wall deformity or subcutaneous emphysema that, in turn, raises the possibility of cardiac injury.[7] Occasionally, findings on physical examination may be absent in patients with severe thoracic trauma. Adding to the confusion is that many patients with significant chest trauma, including sternal fractures, tend not to have any cardiac injury. Although no clear diagnostic test exists, approaches to the workup of

Disclosure Statement: None of the authors have any disclosures.
Mallinckrodt Institute of Radiology, 216 South Kingshighway Boulevard, St Louis, MO 63110, USA
* Corresponding author.
E-mail address: D.raptis@wustl.edu

Radiol Clin N Am 57 (2019) 201–212
https://doi.org/10.1016/j.rcl.2018.08.009

radiologic.theclinics.com

patients with concern for cardiac injury include an electrocardiographic (ECG) evaluation and assessment of cardiac enzymes (troponin-I, CK-MB/CK ratio).[6,7] In hemodynamically stable patients with a normal ECG and cardiac enzyme values, no further workup is required.[5–7] In patients with cardiac arrhythmia, hemodynamic cardiac instability, or elevated enzymes, further workup is often needed. Rarely is the radiologist requested to evaluate for cardiac trauma specifically, but recognition of findings of cardiac trauma on imaging examinations performed for thoracic trauma is essential to avoid misdiagnosis and to provide an explanation for the patient's clinical findings. Furthermore, prompt recognition of cardiac injury can result in a lifesaving intervention.

NORMAL ANATOMY AND IMAGING TECHNIQUE

Although it is infrequent for a radiologist to be requested to specifically evaluate a patient for cardiac injury, findings of cardiac injury may be encountered on routine posttrauma multidetector row computed tomography (MDCT). MDCT is currently the workhorse for evaluation of trauma in the emergent setting because it is can be performed rapidly and provides coverage of multiple regions of the body. MDCT has a high sensitivity for cardiac injury.[8] In cases of suspected cardiac trauma, ECG gating or high pitch scan modes can be used to decrease both cardiac and motion artifact.[9,10] The MDCT protocol used at our institution is our routine trauma examination performed in a single phase with a fixed delay at 70 seconds with the arms raised above the patient's head. Images are obtained in a single pass from the thoracic inlet through the upper abdomen, using a standard 3-mm slice thickness reconstructed at 2-mm intervals, with the option to reconstruct at thinner slices.

Although other modalities may be used in specific instances, they have important limitations. Chest radiography is a useful imaging tool in the initial assessment of patients who have sustained thoracic trauma, but is incapable of providing an in-depth evaluation of the heart.[9] Radiographs may demonstrate more commonly seen injuries, such as rib or clavicular fractures, sternal fractures, pneumothorax, hemothorax, and lung contusion. Transthoracic echocardiography is useful for evaluation of wall motion and structural abnormalities, but transthoracic echocardiography can be technically challenging in the setting of significant chest trauma, especially in the setting of pneumomediastinum or pneumopericardium. Transesophageal echocardiography,

although also useful, is limited by its invasive nature and may be difficult to perform in the setting of severe thoracic injury.[9] Although invasive, catheter angiography can be useful in assessing coronary artery injury, while also providing information about cardiac chamber size, myocardial function, and valve function. Cardiac MR imaging, although providing a potential means for the evaluation of the extent of myocardial injury, infarction, wall motion abnormalities, and valvular dysfunction, is not a practical tool in the setting of acute trauma given its long imaging times. In addition, both angiography and MR imaging remove the patient from the emergency department and may delay other needed interventions.

In the evaluation of aortic and vascular injuries, many reports have pointed to direct and indirect signs of injury. We propose a similar approach to the evaluation of suspected cardiac injury. Direct signs of cardiac injury include decreased myocardial attenuation (typically best appreciated in the portal venous phase), active extravasation of contrast, or a focal outpouching/defect in the myocardium. Indirect signs of cardiac injury include pulmonary edema, cardiac chamber enlargement, pneumopericardium, hemopericardium, and wound path/trajectory.

The right heart, specifically the right ventricle, is the most common location of cardiac injury in blunt and penetrating trauma.[4–6] In blunt trauma, this finding is likely secondary to the close proximity of the right heart to impacts along the anterior chest wall. In penetrating trauma, the right heart is also most vulnerable given its anterior location in the thoracic cavity.[4] Of the patients who experience cardiac injury, only a small percentage make it to the emergency department alive. Awareness of the common locations of cardiac injury and recognition of the direct and indirect findings of cardiac injury can allow for a rapid diagnosis at the time of the initial MDCT. Furthermore, when there is high clinical suspicion for a cardiac abnormality, and a lack of imaging findings to suggest trauma, attention can be directed to an alternative diagnosis (**Fig. 1**).

IMAGING FINDINGS
Blunt Injury

Blunt cardiac injuries can be classified into 2 categories: myocardial concussion and myocardial contusion. Myocardial concussion is defined as having a wall motion abnormality without evidence of anatomic or cellular injury. Myocardial contusion is defined as having an anatomic injury that presents with increased cardiac enzymes or tissue injury diagnosed at surgery or autopsy. Other less

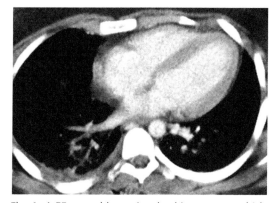

Fig. 1. A 55-year-old man involved in a motor vehicle collision who presented with elevated troponins, increasing upon admission from 0.05 to 0.32 ng/mL. Initial multidetector row computed tomography transaxial images with intravenous contrast showed no evidence of cardiac injury. The patient was treated for a myocardial infarction, unrelated to cardiac injury.

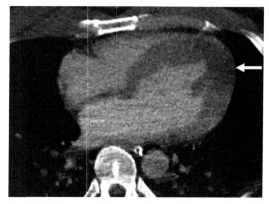

Fig. 2. A 40-year-old man who ran into a pole while playing basketball. Axial postcontrast multidetector row computed tomography image shows hypoenhancement of the left ventricular myocardium (*white arrow*) and papillary muscles. Echocardiography and coronary angiography confirmed left ventricular hypokinesis and findings compatible with myocardial contusion.

commonly encountered cardiac injuries that may occur in the setting of blunt trauma include pericardial injury/rupture, myocardial rupture, papillary muscle injury, atrial or ventricular septal defect, valvular injury, or coronary artery injury.

Myocardial Contusion

In blunt trauma, the incidence of myocardial contusion is unknown with a wide reported range from 10% to 75%.[2] Autopsy and clinical series of patients who have died from cardiac trauma demonstrated contusions in 14% to 100% of patients.[2,5,11] Myocardial contusion involves hemorrhage and necrosis within the myocardium and has a nonspecific clinical presentation ranging. Although no set criteria exist, myocardial contusion should be suspected in the setting of substantial chest trauma with an abnormal EKG, hypotension, and/or elevated cardiac enzymes.[12] The identification of substantial thoracic injuries on MDCT such as multiple rib fractures, sternal fracture, pulmonary contusion, mediastinal hematoma, hemopericardium, great vessel injury, and solid organ injury should raise the suspicion for myocardial injury. It should be noted, however, that myocardial injury may occur in isolation. MDCT may show a decreased enhancement of the myocardium, but this finding is not sensitive.[12] Decreased enhancement of the myocardium is best seen on portal venous phase images (70- to 75-s delay after contrast administration), may be missed on an early arterial phase (<60 s after contrast administration), and can be accentuated with a narrow window (Fig. 2). Although decreased

attenuation of the myocardium is a direct sign of cardiac injury, other indirect signs of cardiac injury may also be present, including pulmonary edema and ventricular enlargement owing to ischemia (Figs. 3 and 4).

Myocardial Rupture

Myocardial rupture is a rare finding seen on MDCT in patients sustaining blunt cardiac injury; a majority of patients with rupture expire in the field. The most common location of chamber rupture is the right ventricle, followed by the right atrium, left ventricle, and left atrium.[5] Clinically, patients may present with profound hypotension and findings of tamponade. On MDCT, findings may be limited to the myocardium and demonstrate a focal aneurysm or posttraumatic ventricular septal defect, a direct finding of myocardial injury (Fig. 5). Other direct findings include complete disruption of the myocardium and extravasation of intravenous contrast outside the heart (Figs. 6 and 7). Indirect imaging findings associated with myocardial rupture include hemopericardium and tamponade. Given the grave consequences of myocardial rupture, early diagnosis is essential to ensure prompt repair.

Pericardial Injury/Rupture

Impact to the anterior chest wall or an acute increase in intraabdominal pressure can result in pericardial injury. The pericardium can rupture along either the diaphragmatic or pleural surface. Clinical presentation is variable ranging from

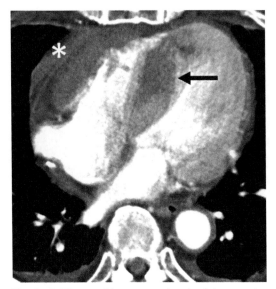

Fig. 3. A 62-year-old man was involved in a motor vehicle collision. Multidetector row computed tomography transaxial images of the chest demonstrate decreased attenuation within the interventricular septum (*black arrow*), consistent with myocardial injury to this location. Hemopericardium (*white asterisk*), an indirect finding, is also seen adjacent to the thickened right ventricular free wall in this patient who also sustained a right ventricular free wall myocardial injury.

hemodynamic instability to cardiac arrest. Rupture of the pericardium has a mortality ranging from 30% to 64%.[13] Pneumopericardium in the setting of blunt thoracic trauma should raise the suspicion for pericardial injury. Pericardial rupture with resultant pneumopericardium can easily be identified on MDCT with gas outlining the heart contained by the pericardial reflections at the root of the great vessels (**Fig. 8**). Distinguishing pneumopericardium from pneumomediastinum relies on identifying strands of fat within pneumomediastinum but not pneumopericardium, because the gas in pneumopericardium is contained within the potential space between the visceral and parietal pericardium and the gas in the pneumomediastinum extends about the mediastinal fat.

Extensive hemopericardium can result in findings of tamponade with early diastolic collapse of the right ventricular free wall with notching (**Fig. 9**A). If images are acquired in late diastole, right atrial flattening may be seen. Non–ECG-gated studies often have a combination of findings. Secondary findings of tamponade include enlarged collateral pathway formation, dilation of the inferior vena cava, a fluid–fluid level in the inferior vena cava, and reflux of contrast into the intrahepatic inferior vena cava (**Fig. 9**B, C).

Contour irregularities, dimpling, and discontinuity of the pericardium should raise suspicion of

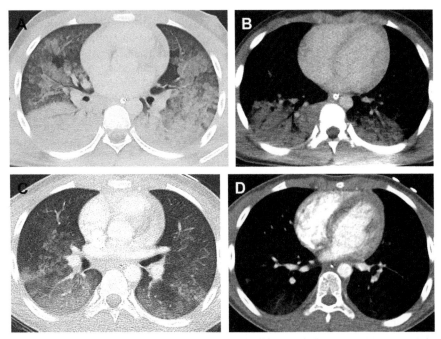

Fig. 4. A 45-year-old man was involved in a motor vehicle collision. multidetector row computed tomography (MDCT) transaxial images at the time of presentation (*A, B*) demonstrate ground glass consistent with pulmonary edema with left ventricular chamber enlargement. Follow-up MDCT imaging (*C, D*) 2 days later shows improved pulmonary edema and reduced size of the left ventricle, suggesting improving findings of myocardial contusion.

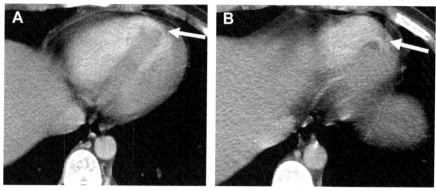

Fig. 5. (A, B) A 36-year-old man was involved in a motor vehicle collision. Multidetector row computed tomography transaxial images with intravenous contrast demonstrate a posttraumatic ventricular septal defect near the apex (*white arrows*). The findings were confirmed during surgery at the time of repair.

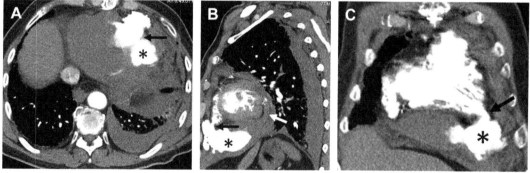

Fig. 6. (A–C) A 37-year-old patients was involved in a motor vehicle collision. Multidetector row computed tomography transaxial (A), sagittal (B), and coronal (C) images with intravenous contrast show complete disruption of the right ventricular myocardium (*black arrows*) with extravasation of contrast (*black asterisks*) outside of the cardiac chamber and extensive hemopericardium (*white arrow*). The findings were confirmed at autopsy.

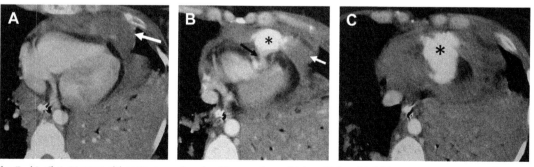

Fig. 7. (A–C) A 44-year-old patient was involved in a motor vehicle collision. Multidetector row computed tomography transaxial images with intravenous contrast show complete disruption of the right ventricular myocardium (*black arrow*) with extravasation of contrast (*black asterisks*) outside of the cardiac chamber and extensive hemopericardium (*white arrows*). The findings were confirmed at autopsy.

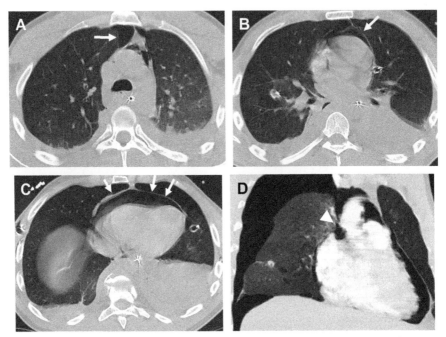

Fig. 8. A 27-year-old patient status post motor vehicle collision. Multidetector row computed tomography trans-axial (*A–C*) and coronal images (*D*) demonstrate extensive pneumopericardium (*white arrows*) that tracks along the great vessels. A suggestion of a pericardial tear is seen along the right side of the pericardium just superior to the right atrium (*white arrowhead*).

injury to the pericardium (see **Fig. 8**). Frank tears of the pericardium are less commonly encountered, but can also be seen on MDCT (see **Fig. 8**). In severe cases, blunt thoracic trauma can result in traumatic diaphragmatic hernias, which can herniate into the pericardial sac or pleural space leading to compression of the ventricles (**Fig. 10**). Cardiac luxation is a rare but serious complication of pericardial rupture leading to cardiac herniation and volvulus, placing the patient at risk for superior

vena cava and right heart obstruction. MDCT may demonstrate displacement of the heart within the thoracic cavity herniating through a pericardial defect with possible leftward bowing of the septum and/or ventricular entrapment.

Coronary Artery Injury

Coronary artery injury is a rare complication of blunt cardiac trauma. The most recent autopsy

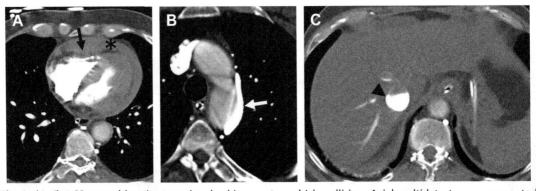

Fig. 9. (*A–C*) A 22-year-old patient was involved in a motor vehicle collision. Axial multidetector row computed tomography images demonstrate extensive hemopericardium (*black asterisk*) and notching of the right ventricular free wall (*black arrow*). Additional findings of cardiac tamponade include contrast within the superior intercostal vein, a collateral pathway (*white arrow*), as well as reflux of contrast into the dilated inferior vena cava with a fluid–fluid level (*black arrowhead*).

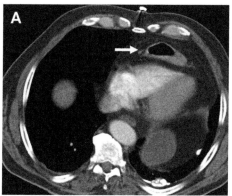
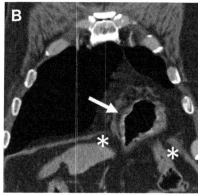

Fig. 10. (*A, B*) A 31-year-old patient was involved in a motor vehicle collision. Axial (*A*) and coronal (*B*) multidetector row computed tomography images with intravenous contrast demonstrate herniation of bowel into the pericardial sac (*white arrows*) secondary to a central tendon defect (*white asterisks*). This patient was taken to the operating room for reduction and repair of the defect.

series demonstrated a 3% incidence of coronary artery injury in the setting of blunt trauma.[5] The most commonly injured coronary vessel is the left anterior descending coronary artery. Given its location posterior to the sternum, injuries to the right coronary artery also may occur. Injuries to the left circumflex coronary artery are rarely encountered. Patients may present with symptoms including arrhythmia and hypotension. ECG may show ST-segment elevation suspicious for myocardial infarction and chest radiograph may demonstrate pulmonary edema. If clinical and EKG findings are suggestive of acute coronary syndrome after sustaining blunt thoracic trauma, coronary artery angiography is the standard of care because interventions such as stenting or angioplasty can be performed at that time. In our practice, there is no primary role for coronary CT angiography in this setting. Findings suggestive of coronary artery injury on routine trauma MDCT injury include pulmonary edema, decreased attenuation of the myocardium in a vascular territory, and ventricular chamber enlargement secondary to ischemia (transient ischemic dilatation; Fig. 11). Although CT examinations in trauma are not routinely ECG gated, if gating or a high-pitch mode is used, direct findings of coronary artery injury including aneurysm or dissection may be identified. Coronary artery injury after blunt trauma may also present in a delayed fashion with findings of an infarct seen on follow-up MDCT or MR imaging (Fig. 12).

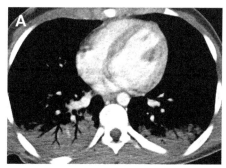
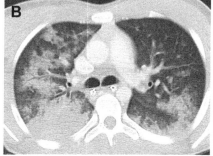

Fig. 11. (*A, B*) A 14-year-old boy was playing baseball when he fell and another player landed with is knee on his chest. The patient went into ventricular tachycardia, ventricular fibrillation, and was pulseless. The patient was resuscitated and intubated and presented in respiratory failure with hypotension. Catheter coronary angiography before the multidetector row computed tomography (MDCT) demonstrated injury to the left main coronary artery extending to the left anterior descending coronary artery. Axial MDCT images with intravenous contrast performed after angiography show left ventricular chamber enlargement and airspace opacities consistent with pulmonary edema, both secondary signs of cardiac injury. Of note, heterogeneous enhancement of the myocardium is secondary to retained contrast from the prior angiography.

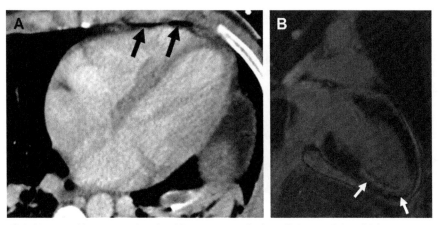

Fig. 12. (A, B) A 28-year-old man was involved in a motor vehicle collision. Axial multidetector row computed tomography image with contrast (A) demonstrates pneumopericardium (*black arrows*), but no direct signs of cardiac injury. At presentation, the patient had elevated troponins and a right coronary artery injury was confirmed on catheter angiography (images not shown). A follow-up cardiac MR imaging study was performed with 2-chamber long axis delayed postcontrast phase sensitive inversion recovery image showing subendocardial and transmural delayed contrast enhancement of the inferior septal wall near the midventricle and apex (*white arrows*), consistent with a resultant myocardial infarct in the right coronary artery territory.

Valvular Dysfunction

Valvular dysfunction is a rare consequence of blunt cardiac injury. At autopsy, the incidence of valvular injury has been reported in about 5% of patients sustaining blunt cardiac trauma.[5] The aortic valve is the most commonly injured valve in the setting of blunt chest injury.[14] The atrioventricular valves are the next most commonly injured followed by the pulmonic valve. Although the exact mechanism is not definitively known, it is proposed that a sudden increase in intracardiac pressure against a closed valve creates a high pressure gradient across the valve and can ultimately result in injury.[15] Echocardiography remains the most useful imaging tool for the evaluation of valvular dysfunction because it allows for dynamic imaging of the valve throughout the cardiac cycle. Valvular injury may present with immediate symptoms or in a delayed fashion several weeks after the injury, particularly in the setting of pulmonic or tricuspid

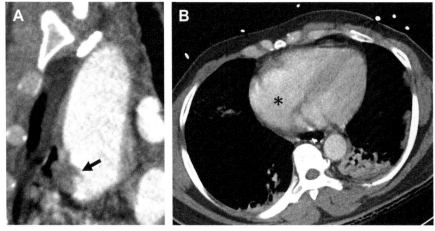

Fig. 13. (A, B) A 28-year-old man was involved in a motor vehicle collision. Axial postcontrast multidetector row computed tomography image (A) demonstrates an aortic injury as noted by the hematoma effacing the fat plate with the ascending aorta (*black arrow*). The patient went to the operating room for repair of the aorta and valve replacement. The patient subsequently developed symptoms of right-sided heart failure with severe tricuspid regurgitation seen on echocardiography. Review of the initial images (B) at time of presentation show enlargement of the right atrium (*black asterisk*), a finding that retrospectively is suggestive of tricuspid valve dysfunction.

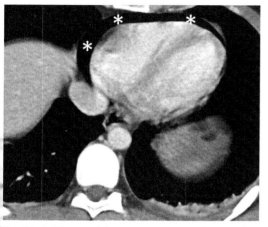

Fig. 14. A 38-year-old man status post stab wound to the chest. Axial multidetector row computed tomography images with intravenous contrast demonstrate extensive pneumopericardium (*white asterisks*), an indirect finding of cardiac injury. At surgery, a right ventricular free wall injury was confirmed.

injury.[16] Evaluation of valvular dysfunction is limited on nongated MDCT examinations obtained in the setting of acute trauma, but the indirect finding of chamber enlargement may be seen at the time of initial evaluation or on follow-up imaging (**Fig. 13**). Traumatic injury to the mitral valve can present with findings of pulmonary edema, which may be localized to the right upper lobe.[17]

Penetrating Cardiac Injury

Penetrating cardiac injury is frequently lethal and has a reported incidence of 0.16% of admissions to trauma centers.[18] Current mortality rates of penetrating cardiac injury vary depending on the mechanism of injury, with gunshot wounds being more fatal than stab wounds. Reported survival rates range from 3% to 84%.[6,19–23] The right ventricle is the most frequently injured cardiac chamber in penetrating trauma.[6,24,25] Injury to the left ventricle has a poor prognosis with a majority

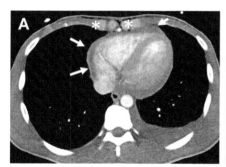
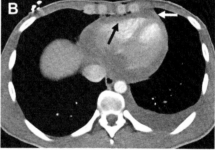

Fig. 15. (*A, B*) A 23-year-old man status post stab wound to the chest. Axial multidetector row computed tomography (MDCT) images with intravenous contrast demonstrate extensive small soft tissue gas overlying the chest wall (*white asterisks*) with small volume hemopericardium (*white arrows*). There is resultant mass effect with dimpling of the right ventricular free wall (*black arrow*). Although no direct sign of myocardial injury was present on the MDCT examination, the suspicion of a right ventricular free wall injury was raised given the hemopericardium. Injury to the right ventricular free wall was confirmed and repaired at time of surgery.

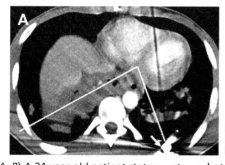
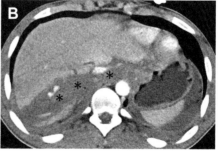

Fig. 16. (*A, B*) A 34-year-old patient status post gunshot wound. Axial multidetector row computed tomography images with intravenous contrast show a bullet located within the posterior left hemithorax (*white arrow*). Evaluation of the bullet tract demonstrates that the bullet took a course (*white line*) from the right hemithorax through the liver ricocheting off of the posterior aspect of the left ventricle. Of note there is an extensive liver laceration (*black asterisks*). These findings raised the suspicion for injury to the posterior wall of the left ventricle, which was confirmed and repaired at surgery.

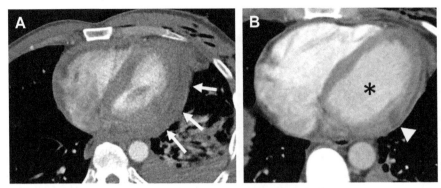

Fig. 17. (*A, B*) A 34-year-old patient status post gunshot wound. Axial multidetector row computed tomography (MDCT) image with intravenous contrast at the time of presentation (*A*) shows hemopericardium (*white arrows*), an indirect finding of cardiac injury. Follow-up axial MDCT image with intravenous contrast several days later (*B*) shows enlargement of the left ventricle (*black asterisk*) and a focal area of myocardial hypoenhancement in the lateral wall of the left ventricle (*white arrowhead*). A cardiac laceration in this location was confirmed at surgery.

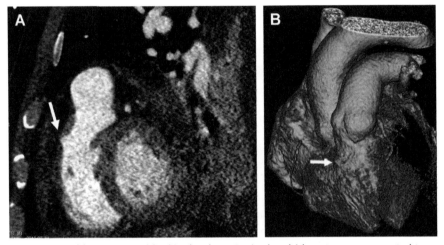

Fig. 18. (*A, B*) A 28-year-old man was stabbed in the chest. Sagittal multidetector row computed tomography images (*A*) and volumetric 3-dimensional reconstructions (*B*) with intravenous contrast demonstrate a contour irregularity and focal outpouching of the right ventricular free wall myocardium (*white arrows*) raising the suspicion for cardiac injury. The findings were confirmed at surgery at the time of repair.

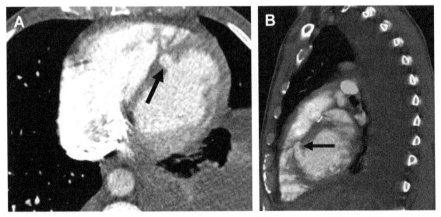

Fig. 19. (*A, B*) A 28-year-old man was stabbed in the chest. Axial (*A*) and sagittal (*B*) multidetector row computed tomography images with intravenous contrast demonstrate a posttraumatic ventricular septal defect (*black arrows*) as a result of the stab wound. The septal defect was repaired at surgery.

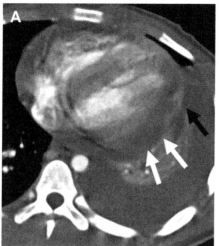
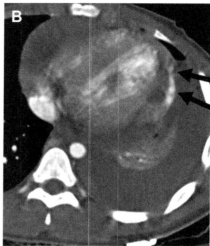

Fig. 20. (*A*, *B*) A 44-year-old man was stabbed in the chest. Axial multidetector row computed tomography images with intravenous contrast demonstrate hemopericardium (*white arrows*), an indirect finding of myocardial injury. Extravasation of contrast (*black arrows*) from the left ventricle, a direct finding of myocardial injury, was also present, consistent with penetrating cardiac injury to the left ventricle. The findings of penetrating injury to the left ventricle were confirmed and repaired at surgery.

of the patients expiring in the field. Trauma to more than 1 cardiac chamber is often seen in penetrating injury, particularly in the setting of gun violence.

Diagnosis of penetrating cardiac injury should begin with a physical examination and evidence of injury to the chest wall. In patients with thoracic gunshot wounds, there should be a high concern for possible cardiac injury. Other clinical findings such as hypotension, jugular venous distension, and muffled heart sounds are suggestive cardiac tamponade and can be used to raise the suspicion of cardiac injury.

In stable patients and those who receive imaging upon presentation to the hospital, MDCT can be a useful imaging tool for the workup of penetrating cardiac injury with a high reported sensitivity, specificity, and accuracy.[26] Findings of penetrating injury may include indirect signs such as pneumopericardium, hemopericardium, intrapericardial herniation, and mediastinal hematoma (**Fig. 14**). These indirect signs can prompt further investigation for possible myocardial injury (**Fig. 15**).

In our experience, the most useful sign in penetrating injury is the trajectory of the projectile. Findings that can be seen in blunt trauma, including hemopericardium or pneumopericardium, may be absent. MDCT is a valuable tool when evaluating potential sites of injury because it allows for the delineation of stab wound and ballistic trajectories, which are not always apparent on physical examination (**Fig. 16A**). Furthermore, bullets that penetrate the thorax can take complex bullet

pathways, causing a great deal of collateral damage (**Fig. 16B**). Bullets that enter cardiac chambers and/or great vessels can embolize distally to other parts of the body and be seen elsewhere on MDCT examinations. Penetrating injury to the myocardium may present in a delayed fashion with indirect findings, such as chamber enlargement and direct findings such as myocardial hypoenhancement seen on follow-up examinations (**Fig. 17**). MDCT may also demonstrate direct signs of cardiac injury, including the presence of a pseudoaneurysm/focal outpouching to the involved ventricles, posttraumatic ventricular septal defect, or frank ventricular rupture (**Figs. 18–20**).

SUMMARY

Although a request to evaluate specifically for cardiac injury in the acute setting rarely occurs, MDCT is a valuable tool for evaluation of both blunt and penetrating thoracic trauma. MDCT offers advantages over other imaging modalities and is the workhorse for evaluation of acute cardiac injury. An understanding of the direct and indirect imaging findings of cardiac injury can help to make a prompt diagnosis and direct life-saving care.

REFERENCES

1. Feghali N, Prisant L. Blunt myocardial injury. Chest 1995;(108):1673–7.
2. Parmley LF, Manion WC, Mattingly TW. Nonpenetrating traumatic injury of the heart. Circulation 1958;18: 371–96.

3. Sigler L. Traumatic injury of the heart: incidence of its occurrence in forty-two cases of severe accidental bodily injury. Am Heart J 1945;30:459–78.

4. Symbas P. Cardiothoracic trauma. Curr Probl Surg 1991;28(11):741–97.

5. Schultz JM, Trunkey DD. Blunt cardiac injury. Crit Care Clin 2004;1:57–70.

6. Bellister S, Dennis B, Guillamondegui O. Blunt and penetrating cardiac trauma. Surg Clin North Am 2017;(5):1065–76.

7. Emet M, Akoz A, Aslan S, et al. Assessment of cardiac injury in patients with blunt chest trauma. Eur J Trauma Emerg Surg 2010;(5):441–7.

8. Mirvis S. Imaging of acute thoracic injury: the advent of MDCT screening. Semin Ultrasound CT MR 2005; 26(5):305–31.

9. Co S, Yong-Hing C, Galea-Soler S, et al. Role of imaging in penetrating and blunt traumatic injury to the heart. Radiographics 2011;31(5):1496.

10. Restrepo C, Gutierrez F, Marmol-Velez J, et al. Imaging patients with cardiac trauma. Radiographics 2012;32(3):633–49.

11. Wisner D, Reed W, Riddick R. Suspected myocardial contusion. Triage and indications for monitoring. Ann Surg 1990;212(1):82–6.

12. Hammer M, Raptis D, Cummings K, et al. Imaging in blunt cardiac injury: computed tomographic findings in cardiac contusion and associated injuries. Injury 2016;47(5):1025–30.

13. Galindo G, Lopez-Cambra M, Fernandez-Acenero M, et al. Traumatic rupture of the pericardium. Case report and literature review. J Cardiovasc Surg (Torino) 1996;37(2):187–91.

14. Kan C, Yang Y. Traumatic aortic and mitral valve injury following blunt chest injury with a variable clinical course. Heart 2005;91(5):568–70.

15. Saric P, Ravaee B, Patel T, et al. Acute severe mitral regurgitation after blunt chest trauma. Echocardiography 2017;35(2):272–4.

16. van Son J, Danielson G, Schaff H, et al. Traumatic tricuspid valve insufficiency. Experience in thirteen patients. J Thorac Cardiovasc Surg 1994;108(5): 893–8.

17. Murakami S, Michihiro S, Hideaki M, et al. Localized pulmonary edema after blunt chest trauma. Circulation 2007;115(8):e206–7.

18. Asensio JA, Garcia-Nunez LM, Petrone P. Trauma to the Heart. In: Feliciano DV, Mattox KL, Moore EE, editors. Trauma. New York: McGraw Hill; 2008.

19. Barleben A, Huerta S, Mendoza R, et al. Left ventricle injury with a normal pericardial window: case report and review of the literature. J Trauma 2007;63(2):414–6.

20. Demetriades D, van der Veen B. Penetrating injuries of the heart: experience over two years in South Africa. J Trauma 1983;23(12):1034–41.

21. Kang N, Hsee L, Rizoli S, et al. Penetrating cardiac injury: overcoming the limits set by nature. Injury 2009;40:919–27.

22. Naughton M, Brissie R, Bessey P, et al. Demography of penetrating cardiac trauma. Ann Surg 1989;(209): 676–81.

23. Rhee P, Foy H, Kaufman C. Penetrating cardiac injuries: a population based study. J Trauma 1988; 45(2):366–70.

24. Morse B, Mina M, Carr J. Penetrating cardiac injuries: a 36 year perspective at an urban, level I trauma center. J Trauma Acute Care Surg 2016; 81(4):623–31.

25. Topal A, Celik Y, Eren M. Predictors of outcome in penetrating cardiac injuries. J Trauma 2010;69(3): 574–8.

26. Nagy K, Gilkey S, Roberts R, et al. Computed tomography screens stable patients at risk for penetrating cardiac injury. Acad Emerg Med 1996; 3(11):1024–7.

Postcardiovascular Surgery Findings of the Thoracic Aorta

Sherief Garrana, MD[a],*, Santiago Martínez-Jiménez, MD[b]

KEYWORDS

- Aorta • Postsurgical aorta • Supracoronary graft • Composite graft • Ross procedure
- Pseudoaneurysm • TEVAR • Endoleak

KEY POINTS

- Various disease processes may affect the ascending thoracic aorta, aortic arch, and/or descending thoracic aorta, including aneurysms, dissections, intramural hematomas, penetrating atherosclerotic ulcers, and aortic transection/rupture.
- Many of those conditions require surgical intervention for repair.
- Multiple open and endovascular techniques are used for treatment of thoracic aortic pathology.
- It is imperative that the cardiothoracic radiologist have a thorough knowledge of the surgical techniques available, the expected postoperative imaging findings, and the complications that may occur, to accurately diagnose life-threatening pathology when present, and avoid common pitfalls of misinterpreting normal postoperative findings as pathologic conditions.

INTRODUCTION

Various disease processes may affect the ascending thoracic aorta, aortic arch, and/or descending thoracic aorta, including aneurysms, dissections, intramural hematomas, penetrating atherosclerotic ulcers, and aortic transection/rupture. Many of those conditions require surgical intervention for repair. This article focuses on the surgical and/or endovascular interventions used to treat the diseased thoracic aorta, the indications for those surgical procedures, the expected imaging appearance, and the appearance of complications that may arise, particularly as seen on computed tomography angiography (CTA).

IMAGING TECHNICAL CONSIDERATIONS

CTA is the modality of choice for imaging of the postsurgical aorta, because it is noninvasive and

provides optimal image quality, and capability to reconstruct multiplanar and three-dimensional reformatted images.[1] Although there is interinstitutional variability when it comes to the protocol used for aortic imaging, generally two computed tomography (CT) acquisitions are recommended: an initial acquisition without intravenous contrast; followed by a second acquisition after the administration of contrast, ideally obtained during the arterial phase of imaging. The nonenhanced CT is important to identify postoperative material that may have a hyperdense appearance, therefore avoiding the pitfall of misinterpreting a normal postoperative appearance as extraluminal contrast on contrast-enhanced CT (eg, anastomotic felt along the anastomoses, pledgets). Furthermore, nonenhanced CT is important to identify intramural hematomas within the aortic wall, which otherwise may be obscured by

Disclosure Statement: No relevant disclosures (S. Garrana). Author for Elsevier (S. Martínez-Jiménez).
[a] Department of Radiology, University of Missouri in Kansas City (UMKC), St Luke's Hospital of Kansas City, 4401 Wornall Road, Kansas City, MO 64111, USA; [b] Department of Radiology, St Luke's Hospital of Kansas City, 4401 Wornall Road, Kansas City, MO 64111, USA
* Corresponding author. 318 West 7th Street, #108, Kansas City, MO 64105.
E-mail address: sherief.garrana@gmail.com

Radiol Clin N Am 57 (2019) 213–231
https://doi.org/10.1016/j.rcl.2018.08.005
0033-8389/19/© 2018 Elsevier Inc. All rights reserved.

radiologic.theclinics.com

adjacent contrast material after contrast administration. Acquiring images during the arterial phase is particularly important because several serious complications, such as pseudoaneurysms and aortic dissections, are best seen during this phase of imaging.[2] Cardiac motion artifacts may interfere in evaluation of the ascending thoracic aorta, especially at the level of the coronary sinuses, and therefore cardiac gating is helpful when detailed evaluation of the aortic valve, coronary sinuses, coronary arteries, and coronary bypass grafts is needed.[3,4] Most aortic assessments, however, are achieved without cardiac gating, because most complications are readily identified without the use of gating techniques.[1,5] Ultimately, the choice of imaging technique for assessment of the postoperative aorta requires an understanding of the surgical procedure and its possible complications.

INDICATIONS FOR TREATMENT

Surgical repair of the aorta is most commonly performed for aortic aneurysms and acute aortic syndromes (eg, intramural hematoma, dissection). Aortic intramural hematomas are within the spectrum of the acute aortic syndrome, sometimes considered a noncommunicating variant of aortic dissection, and therefore are classified and managed in a similar fashion.[6] Open surgical approaches are typically used for pathology affecting the ascending thoracic aorta and aortic arch, whereas endovascular approaches are increasingly being used in certain conditions involving the descending thoracic aorta in cases where intervention is required.[7] Surgical management of ascending thoracic aortic dissections, intramural hematomas, incomplete dissections, and penetrating aortic ulcers is the treatment of choice given the risk of progression, rupture, coronary artery dissections, and cardiac tamponade. Regarding ascending aortic aneurysms, current indications for surgical intervention include:

1. Evidence of rupture
2. End-diastolic aortic diameter exceeding 5.5 cm in the general population, or aortic size index (aortic diameter [centimeters] divided by body surface area [square meters]) greater than or equal 2.75 cm/m^2
3. End-diastolic aortic diameter greater than 4.5 cm in patients with syndromic connective tissue diseases (eg, Marfan syndrome, Loeys-Dietz, Ehlers-Danlos) or bicuspid aortic valves
4. Aneurysms with annual growth greater than 0.5 cm per year

5. Any aneurysm that is symptomatic, regardless of size

Current indications for surgical intervention in aneurysms of the descending thoracic aorta are similar to those in the ascending aorta except for size cutoffs, which include aortic diameter exceeding 5.5 cm in the general population or greater than 5.0 cm in patients with connective tissue diseases. In patients with high surgical risk (Society of Thoracic Surgeons predicted rate of mortality score >8%, frailty score index >2, two compromised organ systems) a diameter equal to or greater than 7 cm is used. For smaller patients, including many women, a diameter greater than twice the diameter of the nonaneurysmal aorta or the aorta size index is used.[7–9]

GENERAL OVERVIEW OF SURGICAL PROCEDURES OF THE THORACIC AORTA

Various surgical procedures are used for aortic repair. Depending on the specific procedure, synthetic or biologic grafts may be used, and the native aortic valve may be spared or may be replaced with an aortic valve prosthesis. In general, most aortic graft repairs excise the diseased native aorta and replace the diseased segment with a synthetic or biologic graft that is reanastomosed to the native anatomic structures, which is known as an "interposition graft." An alternative technique that is no longer frequently used because of superior outcomes with interposition grafts is the "inclusion graft," where the synthetic graft is placed within the diseased aortic lumen, and the native aorta wrapped around the graft, therefore leaving a potential space between the graft and native aortic wall. From a technical standpoint, inclusion grafts are faster to perform (ie, decreasing surgical times), which is important in severely ill patients (Fig. 1).[5]

Synthetic grafts, which are often made from polyethylene terephthalate (Dacron), are smooth walled rounded grafts that appear slightly hyperdense in comparison with the native aortic wall on noncontrast CT; however, after the administration of contrast on arterial phase imaging they appear hypodense relative to the enhanced blood pool and the surrounding surgical felt ring (Fig. 2).[1] The position of the graft can usually be identified by noting the sharply demarcated change in caliber and/or contour of the aorta, which are most easily identified on multiplanar reformatted images, especially those demonstrating the vessel in long-axis (Fig. 3). The graft anastomoses can frequently be identified by noting felt pledgets, rings, or strips at the anastomotic sites, all of

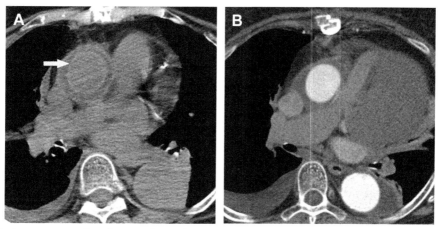

Fig. 1. Inclusion reconstruction. (*A*) Unenhanced CT, axial image, shows features of ascending aortic inclusion technique. A hyperdense synthetic aortic graft is within the lumen of an aneurysmal ascending thoracic aorta (*arrow*). Note fluid collection between the graft and the native aorta. (*B*) Contrast-enhanced CT, axial image, shows enhancement of the graft lumen. The space between the graft and the thoracic aorta should not enhance normally.

which appear hyperdense on unenhanced and contrast-enhanced images. It is crucial to confirm that the areas of the felt pledgets appear hyperdense on the unenhanced images, to avoid mistaking those areas for pseudoaneurysms, which would appear as hypodense or isodense on unenhanced images, a common pitfall. In addition, felt rings and strips are usually located along the entire circumference of the anastomosis, as opposed to a pseudoaneurysm, which would be eccentric along a single wall. A false intimomedial defect (or "pseudoflap") is frequently seen where there is mild angulation graft and should not be mistaken for a dissection (**Fig. 4**).[1,4]

EXPECTED POSTOPERATIVE IMAGING FINDINGS AND COMPLICATIONS

Postoperative perigraft fluid collection/soft tissue attenuation may be seen following open surgical aortic repair and could represent inflammatory reaction from the synthetic graft material, evolving hematoma or seroma. Sterile fluid collections (seromas) are commonly seen and can resolve or remain stable over time (**Fig. 5**). However, some findings should raise concern for specific complications, such as:

1. A perigraft hematoma greater than 1.5 cm in thickness on initial postoperative imaging is

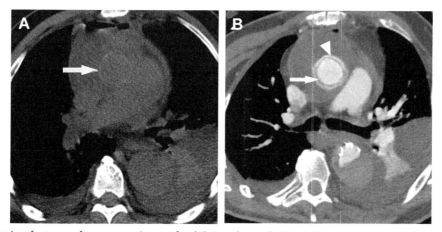

Fig. 2. Imaging features of reconstruction grafts. (*A*) Unenhanced CT, axial image, shows a slightly hyperdense synthetic aortic graft (*arrow*). (*B*) Contrast-enhanced CT, axial image, shows the aortic graft (*arrow*), which appears hypodense relative to the enhanced blood pool and the surrounding surgical felts (*arrowhead*).

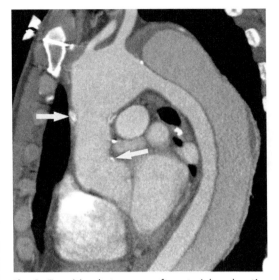

Fig. 3. Transition between graft material and native aorta. Contrast-enhanced CT, double oblique sagittal reformation, shows discrete change in caliber between the reconstructed ascending aorta and the distal native aortic arch. Notice the high attenuation material at the proximal and distal anastomotic sites (*arrows*), indicating surgical felts.

associated with increased risk of pseudoaneurysm formation at the anastomosis.

2. Superinfection of the perigraft fluid should be suspected if there is postcontrast rim enhancement, increasing air within the fluid, fistulous communication to neighboring structure, or extension into other mediastinal compartments (**Fig. 6**).

Small amount of perigraft air is an expected postoperative finding; however, persistence of air

for more than 6 to 8 weeks or progressively increasing air is highly concerning for infection with gas-forming organisms or fistula formation with the esophagus or tracheobronchial tree.[1,2,5]

Finally, sternal osteomyelitis is a common complication following median sternotomy, and direct extension in the mediastinum could result in mediastinitis and abscess formation. CT findings include osseous destruction, periosteal reaction, reactive sclerosis, demineralization, change in alignment of sternal wires or sternal dehiscence, and adjacent fluid collections.[1,2,5]

SPECIFIC SURGICAL PROCEDURES OF THE ASCENDING THORACIC AORTA
Supracoronary Grafts

Any type of surgical repair that spares the aortic root (sinuses of Valsalva) and placed distal to the coronary ostia is called a supracoronary graft. The Wheat procedure, first described by Wheat and colleagues[10] in 1964, refers to a simultaneous supracoronary graft repair and an aortic valve replacement (**Figs. 7** and **8**). A supracoronary graft maintains the normal integrity of the coronary arteries because the aortic root is spared, and thus is technically less complicated and minimizes the risk of developing complications related to the coronary arteries, such as pseudoaneurysms, stenosis, thrombosis, or kinking at the coronary anastomoses.[1,10] Supracoronary grafts are indicated in patients who have an ascending thoracic aortic aneurysm (usually of atherosclerotic origin) with normal sinuses of Valsalva.[11] One of the most commonly recognized complications of supracoronary graft repair is development of dissection or aneurysm of the native aortic root

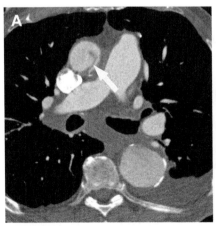
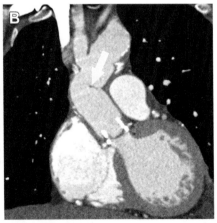

Fig. 4. Pseudoflap (false intimomedial flap). (*A*) Contrast-enhanced CT, axial image, shows a false intimomedial defect (*arrow*). This occurs because of mild angulation of the graft and should not be mistaken for an aortic dissection. (*B*) Contrast-enhanced CT, coronal reformation, further shows the aortic graft angulation responsible for the pseudoflap (*arrow*).

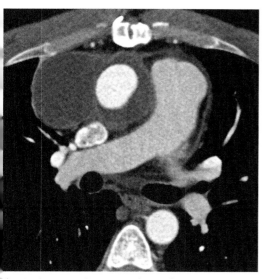

Fig. 5. Seroma. Contrast-enhanced CT, axial image, shows a large hypoattenuating nonenhancing fluid collection surrounding to aortic graft, consistent with a seroma. No contrast extravasation should be present within the collection, which otherwise would suggest pseudoaneurysm.

proximal to the graft, which most frequently occurs in patients with annuloaortic ectasia, usually with connective tissue disorders (eg, Marfan) or patients with inflammatory conditions, such as aortitis. Another potential complication is pseudoaneurysm formation at the anastomoses (Fig. 9), caused by weakening at anastomosis, which can be caused by infection.[1,5,11]

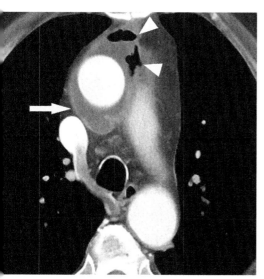

Fig. 6. Graft infection. Contrast-enhanced CT, axial image, shows a fluid collection around the graft. Note rim-enhancement (arrow) and foci of air (arrowheads), findings highly concerning for infection.

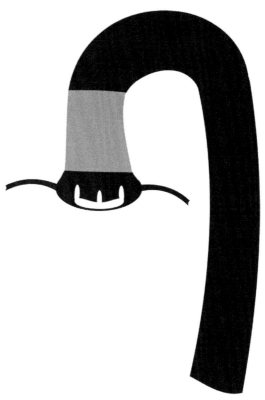

Fig. 7. Illustration of Wheat procedure. The Wheat procedure includes a supracoronary ascending aortic graft (gray) and an aortic valve replacement (white). The native aortic root and coronary arteries (black) are spared.

Complications of supracoronary graft repair are usually identified in asymptomatic patients during routine imaging surveillance. Identifying aortic root aneurysms is challenging because of variation in aortic root size depending on age and gender, which emphasizes the importance of serial imaging examinations, where progressive enlargement of the aortic root size should raise suspicion for aneurysm. Dissection involving the aortic root/sinuses of Valsalva is identified by an intimal flap seen on CTA or MR imaging and constitutes a surgical emergency because of risk of coronary artery involvement and myocardial infarction. Pseudoaneurysm at the anastomotic site usually appears as an extraluminal mass on unenhanced CT, with marked postcontrast enhancement after contrast administration; nonenhancing components within the pseudoaneurysm can also be seen and indicate the presence of peripheral thrombus (Fig. 10).[1,2,5]

Composite Artificial Grafts

Composite artificial grafts are used when the surgical repair also involves the aortic root and are

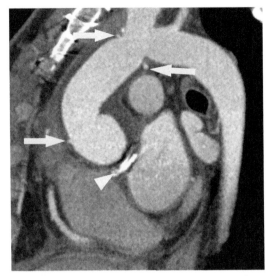

Fig. 8. Imaging findings of Wheat procedure. Contrast-enhanced CT, double oblique sagittal reformation, shows the normal appearance following a Wheat procedure. Discrete changes in caliber are seen between the aortic root and proximal anastomosis, and at the distal anastomotic sites. High-attenuation surgical felt is seen along the proximal and distal anastomotic sites (*arrows*). An aortic valve prosthesis is present (*arrowhead*).

usually used in patients with annuloaortic ectasia and/or patients with aortic valvular disease or severely atherosclerotic ascending aorta, which precludes appropriate healthy tissue to be left in place. The two most common procedures are the modified Bentall and the Cabrol procedures (**Fig. 11**). In both of these procedures, a prosthetic aortic valve is incorporated into the synthetic aortic graft, and both are implanted as a single unit. Because the sinuses of Valsalva are replaced, the coronary arteries are reimplanted onto the graft.[12–14] The modified Bentall and Cabrol procedures differ in the manner that the coronary arteries are anastomosed onto the graft.

In the original Bentall procedure the coronary arteries are directly implanted onto the ascending aortic graft; however, because of the high rate of complications involving the coronary artery anastomoses, particularly pseudoaneurysms, the modified "button Bentall" or "Carrel patch" procedure was created, in which a rim or "button" of native aorta encircling the coronary ostia is removed with the coronary artery, which is then sutured onto the graft.[14,15] This technique has become the most common method for attaching the coronary arteries to the aortic graft. The button technique may cause the origin of the coronary arteries to appear dilated or bulbous-like on CT, which could commonly be mistaken for an aneurysm or pseudoaneurysm at the origin of the coronary arteries (**Figs. 12** and **13**).[1] The incidence of ostial pseudoaneurysm is significantly reduced with the button Bentall technique; however, some authors have reported persistent high frequency of ostial pseudoaneurysms in patients with connective tissue disorders (eg, Marfan).[15–17] Another potential complication of the original and button Bentall procedures is pseudoaneurysm formation at the aortic anastomosis (**Fig. 14**).

In the Cabrol procedure, the coronary ostia are anastomosed onto a prosthetic conduit in an end-to-end fashion, and this conduit is then anastomosed to the aortic graft in a side-to-side fashion, typically posterior to the graft (**Fig. 15**).[13] This procedure was developed as an alternative

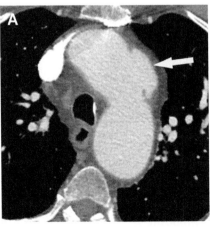
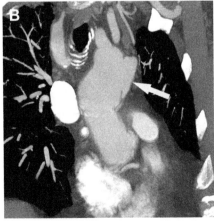

Fig. 9. Wheat procedure with pseudoaneurysm of the distal anastomosis. (*A, B*) Contrast-enhanced CT, axial image (*A*) and coronal oblique maximum intensity projection (MIP) (*B*) show an enhancing outpouching at the distal graft anastomosis consistent with pseudoaneurysm (*arrows*).

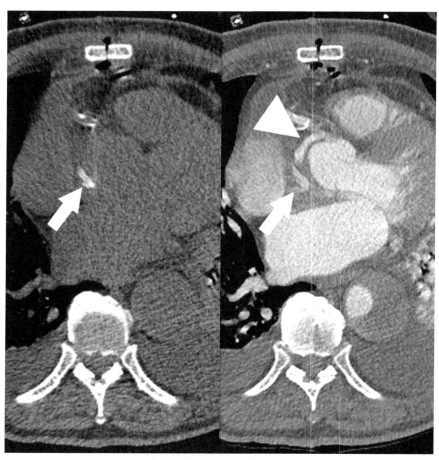

Fig. 10. Supracoronary reconstruction with pseudoaneurysm of the proximal anastomosis. CT, composite image with unenhanced CT (*left*) and contrast-enhanced CT (*right*) at the same level at proximal ascending aorta shows hyperdense felt at the anastomosis (*arrows*) and small outpouching only seen after administration of contrast consistent with pseudoaneurysm (*arrowhead*). Note that the surgical felt could be mistaken for a pseudoaneurysm, if noncontrast imaging was unavailable for correlation (*arrows*).

for patients who were not suitable candidates for the button Bentall procedure (eg, severe atherosclerosis of the ascending aorta near the coronary ostia or proximal coronary arteries, redo procedures, patients in whom the coronary arteries cannot be mobilized sufficiently to achieve tension-free anastomosis to the graft).[13,18] The common imaging pitfall is that the normal imaging appearance of the retroaortic conduit could be misinterpreted as an intimomedial flap related to an aortic dissection or pseudoaneurysm.[13,19] Complications of this procedure also include pseudoaneurysms at the distal anastomotic sites, and early postoperative death in patients with aortic dissection, anastomotic leak, coronary graft insufficiency from intimal hyperplasia or kinking, coronary graft thrombosis, and endocarditis.[13] On CTA, thrombosis within the coronary graft conduit may be diagnosed when there is lack of enhancement within the graft. Intimal hyperplasia

is identified as low-attenuation thickening along the conduit wall. Kinking, with or without thrombosis, can also be seen (**Fig. 16**). Comparison with prior imaging is useful in identifying variation in enhancement or conduit configuration.[1]

Biologic Grafts

Cadaveric (homografts) and autologous grafts can be used as an alternative to synthetic grafts. Common examples using a biologic graft include ascending aortic homografts and the Ross procedure, the latter used to repair a dilated aortic root and aortic valve pathology in children and young individuals (eg, pregnant women). The Ross procedure consists of an autograft that includes the pulmonic valve and proximal pulmonary trunk is used to replace the native aortic valve and aortic root, followed by placement of a cadaveric or synthetic pulmonary graft to

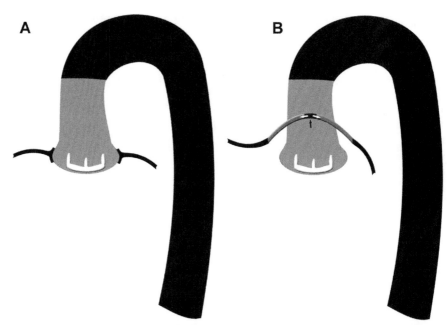

Fig. 11. Illustration of modified Bentall and Cabrol procedures. (*A*) Illustration modified Bentall procedure shows a single graft unit in which a prosthetic aortic valve is incorporated. The sinuses of Valsalva are replaced, and the coronary arteries reimplanted onto the graft, with a rim and native aortic tissue (the "button"). (*B*) Illustration of Cabrol procedure shows a single graft unit where the coronary arteries are anastomosed to a prosthetic conduit, which is then attached to the graft in a laterolateral fashion.

reconstruct the pulmonary artery trunk.[20] Advantages of this technique in children include growth potential of the autograft aortic annulus and valve, improved hemodynamics, lower risk of thrombosis, lack of need for long-term anticoagulation, and lower risk of endocarditis. The most common complication is aortic root dilatation and subsequent aortic valve insufficiency (**Fig. 17**). Other less common complications of the Ross procedure and homografts include pseudoaneurysms at the anastomotic sites and ascending aortic dissection. These complications are readily identified on cross-sectional imaging.[1,20]

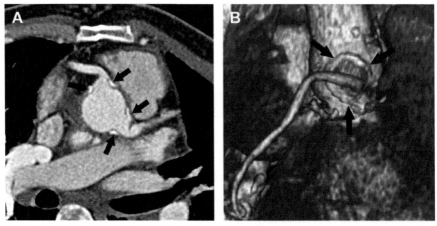

Fig. 12. Imaging findings of the modified Bentall procedure. (*A*) Contrast-enhanced CT, axial image, shows hyperdense felts (*arrows*) and expected bulbous appearance of the take-off of coronary arteries. This morphologic appearance should not be confused with pseudoaneurysm at the coronary anastomosis. (*B*) Contrast-enhanced CT, three-dimensional reformation, shows the tridimensional appearance of the button (*arrows*).

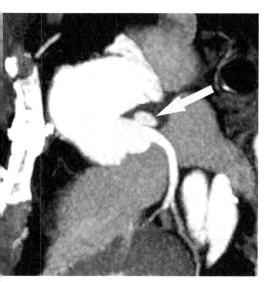

Fig. 13. Pseudonaeurysm of the coronary anastomosis in a modified Bentall procedure. Contrast-enhanced CT, sagittal oblique reformation, shows outpouching (ie, pseudoaneurysm) (*arrow*) at the anastomosis of the left coronary artery.

Aortic Valve–Sparing Procedures

Aortic valve–sparing procedures implement techniques that allow surgical repair of the aortic root with preservation of the patient's native aortic valve. These procedures are particularly useful in patients with annuloaortic ectasia, but with normal aortic valve leaflets (eg, Marfan), especially because these patients are prone to coronary pseudoaneurysm formation after button Bentall procedures. These procedures recreate the sinuses of Valsalva and sinotubular junction, with

the goal of improving hemodynamics and allowing for nearly normal valvular cusp motion. The two main categories of valve-sparing aortic root repair are the remodeling technique developed by Yacoub, and the reimplantation technique developed by David.[21–23] The coronary arteries are reimplanted onto the aortic graft in both techniques.

In the remodeling technique, the native aorta is resected down to the level of valve insertions within the sinuses of Valsalva, while leaving the native aortic valve intact. The sinuses are reconstructed with a scalloped polyethylene (Dacron) graft, which is then attached to the remaining aortic tissue above the valve insertions.[24]

In the reimplantation technique, the native aorta is resected down to the level of the valve insertions. The proximal anastomosis of the polyethylene graft is made to the aortic annulus, below the level of the native aortic valve. A second proximal suture line along the edge of the resected tissue above the valve insertions is then used to resuspend the native aortic valve within the graft, rather than reconstructing the sinuses of Valsalva around the valve.[24]

A modification of the reimplantation technique (David-V, Stanford modification), is when two separate grafts are used for the aortic root and the ascending aortic reconstruction, thus allowing flexibility to individualize the dimensions and configuration of the neosinuses, which mimic the sinuses of Valsalva.[24,25]

The most common complication of valve-sparing procedures is aortic insufficiency, which is easily assessed with echocardiography or cardiac MR imaging. Some authors report a

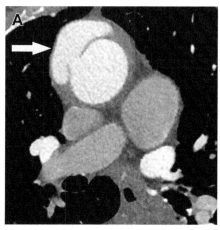
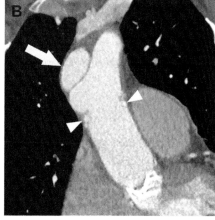

Fig. 14. Modified Bentall procedure with pseudoaneurysm of the distal anastomosis. (*A*, *B*) Contrast-enhanced CT, axial image and coronal reformation shows a pseudoaneurysm (*arrow*) arising at the distal graft anastomosis (*arrowheads*).

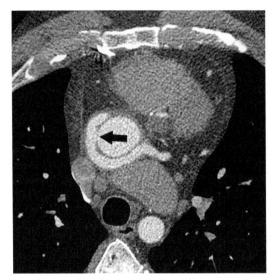

Fig. 15. Imaging findings of the Cabrol procedure. Contrast-enhanced CT, axial image, shows coronary artery prosthetic conduit, with a retroaortic course, anastomosed to the aortic graft in a side-to-side fashion (*arrow*). This can sometimes be misinterpreted as an intimomedial flap related to an aortic dissection.

decreased incidence of aortic insufficiency with the reimplantation technique. Aortic dissection and pseudoaneurysms may also occur. When CTA is used for postoperative evaluation, cardiac gating techniques must be implemented to allow thorough evaluation of the coronary artery anastomoses or other anastomotic complications.[22,24,26]

SPECIFIC SURGICAL PROCEDURES OF THE AORTIC ARCH

Total arch replacement is indicated in patients with extensive thoracic aortic aneurysms that involve the ascending, transverse, and descending thoracic aorta. A commonly used technique known as the elephant trunk (ET) procedure is a two-stage procedure that eventually results in total arch replacement.[27,28] In stage I, the ascending thoracic aorta and aortic arch are replaced by a synthetic graft. An anastomosis is made proximally with the ascending thoracic aorta. The arch vessels are also relocated by debranching from the native aortic arch and reattachment to a trifurcated synthetic graft, which is then anastomosed at its proximal end to the ascending aortic graft, while the distal end is left unattached and free-floating within the lumen of the descending thoracic aorta (**Fig. 18**). In stage II, often performed when the patient is fully recovered from prior stage I, a second graft is placed with the descending thoracic aorta via an open or endovascular approach, and then anastomosed with the distal graft from stage I.[27,28] When an endovascular approach is used for stage II, the surgical procedure is known as a hybrid ET procedure (**Fig. 19**).[29] A one-stage version of the ET procedure known as the frozen ET procedure can be used, with the initial portion of the procedure repairing the ascending thoracic aorta and the arch in a similar fashion to the traditional ET procedure. However, instead of terminating the procedure after the proximal arch repair, the distal arch and descending thoracic aorta are also repaired by using a

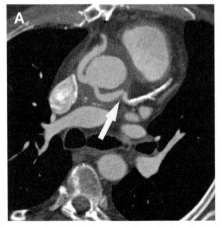
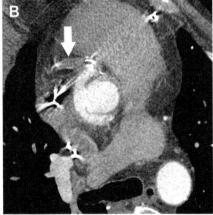

Fig. 16. Coronary limb kinking and obstruction in Cabrol procedure. (*A*) Contrast-enhanced CT, axial image, shows kinking at the left coronary anastomosis (*arrow*) without overt stenosis or obstruction. Note dense calcified atherosclerosis is seen within the native left coronary artery distal to the conduit. (*B*) Contrast-enhanced CT, axial image, shows kinking and lack of opacification of the right coronary limb (*arrow*) consistent with complete obstruction.

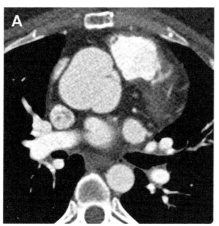
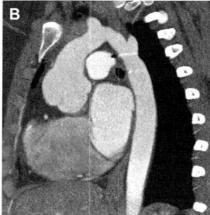

Fig. 17. Aortic root dilatation in Ross procedure. (*A*, *B*) Contrast-enhanced CT, axial (*A*) and sagittal oblique MIP (*B*) images show a dilated aortic root in a patient who has undergone the Ross procedure. Aortic insufficiency and aortic root dilatation are the most common complications encountered after Ross reconstruction of the ascending aorta.

composite graft consisting of a distal aortic stent graft that is sutured to a more proximal conventional tubular graft. The tubular graft is anastomosed to the proximal aortic arch repair, and the distal stent graft is deployed by an anterograde approach.[30–32]

Complications of the ET procedure after the first stage include aneurysm rupture, air embolism into the distal aorta, stroke, and left recurrent laryngeal nerve injury causing vocal cord paralysis. After the second stage, the most serious complication is spinal cord ischemia and subsequent paraplegia. Aortic rupture and death may occur in the interval between the first and second stages of the procedure. Although the one-stage hybrid techniques may decrease the risk of aortic rupture that may occur between the procedural stages, the risk of spinal cord ischemia remains a significant risk for the conventional and one-stage hybrid methods.[1,29,33]

On CTA, the free-floating edge of the graft after the first stage is well demarcated and surrounded by contrast within the lumen of the descending thoracic aorta, and may be mistaken for dissection or pseudoaneurysm. Furthermore, the appearance of the debranched arch vessels now originating from a conduit arising from the ascending aortic graft should be accurately identified (**Fig. 20**).[1]

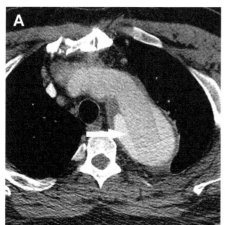
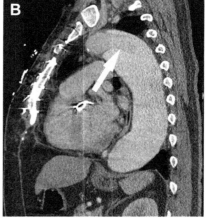

Fig. 18. Imaging findings of the elephant trunk procedure, stage I. (*A*, *B*) Contrast-enhanced CT, axial (*A*) and sagittal oblique MIP (*B*) show a normal postoperative appearance following stage I of the elephant trunk procedure, with the distal end of the graft free floating within the lumen of the aneurysmal descending thoracic aorta (*arrows*), which should not be misinterpreted as abnormal intimomedial flap.

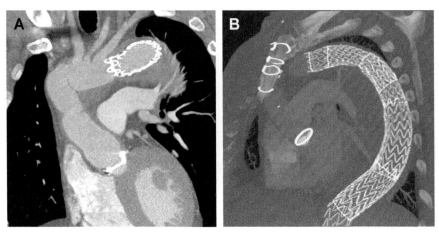

Fig. 19. Imaging findings of the hybrid elephant trunk procedure, stage II. (*A, B*) Contrast-enhanced CT, coronal oblique reformation (*A*) and sagittal oblique MIP (*B*) show the normal postoperative appearance after the completion of stage II of the hybrid elephant trunk procedure. Note the ascending and transverse thoracic aorta have been repaired using a conventional graft, and the descending aorta has been repaired by deploying an endovascular stent, just distal to the origin of the left subclavian artery.

The arch-first technique is a one-stage procedure that replaces the entire aorta through multiple incisions. The arch vessels are debranched from the native arch and attached to a tubular graft with branches onto which those vessels are anastomosed. This allows early anterograde perfusion of the arch vessels and therefore minimizing cerebral ischemia. The distal end of the branch graft is then attached onto a normal portion of the descending thoracic aorta, and distal perfusion to the body is established. Finally, the proximal portion of the branched graft is

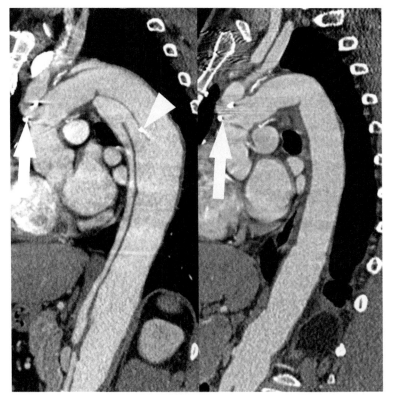

Fig. 20. Imaging findings of the elephant trunk procedure, stage I and II. Contrast-enhanced CT, composite image with double oblique sagittal stage I (*left*) and stage II (*right*) of the elephant trunk procedure. The free end of the graft (*arrowhead*) is seen floating within the lumen of the descending thoracic aorta. An intimomedial dissection flap is also seen within the descending aorta. Note the appearance of the arch vessels, now arising off a conduit arising the ascending aortic graft (*arrows*).

anastomosed to a normal caliber aortic root, to a preexisting ascending aortic synthetic graft, or a newly placed interposition graft. The arch-first technique virtually eliminates the risk of aneurysm rupture and the risks associated with a second surgical procedure, and is also associated with a lower rate of reintervention. It has a lower rate of morbidity and mortality when compared with the ET procedure, particularly with neurologic complications.[34–37]

Disease limited to the transverse aorta is exceptionally rare. However, when an ascending thoracic aortic aneurysm extends into the proximal aortic arch sparing the arch vessels and distal arch, a hemiarch procedure can be performed, where the distal ascending thoracic aorta and proximal transverse aorta are resected, and the remaining transverse aorta carved to leave the arch vessels attached and intact. A graft extending from the ascending thoracic aorta is then anastomosed onto the residual native aortic cuff of the transverse aorta.[5,38,39]

SPECIFIC SURGICAL PROCEDURES OF THE DESCENDING THORACIC AORTA

Although more commonly disease limited to the descending thoracic aorta is treated medically rather than surgically, there are several indications for surgical interventions as described previously. When open surgical approaches are used, the most common complications are left recurrent laryngeal nerve injury resulting in left vocal cord paralysis, renal failure, paraplegia from spinal cord ischemia, stroke, and hemorrhage.[7,40]

With the advent of endovascular stent grafting in the 1990s, known as thoracic endovascular aortic repair (TEVAR), it has been increasingly used for treatment of the diseased descending thoracic aorta. The lack of curvature and presence of few branch vessels render endovascular approaches a convenient alternative to conventional open surgical repair. Some studies have suggested that TEVAR may have a lower early complication rate in comparison with open surgical repair, such as early death, paraplegia, renal insufficiency, and length of hospital stay. Long-term studies regarding survival will provide more comprehensive understanding.[7,40–42]

In general, deployment of stent grafts requires a 2-cm proximal and distal landing zone. The left subclavian artery may be intentionally sacrificed in cases with an insufficient proximal landing zone, with flow to the left upper extremity restored via retrograde flow from the vertebral artery or via bypass grafting. As expected, if the left subclavian artery is sacrificed, such complications as upper extremity ischemia and vertebrobasilar insufficiency may occur.

TEVAR should be avoided in patients with connective tissue diseases (eg, Marfan) because of the risk of retrograde dissection, pseudoaneurysms, or endoleaks at the landing zones.[40–42]

Imaging with CTA or conventional angiography should be performed shortly after stent graft placement to establish a baseline appearance of the graft and detect early complications. Follow-up is then obtained at 6- to 12-month intervals. Imaging protocols usually include unenhanced and contrast-enhanced arterial phase image acquisitions; however, some institution obtain triphasic CTA, with additional delayed images approximately 60 seconds after contrast administration, which could help detect certain subtypes of endoleaks.

Wireless pressure sensor devices are also available, which are placed in the excluded portion of the aortic aneurysm at the time of endograft deployment. Sensing continued high pressures in the excluded aorta may help identify persistent communication between the systemic circulation and excluded aorta.[40–43]

Specific complications specific to TEVAR include endoleaks, stent collapse, retrograde dissection, stent migration, infection, and fistula formation.

Endoleaks

Endoleak is the most common complication following TEVAR, and it indicates ongoing perfusion of the excluded portion of the aorta following stent placement. Endoleaks are usually found incidentally on routine postoperative imaging surveillance in asymptomatic patients.[43–45] Five main types of endoleaks are described, in addition to a mixed type:

1. Type I: leaks at the attachment sites caused by inadequate seal; IA proximal, IB distal (**Figs. 21 and 22**).
2. Type II: leaks caused by supply by collateral vessels; IIA single vessel, IIB two or more vessels (**Fig. 23**).
3. Type III: leak through the body of the stent graft/graft failure. May be related to poor apposition or separation of the stent-graft components, junctional leak between two overlying stents, or rupture/tear of the graft material (**Fig. 24**).
4. Type IV: leak that occurs immediately after placement of a stent graft, where opacification of the aneurysm sac is seen without an identifiable source of leakage. Occurs because of porosity of some graft material. These occur intraprocedurally, are transient, and usually resolve after withdrawal of anticoagulation.

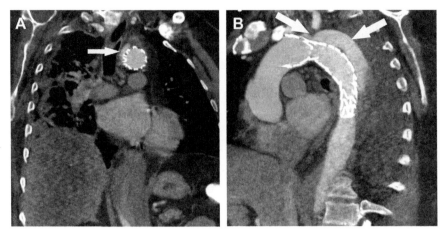

Fig. 21. Endoleak type IA. (*A, B*) Contrast-enhanced CT, coronal (*left*) and sagittal oblique (*right*) reformations, show type IA endoleak, with contrast extravasation into the false lumen along an incompletely apposed proximal landing zone (*arrows*).

5. Type V: poorly understood phenomenon, identified on imaging by increasing aneurysm size, without identifiable endoleaks. Thought to occur when increased graft permeability allows increased pressure to be transmitted through the aneurysm sac, affecting the native aortic wall. Also known as "endotension."
6. Mixed types of endoleaks

Type I and type III endoleaks are considered "high-pressure" endoleaks and require prompt reintervention. Type II endoleaks are treated conservatively with serial monitoring; however, they occasionally require intervention if the excluded aneurysm sac continues to enlarge on serial imaging, and/or if the collateral vessels supplying the excluded aneurysm sac are large,

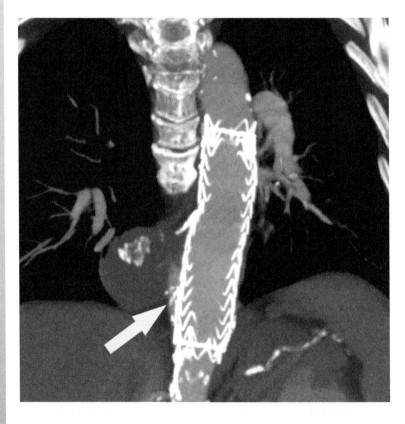

Fig. 22. Endoleak type IB. Contrast-enhanced CT, coronal oblique MIP, shows type IB endoleak, with contrast extending into the excluded aneurysm sac, near the distal landing zone of the stent along an incompletely apposed distal landing zone (*arrow*).

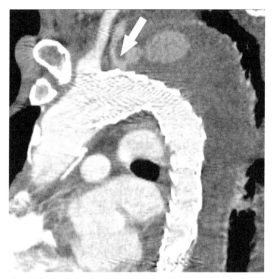

Fig. 23. Endoleak type IIA. Contrast-enhanced CT, sagittal reformation, shows type IIA endoleak, with contrast opacifying the excluded portion of the aorta via retrograde filling from the left subclavian artery (*arrow*).

therefore causing elevated pressures. On triphasic CTA, the excluded portion of the aneurysm sac enhances in a similar fashion to the enhanced blood pool on the arterial phase and delayed imaging for type I and III endoleaks. Low-flow type II endoleaks may sometimes only be identified on delayed imaging.[42,43,45,46]

"Bird beaking" is a common pitfall that is mistaken for type Ia endoleak and occurs when the seal at the proximal landing zone of the stent graft is incomplete against the aortic wall; however, the remainder of the graft is sufficiently aligned against the aortic wall. On CTA, a beaked appearance is seen when contrast material undermines the proximal aspect of the stent graft (**Fig. 25**). Although bird-beaking is not a true endoleak because contrast does not reach the excluded aneurysm sac, it does require serial monitoring because of risk of progression to type Ia endoleak.[5,42,43]

Endograft Collapse

Endograft collapse is an uncommon complication that may occur soon after stent deployment. It

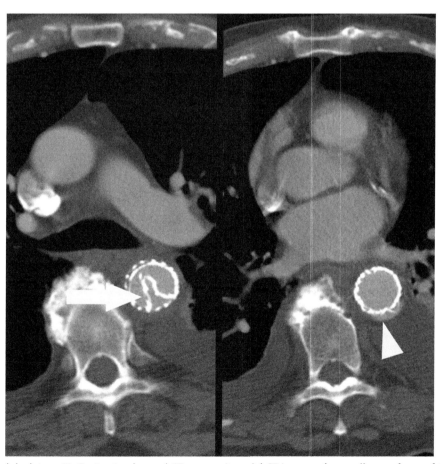

Fig. 24. Endoleak type III. Contrast-enhanced CT, composite axial CT Images, show collapse of one of two endovascular stents (*arrow*), with associated type III junctional endoleak (*arrowhead*).

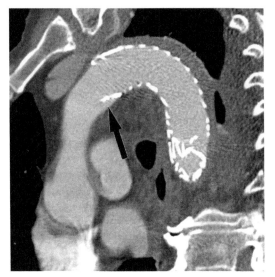

Fig. 25. Bird beaking. Contrast-enhanced CT, oblique sagittal reformation, shows small contrast extending underneath the proximal anastomosis (*arrow*) from incomplete apposition of the proximal stent. Although this per se is not abnormal nor constitutes an endoleak, it should be followed up because it can sometimes result in formation of endoleak.

may also occur months to years later often leading to type I or III endoleak (see **Fig. 24; Fig. 26**). Collapsed appearance of the stent is readily identified on CT, and occasionally on radiography. Collapsed stent is a surgical complication requiring priority treatment. If two or more endografts are overlapping and one collapses, this often results in type IIIB endoleak and requires emergent intervention (ie, deployment of a more rigid stent, such as a Palmaz stent).[5,42]

Dissection and Pseudoaneurysm

Injury of the aortic intima with subsequent dissection in an anterograde or retrograde fashion or pseudoaneurysm formation may be complications occurring after stent deployment. Patients who have underlying connective tissue disorders in particular are at risk for this complication, and therefore should not undergo TEVAR. It usually occurs in the early postoperative period, but may occur up to several weeks later. Imaging findings and therapeutic considerations are identical to those described in dissection or pseudoaneurysm formation in other settings.[5,42]

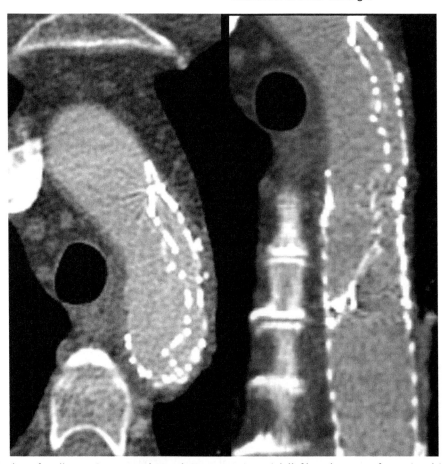

Fig. 26. Endograft collapse. Contrast-enhanced CT, composite axial (*left*) and curve reformation (*right*), show collapse of the proximal endovascular stent.

Stent Migration

Stent migration is an uncommon complication that can occur as a result of type I endoleaks, where increasing systemic pressure around the edges of the stent results in cranial or caudal migration. Changes in stent position are readily identified on radiography or cross-sectional imaging, and it is important to compare the stent position in relation to adjacent static landmarks on serial imaging.[5,42,47]

Endograft Infection/Fistula Formation

Endograft infection is an uncommon but often fatal complication. When infection does occur, it usually happens several months after stent placement. CT findings that suggest infection include air/fluid around the stent, irregular soft tissue thickening around the graft, and irregular enhancement adjacent to the graft. Although a small amount of air and fluid is a normal postoperative finding with open surgical approaches, these findings should never be seen when an endovascular technique is used. When air is present because of an infection, that amount of air is usually small. Fistula formation between the graft and esophagus or tracheobronchial tree may occur in one of two ways: as a complication of graft infection; or may occur primarily if the stent struts perforate the aorta and adjacent structures at the time of deployment, which ultimately also results in secondary infection. CT findings that suggest fistula include a large amount of air around the graft, air-fluid level near the graft, air within the excluded part of the aorta, and/or obliteration of distinct fat planes between the aorta and esophagus or tracheobronchial tree (**Fig. 27**).[47–51]

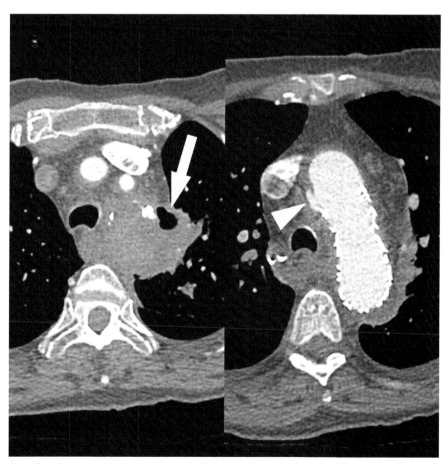

Fig. 27. Endograft infection. Contrast-enhanced CT, composite axial images, show an endovascular stent extending along the distal aortic arch and proximal ascending aorta with associated soft tissue mass with intrinsic air from infection and abscess (*arrow*). Note the presence of a small pseudoaneurysm (*arrowhead*) at the junction of the native aorta and the endograft. Not infrequently pseudoaneurysm can result from infection.

SUMMARY

Various open and endovascular techniques are used for treatment of thoracic aortic pathology. It is imperative that the cardiothoracic radiologist have a thorough knowledge of the different surgical techniques available, the normal postoperative imaging findings, and the various complications that may occur, to accurately and promptly diagnose life-threatening pathology when present, and to avoid common pitfalls of misinterpreting normal postoperative findings as pathologic conditions.

REFERENCES

1. Prescott-Focht JA, Martinez-Jimenez S, Hurwitz LM, et al. Ascending thoracic aorta: postoperative imaging evaluation. Radiographics 2013;33(1):73–85.
2. Hoang JK, Martinez S, Hurwitz LM. MDCT angiography after open thoracic aortic surgery: pearls and pitfalls. AJR Am J Roentgenol 2009;192(1):W20–7.
3. Roos JE, Willmann JK, Weishaupt D, et al. Thoracic aorta: motion artifact reduction with retrospective and prospective electrocardiography-assisted multi-detector row CT. Radiology 2002;222(1):271–7.
4. Sundaram B, Quint LE, Patel HJ, et al. CT findings following thoracic aortic surgery. Radiographics 2007;27(6):1583–94.
5. Abbara S, Kalva SP. Problem solving in radiology: cardiovascular imaging. Elsevier Health Sciences; 2013.
6. Gutschow SE, Walker CM, Martinez-Jimenez S, et al. Emerging concepts in intramural hematoma imaging. Radiographics 2016;36(3):660–74.
7. Coady MA, Ikonomidis JS, Cheung AT, et al. Surgical management of descending thoracic aortic disease: open and endovascular approaches: a scientific statement from the American Heart Association. Circulation 2010;121(25):2780–804.
8. Erbel R, Aboyans V, Boileau C, et al. 2014 ESC guidelines on the diagnosis and treatment of aortic diseases: document covering acute and chronic aortic diseases of the thoracic and abdominal aorta of the adult. The task force for the diagnosis and treatment of aortic diseases of the European Society of Cardiology (ESC). Eur Heart J 2014;35(41):2873–926.
9. Hiratzka LF, Creager MA, Isselbacher EM, et al. Surgery for aortic dilatation in patients with bicuspid aortic valves: a statement of clarification from the American College of Cardiology/American Heart Association task force on clinical practice guidelines. J Am Coll Cardiol 2016;67(6):724–31.
10. Wheat MW, Wilson JR, Bartley TD. Successful replacement of the entire ascending aorta and aortic valve. JAMA 1964;188:717–9.
11. Yoda M, Nonoyama M, Shimakura T, et al. Surgical case of aortic root and thoracic aortic aneurysm after the wheat procedure. Ann Thorac Cardiovasc Surg 2002;8(2):115–8.
12. Bentall H, De Bono A. A technique for complete replacement of the ascending aorta. Thorax 1968;23(4):338–9.
13. Gelsomino S, Frassani R, Da Col P, et al. A long-term experience with the Cabrol root replacement technique for the management of ascending aortic aneurysms and dissections. Ann Thorac Surg 2003;75(1):126–31.
14. Cherry C, DeBord S, Hickey C. The modified Bentall procedure for aortic root replacement. AORN J 2006;84(1):52–5, 58–70. [quiz: 71–4].
15. Milano AD, Pratali S, Mecozzi G, et al. Fate of coronary ostial anastomoses after the modified Bentall procedure. Ann Thorac Surg 2003;75(6):1797–801 [discussion: 1802].
16. Erkut B, Ceviz M, Becit N, et al. Pseudoaneurysm of the left coronary ostial anastomoses as a complication of the modified Bentall procedure diagnosed by echocardiography and multislice computed tomography. Heart Surg Forum 2007;10(3):E191–2.
17. Okamoto K, Casselman FP, De Geest R, et al. Giant left coronary ostial aneurysm after modified Bentall procedure in a Marfan patient. Interact Cardiovasc Thorac Surg 2008;7(6):1164–6.
18. García À, Ferreirós J, Santamaría M, et al. MR angiographic evaluation of complications in surgically treated type A aortic dissection. Radiographics 2006;26(4):981–92.
19. Kruser TJ, Osaki S, Kohmoto T, et al. Computed tomography finding mimicking aortic dissection after Cabrol procedure. Asian Cardiovasc Thorac Ann 2009;17(1):108–9.
20. Kouchoukos NT, Masetti P, Nickerson NJ, et al. The Ross procedure: long-term clinical and echocardiographic follow-up. Ann Thorac Surg 2004;78(3):773–81 [discussion: 773–81].
21. David TE, Feindel CM. An aortic valve-sparing operation for patients with aortic incompetence and aneurysm of the ascending aorta. J Thorac Cardiovasc Surg 1992;103(4):617–21 [discussion: 622].
22. David TE, Ivanov J, Armstrong S, et al. Aortic valve-sparing operations in patients with aneurysms of the aortic root or ascending aorta. Ann Thorac Surg 2002;74(5):S1758–61 [discussion: S1792–9].
23. Fleischmann D, Liang DH, Mitchell RS, et al. Pre- and postoperative imaging of the aortic root for valve-sparing aortic root repair (V-SARR). Semin Thorac Cardiovasc Surg 2008;20(4):365–73.
24. Hanneman K, Chan FP, Mitchell RS, et al. Pre- and postoperative imaging of the aortic root. Radiographics 2016;36(1):19–37.
25. Demers P, Miller DC. Simple modification of "T. David-V" valve-sparing aortic root replacement to create graft pseudosinuses. Ann Thorac Surg 2004;78(4):1479–81.

26. David TE, Feindel CM, Webb GD, et al. Long-term results of aortic valve-sparing operations for aortic root aneurysm. J Thorac Cardiovasc Surg 2006; 132(2):347–54.

27. Schepens MA, Dossche KM, Morshuis WJ, et al. The elephant trunk technique: operative results in 100 consecutive patients. Eur J Cardiothorac Surg 2002;21(2):276–81.

28. LeMaire SA, Carter SA, Coselli JS. The elephant trunk technique for staged repair of complex aneurysms of the entire thoracic aorta. Ann Thorac Surg 2006;81(5):1561–9 [discussion: 1569].

29. Azizzadeh A, Estrera AL, Porat EE, et al. The hybrid elephant trunk procedure: a single-stage repair of an ascending, arch, and descending thoracic aortic aneurysm. J Vasc Surg 2006;44(2):404–7.

30. Roselli EE, Isabella MA. Frozen elephant trunk procedure. Operative Techniques in Thoracic and Cardiovascular Surgery: A Comparative Atlas 2013; 18(2):87–100.

31. Roselli EE, Bakaeen FG, Johnston DR, et al. Role of the frozen elephant trunk procedure for chronic aortic dissection. Eur J Cardiothorac Surg 2017; 51(suppl 1):i35–9.

32. Folkmann S, Weiss G, Pisarik H, et al. Thoracoabdominal aortic aneurysm repair after frozen elephant trunk procedure. Eur J Cardiothorac Surg 2015; 47(1):115–9 [discussion: 119].

33. Kouchoukos NT. Complications and limitations of the elephant trunk procedure. Ann Thorac Surg 2008; 85(2):690–1 [author reply: 691–2].

34. Kouchoukos NT, Mauney MC, Masetti P, et al. Single-stage repair of extensive thoracic aortic aneurysms: experience with the arch-first technique and bilateral anterior thoracotomy. J Thorac Cardiovasc Surg 2004;128(5):669–76.

35. Kouchoukos NT. One-stage repair of extensive thoracic aortic disease. J Thorac Cardiovasc Surg 2010;140(6 Suppl):S150–3 [discussion: S185–90].

36. Sasaki M, Usui A, Yoshikawa M, et al. Arch-first technique performed under hypothermic circulatory arrest with retrograde cerebral perfusion improves neurological outcomes for total arch replacement. Eur J Cardiothorac Surg 2005;27(5):821–5.

37. Usui A, Ueda Y. Arch first technique under deep hypothermic circulatory arrest with retrograde cerebral perfusion. Multimed Man Cardiothorac Surg 2007; 2007(102). mmcts.2006.001974.

38. Rylski B, Milewski RK, Bavaria JE, et al. Long-term results of aggressive hemiarch replacement in 534 patients with type A aortic dissection. J Thorac Cardiovasc Surg 2014;148(6):2981–5.

39. Poon SS, Theologou T, Harrington D, et al. Hemiarch versus total aortic arch replacement in acute type A dissection: a systematic review and meta-analysis. Ann Cardiothorac Surg 2016;5(3):156–73.

40. Bavaria JE, Appoo JJ, Makaroun MS, et al. Endovascular stent grafting versus open surgical repair of descending thoracic aortic aneurysms in low-risk patients: a multicenter comparative trial. J Thorac Cardiovasc Surg 2007;133(2):369–77.

41. Lin PH, Sayed El HF, Kougias P, et al. Endovascular repair of thoracic aortic disease: overview of current devices and clinical results. Vascular 2007;15(4): 179–90.

42. Wang GJ, Fairman RM. Endovascular repair of the thoracic aorta. Semin Intervent Radiol 2009;26(1): 17–24.

43. Reginelli A, Capasso R, Ciccone V, et al. Usefulness of triphasic CT aortic angiography in acute and surveillance: our experience in the assessment of acute aortic dissection and endoleak. Int J Surg 2016; 33(Suppl 1):S76–84.

44. Le TB, Park K-M, Jeon YS, et al. Evaluation of delayed endoleak compared with early endoleak after endovascular aneurysm repair. J Vasc Interv Radiol 2018;29(2):203–9.

45. Sommer WH, Becker CR, Haack M, et al. Time-resolved CT angiography for the detection and classification of endoleaks. Radiology 2012;263(3):917–26.

46. Flors L, Leiva-Salinas C, Norton PT, et al. Endoleak detection after endovascular repair of thoracic aortic aneurysm using dual-source dual-energy CT: suitable scanning protocols and potential radiation dose reduction. AJR Am J Roentgenol 2013; 200(2):451–60.

47. Pandey N, Litt HI. Surveillance imaging following endovascular aneurysm repair. Semin Intervent Radiol 2015;32(3):239–48.

48. Murphy DJ, Keraliya AR, Agrawal MD, et al. Cross-sectional imaging of aortic infections. Insights Imaging 2016;7(6):801–18.

49. Smeds MR, Duncan AA, Harlander-Locke MP, et al. Treatment and outcomes of aortic endograft infection. J Vasc Surg 2016;63(2):332–40.

50. Cernohorsky P, Reijnen MMPJ, Tielliu IFJ, et al. The relevance of aortic endograft prosthetic infection. J Vasc Surg 2011;54(2):327–33.

51. Heyer KS, Modi P, Morasch MD, et al. Secondary infections of thoracic and abdominal aortic endografts. J Vasc Interv Radiol 2009;20(2):173–9.

Printed and bound by CPI Group (UK) Ltd, Croydon, CR0 4YY

08/05/2025

01864741-0003